OXFORD MEDICAL PUBLICATIONS

Oxford Handbook of
Emergency Nursing

Oxford Handbook of
Emergency Nursing

SECOND EDITION

Edited by

Robert Crouch

Consultant Nurse and Honorary Professor of
Emergency Care
Emergency Department
University Hospital Southampton NHS Foundation Trust and
Faculty of Health Sciences
University of Southampton, Southampton, UK

Alan Charters

Consultant Nurse
Emergency Department
Portsmouth Hospitals NHS Trust, Hampshire, UK

Mary Dawood

Consultant Nurse
Emergency Directorate, Imperial College NHS Trust
and Honorary Lecturer, Imperial College London, UK

Paula Bennett

Consultant Nurse
Emergency Department
Stockport NHS Foundation Trust
and Honorary Lecturer
University of Manchester School of Nursing,
Midwifery and Social Work
Manchester, UK

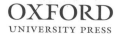

OXFORD
UNIVERSITY PRESS

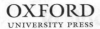

OXFORD
UNIVERSITY PRESS

Great Clarendon Street, Oxford, OX2 6DP,
United Kingdom

Oxford University Press is a department of the University of Oxford.
It furthers the University's objective of excellence in research, scholarship,
and education by publishing worldwide. Oxford is a registered trade mark of
Oxford University Press in the UK and in certain other countries

© Oxford University Press 2017

The moral rights of the authors have been asserted

First Edition published in 2009
Second Edition published in 2017

Impression: 1

Published in the United States of America by Oxford University Press
198 Madison Avenue, New York, NY 10016, United States of America

British Library Cataloguing in Publication Data
Data available

Library of Congress Control Number: 2015942563

ISBN 978–0–19–968886–9

Printed and bound in China by
C&C Offset Printing Co., Ltd.

This handbook is dedicated to the late Kate O'Hanlon, Sister in Charge, Royal Victoria Hospital, Belfast, for her dedication to serving the people of Northern Ireland and her inspirational leadership of emergency nurses.

Foreword

There is a lot to learn in emergency care! I never managed to get a placement in 'Casualty' when I was training, so was very shocked when someone on the recruitment panel for my first job thought I would be suited to the emergency department (ED). Twenty-five years later and I am still learning. Unlike other fields of care, pre-registration education prepares clinical staff poorly for emergency care, for the sheer volume and nature of work, for the complexity and often simplicity of the patients' problems, or for the inter-dependency of the professionals working within it. There is little that can prepare us, other than immersion in the work and a personal commitment to continuing development. Every clinical shift or project provides an opportunity to understand better a diagnosis or care process. A simple audit of pain management can enable staff to challenge the quality of care delivered and/or to enhance patient-centred treatment models.

Clinicians in the ED must generate knowledge and skill across every health-care specialty. They are the textbook generalists—experts in the frontline management of any presentation, but also skilled in accessing specialist help. They assess patients, their families, and the situation around them constantly, in order to make sense of their patients' needs. They must use this skill to ask the right questions, in order to compare and prioritize patients effectively, so that everyone receives treatment which is safe and effective. Increasingly, they practise autonomously across the full spectrum of the patient workload, expanding their scope and impact within the emergency care field. In addition, they must respond quickly to public health emergencies, whilst still being committed to developing their services for the chronic shift in population health needs.

Access to applicable and realistic information is essential for care, as patient treatment must be evidence-based for staff to make effective decisions. Information has never been more accessible than it is today, yet there is often a lack of concise and precise data that enable our practitioners to make timely decisions and to learn as they practise. This text makes all the information needed to practise in the ED readily available. It contextualizes care in that setting, and it provides a concise overview of the vast range of presentations and skills needed to practise safely, whilst providing plenty of opportunities for further learning. Wherever you are in the world, you are providing emergency care, and you should keep this handbook within reach.

Heather McClelland RGN MSc
Nurse Consultant, Emergency Care
Calderdale and Huddersfield NHS Foundation Trust
Editor, *International Emergency Nursing*

Preface

When we wrote the first edition of this handbook, it was with the primary aim of supporting clinical practice at the bedside or trolley side. We wanted to write a comprehensive, easily accessible text that provided valuable information for every question or query that may arise in the course of a shift. The vast array of clinical presentations in emergency care can be daunting for those new to the specialty. Prioritizing care in a fast-paced environment is a unique skill that has to be underpinned by a sound knowledge base.

This handbook covers the whole range of adult and paediatric emergency presentations. Each chapter covers a physiological system and starts with a review of anatomy and physiology (where appropriate). The chapter's format allows the clinician to quickly review the associated presentations, priorities, and red flags. The final skills chapter details the multitude of clinical skills and procedures encountered in emergency care.

This second edition has continued with the primary aim. Now available in digital format (smartphone application), it can support clinical practice in any setting. The provision of emergency care has changed significantly since the first edition, and the new edition reflects this. All of the chapters have been reviewed, revised, and updated. There are two new chapters, on major trauma and elderly care, which cover all the essential elements of these priority areas. Several chapters have been written by experts in their respective fields, and both editions have been enhanced by their contribution.

We hope that this handbook, in either its written or digital form, provides you with immediate access to the knowledge and skills you require. We believe that this second edition is a significant improvement on the first, and we are keen to hear your views via ✒ https://global.oup.com/academic/category/medicine-and-health/ohfeedback.

Contents

Contributors

Nicola Adams
(Chapter 20, 1e) Imperial College NHS Trust, St Mary's Hospital, London, UK

Nicola Adshead
(Chapter 20, 1e) (Formerly) Emergency Department, Stockport NHS Foundation Trust, Stockport, UK

Bruce Armstrong
(Chapter 15, 2e) Lead Clinical Educator, Emergency Department, Southampton University Hospital NHS Foundation Trust, Southampton, UK

Dawn Atkinson
(Chapter 21, 2e) Emergency Department, Stockport NHS Foundation Trust, Stockport, UK

Anne Baileff
(Chapter 14, 1e) Faculty of Health Sciences, University of Southampton, Southampton, UK

Sarah Blair
(Chapter 20, 2e) Emergency Department, Stockport NHS Foundation Trust, Stockport, UK

Carrie Boydell
(Chapter 20, 2e) Emergency Department, Stockport NHS Foundation Trust, Stockport, UK

Louise Bratt
(Chapter 20, 1e) (Formerly) Emergency Department, Stockport NHS Foundation Trust, Stockport, UK

Jenna Burnett
(Chapter 20, 2e) Emergency Department, Stockport NHS Foundation Trust, Stockport, UK

Clare Carrie
(Chapter 21, 2e) Emergency Department, Stockport NHS Foundation Trust, Stockport, UK

Mark Case
(Chapter 8, 2e) Charge Nurse, Emergency Department, Southampton University Hospital NHS Foundation Trust, Southampton, UK

Nick Castle
(Chapter 8, 1e; Chapter 20, 1e) Frimley Park Hospital NHS Foundation Trust, Frimley, UK, Honorary Research Fellow, Durban University of Technology, South Africa

Sarah Charters
(Chapter 3, 1e; Chapter 2, 2e) Emergency Department, Southampton General Hospital, Southampton, UK

Andrea Chatterton
(Chapter 20, 2e) Emergency Department, Stockport NHS Foundation Trust, Stockport, UK

Denise Conyard
(Chapter 21, 2e) Emergency Department, Stockport NHS Foundation Trust, Stockport, UK

Nicola Davies
(Chapter 21, 2e) Emergency Department, Stockport NHS Foundation Trust, Stockport, UK

Harriet Deighton
(Chapter 20, 2e) Emergency Department, Stockport NHS Foundation Trust, Stockport, UK

Charlotte Elliott
(Chapter 20, 2e) Emergency Department, Stockport NHS Foundation Trust, Stockport, UK

Aidan Foley
(Chapter 20, 1e) Imperial College NHS Trust, St Mary's Hospital, London, UK

Gerry Gallagher
(Chapter 20, 1e) Imperial College NHS Trust, St Mary's Hospital, London, UK

Rebecca Guest
(Chapter 21, 2e) Emergency Department, Stockport NHS Foundation Trust, Stockport, UK

Debbie Hancock
(Chapter 20, 1e) (Formerly) Emergency Department, Stockport NHS Foundation Trust, Stockport, UK

John Henry
(Chapter 18, 1e) Late Professor of Accident and Emergency Medicine, Imperial College NHS Trust, St Mary's Hospital, London, UK

Laura Henshall
(Chapter 20, 2e) Emergency Department, Stockport NHS Foundation Trust, Stockport, UK

Rebecca Hodgetts
(Chapter 20, 2e) Emergency Department, Stockport NHS Foundation Trust, Stockport, UK

Caroline Hodnett
(Chapter 20, 1e) Imperial College NHS Trust, St Mary's Hospital, London, UK

Joanna Jarvis
(Chapter 21, 2e) Emergency Department, South Manchester University Hospital NHS Foundation Trust, Manchester, UK

Katie Judge
(Chapter 20, 2e) Emergency Department, South Manchester University Hospital NHS Foundation Trust, Manchester, UK

Cara Lawrence
(Chapter 20, 2e) Emergency Department, Stockport NHS Foundation Trust, Stockport, UK

Stephanie Lockwood
(Chapter 4, 1e) Emergency Department, Queen Alexandra's Hospital, Portsmouth, UK

Janet Marsden
(Chapters 13 and 21, 1e and 2e) Professor of Ophthalmology and Emergency Care, Manchester Metropolitan University, Manchester, UK

Cathie Marsland
(Chapter 20, 1e) (Formerly) Emergency Department, Stockport NHS Foundation Trust, Stockport, UK

Jenny Mather
(Chapter 20, 2e) Emergency Department, Stockport NHS Foundation Trust, Stockport, UK

Gemma Parr
(Chapter 20, 1e) (Formerly) Emergency Department, Stockport NHS Foundation Trust, Stockport, UK

Rachael Pilkington
(Chapter 21, 2e) Emergency Department, Stockport NHS Foundation Trust, Stockport, UK

Paula Roderick
(Chapter 20, 1e) (Formerly) Emergency Department, Stockport NHS Foundation Trust, Stockport, UK

Audrey Ryan
(Chapter 11, 1e) Imperial College
NHS Trust, St Mary's Hospital,
London, UK

Russell Shaw
*(Illustrations Figs. 7.6, 7.8, and 7.9,
1e)* Outpatients Department,
Stockport NHS Foundation Trust,
Stockport, UK

Clare Taylor
(Chapter 20, 1e) (Formerly)
Emergency Department,
Stockport NHS Foundation Trust,
Stockport, UK

Iain Taylor
(Chapter 19, 1e) Imperial College
NHS Trust, St Mary's Hospital,
London, UK

Paul Thirlwell
(Chapter 8, 1e and 2e) Coronary
Care Unit, Southampton University
Hospital NHS Foundation Trust,
Southampton, UK

Raynie Thomson
(Chapter 20, 1e) (Formerly)
Emergency Department,
Stockport NHS Foundation Trust,
Stockport, UK

Andrew Turvey
(Chapter 20, 1e) (Formerly)
Emergency Department,
Stockport NHS Foundation Trust,
Stockport, UK

Chris Walker
(Chapter 16, 1e and 2e) Consultant
Nurse, Emergency Department,
Portsmouth Hospitals NHS Trust,
Hampshire, UK

Symbols and abbreviations

↓	decrease
↑	increase
→	leading to
◆	cross reference
☞	website
▶	important
▶▶	act quickly
❶	warning
⚠	warning
~	approximately
β	beta
x	multiplication
°C	degree Celsius
°F	degree Fahrenheit
±	plus/minus
☻	paediatric considerations
♀	female
♂	male
1°	primary
2°	secondary
=	equal to
∴	therefore
®	registered trademark
™	trademark
>	greater than
<	less than
≥	greater than or equal to
≤	less than or equal to
%	per cent
£	pound sterling
AAA	abdominal aortic aneurysm
AAP	American Academy of Pediatrics
ABC	airway, breathing, circulation
ABCDE	airway, breathing, circulation, disability, exposure
ABG	arterial blood gas
ACF	antecubital fossa

ACJ	acromioclavicular joint
ACL	anterior cruciate ligament
ACP	advanced clinical practitioner
ACS	acute coronary syndrome
ACTH	adrenocorticotrophic hormone
ADL	activity of daily living
AED	automated external defibrillator
AF	atrial fibrillation
AGE	arterial gas embolism
AIDS	acquired immune deficiency syndrome
ALD	alcoholic liver disease
ALP	alkaline phosphatase
ALS	advanced life support
ALT	alanine aminotransferase
ALTE	apparent life-threatening episode
AMD	age-related macular degeneration
AMI	acute myocardial infarction
AMS	acute mountain sickness
ANP	advanced nurse practitioner
AOM	acute otitis media
AP	anteroposterior
APGAR	American Pediatric Gross Assessment Record
aPTT	activated partial thromboplastin time
ARDS	acute respiratory distress syndrome
AST	aspartate aminotransferase
ATLS	advanced trauma life support
AV	atrioventricular
AVM	arteriovenous malformation
AXR	abdominal X-ray
BAC	blood alcohol concentration
bd	twice daily
BiPAP	bilevel positive airway pressure
BLS	basic life support
BMI	body mass index
BNF	*British National Formulary*
BP	blood pressure
bpm	beats per minute
BTS	British Thoracic Society
BVM	bag–valve–mask
Ca^{2+}	calcium

CAADA	Coordinated Action Against Domestic Abuse
$CaCl_2$	calcium chloride
CAD	coronary artery disease
CAP	community-acquired pneumonia
CBG	capillary blood glucose
cc	cubic centimetre
CCF	congestive cardiac failure
CCU	coronary care unit
CGCS	children's Glasgow Coma Score
Ch	Charrière
CHD	coronary heart disease
CJD	Creutzfeldt–Jakob disease
CK	creatine kinase
Cl^-	chloride ion
cm	centimetre
cmH_2O	centimetre of water
CN	cranial nerve
CNS	central nervous system
CO	cardiac output; carbon monoxide
CO_2	carbon dioxide
COHb	carboxyhaemoglobin
COPD	chronic obstructive pulmonary disease
CPAP	continuous positive airway pressure
CPR	cardiopulmonary resuscitation
CRF	capillary refill
CRP	C-reactive protein
C&S	culture and sensitivity
CSF	cerebrospinal fluid
CSM	Committee on Safety of Medicines
C-spine	cervical spine
CSR	central serous retinopathy
CT	computed tomography
cTnI	cardiac-specific troponin I
cTnT	cardiac-specific troponin T
CTPA	computed tomographic pulmonary angiogram
CTS	carpal tunnel syndrome
CVA	cerebrovascular accident
CVP	central venous pressure
CXR	chest X-ray
DASH	Domestic Abuse, Stalking and Honour-Based Violence

DBD	donation after brainstem death
DC	direct current
DCD	donation after circulatory death
DCS	decompression sickness
DIC	disseminated intravascular coagulation
DIPJ	distal interphalangeal joint
DKA	diabetic ketoacidosis
dL	decilitre
DNAR	do not attempt resuscitation
DPL	diagnostic peritoneal lavage
DSH	deliberate self-harm
DU	duodenal ulcer
DVT	deep vein thrombosis
ECG	electrocardiogram
ED	emergency department
EF	ejection fraction
ENP	emergency nurse practitioner
ENT	ear, nose, and throat
EOM	extraocular movement
EPAP	end-positive airway pressure
ESR	erythrocyte sedimentation rate
$EtCO_2$	end-tidal carbon dioxide
ETT	endotracheal tube
EWS	early warning score
FAST	focused assessment with sonography for trauma; Face Arm Speech Test
FB	foreign body
FBC	full blood count
FEV_1	forced expiratory volume in 1s
FFP	fresh frozen plasma
FG	French gauge
FGM	female genital mutilation
FOOSH	fall on to the outstretched hand
g	gram
G	gauge
GABHS	group A β-haemolytic Streptococcus
GCS	Glasgow Coma Scale (score)
GFR	glomerular filtration rate
GGT	gamma-glutamyl transferase
GI	gastrointestinal
GMC	General Medical Council

GP	general practitioner
GTN	glyceryl trinitrate
GU	genitourinary
GUM	genitourinary medicine
h	hour
H^+	hydrogen ion
HACO	high-altitude cerebral oedema
HAPO	high-altitude pulmonary oedema
Hb	haemoglobin
HBV	hepatitis B virus
HCG	human chorionic gonadotrophin
HCO_3^-	bicarbonate
H_2CO_3	carbonic acid
Hct	haematocrit
HCV	hepatitis C virus
HDL	high-density lipoprotein
HDL-C	high-density lipoprotein cholesterol
HDU	high dependency unit
HELLP	haemolysis, elevated liver enzymes, low platelet count
Hib	*Haemophilus influenzae* type b
HIV	human immunodeficiency virus
HME	heat and moisture exchanger
HPC	history of presenting complaint
HR	heart rate
HSE	herpes simplex encephalitis
hs-cTnI	high-sensitivity cardiac-specific TnI
hs-cTnT	high-sensitivity cardiac-specific TnT
HSV	herpes simplex virus
HTS	hypertonic sodium solution
HUS	haemolytic uraemic syndrome
HVR	hypoxic ventilatory response
IBD	inflammatory bowel disease
ICD	implantable cardioverting defibrillator
ICP	intracranial pressure
ICS	intercostal space
ICU	intensive care unit
IDC	indwelling catheter
IDL	intermediate-density lipoprotein
IDVA	Independent Domestic Violence Advocate
I:E	inspiration time:expiration time ratio

Ig	immunoglobulin
IM	intramuscular
in	inch
INR	international normalized ratio
IO	intraosseous
IPAP	intermittent positive airway pressure
IPJ	interphalangeal joint
IRMER	Ionising Radiation (Medical Exposure) Regulations
ISVA	Independent Sexual Violence Advisor
ITP	idiopathic thrombocytopenic purpura
IU	international unit
IUCD	intrauterine contraceptive device
IUD	intrauterine device
IV	intravenous
IVIG	intravenous immunoglobulin
IVU	intravenous urogram
J	joule
K^+	potassium
kg	kilogram
kPa	kilopascal
KUB	kidneys, urine, bladder (X-ray)
L	litre
LA	left atrium; local anaesthetic
lb	pound
LBBB	left bundle branch block
LDL	low-density lipoprotein
LDL-C	low-density lipoprotein cholesterol
LFT	liver function test
LLQ	left lower quadrant (of abdomen)
LMA	laryngeal mask airway
LMP	last menstrual period
LMWH	low-molecular-weight heparin
LRTI	lower respiratory tract infection
LSD	lysergic acid dimethylamide
LUQ	left upper quadrant (of abdomen)
LV	left ventricle
LVF	left ventricular failure
m	metre
mA	milliampere
MAOI	monoamine oxidase inhibitor

MAP	mean arterial pressure
MARAC	Multi-Agency Risk Assessment Conference
MASH	Multi-Agency Safeguarding Hub
MCPJ	metacarpal phalangeal joint
M, C & S	microscopy, culture, and sensitivity
MDI	metered-dose inhaler
MDR	multi-drug-resistant
mEq	milliequivalent
mg	milligram
Mg^{2+}	magnesium
MI	myocardial infarction
MIG	metal inert gas
min	minute
mL	millilitre
mm	millimetre
mmHg	millimetre of mercury
mmol	millimole
MMR	measles, mumps, rubella (vaccine)
mph	miles per hour
MRI	magnetic resonance imaging
MRSA	meticillin-resistant *Staphylococcus aureus*
MS	multiple sclerosis
MSU	midstream urine
MUA	manipulation under anaesthetic
mV	millivolt; minute volume
Na^+	sodium
NAI	non-accidental injury
NBM	nil by mouth
NEWS	National Early Warning Score
NG	nasogastric
NHS	National Health Service
NICE	National Institute for Health and Care Excellence
NIPPV	non-invasive positive pressure ventilation
NIV	non-invasive ventilation
nmol	nanomole
NPA	nasopharyngeal airway
NSAID	non-steroidal anti-inflammatory drug
NSTEMI	non-ST-elevation myocardial infarction
O_2	oxygen
OCD	obsessive–compulsive disorder

OCP	oral contraceptive pill
OE	otitis externa
OPA	oropharyngeal airway
OPG	orthopantomogram
ORIF	open reduction and internal fixation
PaO_2	arterial oxygen tension
$PaCO_2$	arterial carbon dioxide tension
PAT	Paddington Alcohol Test
PC	presenting complaint
PCI	percutaneous coronary intervention
PCL	posterior cruciate ligament
PCO_2	carbon dioxide tension
PCR	polymerase chain reaction
PE	pulmonary embolism
PEA	pulseless electrical activity
PEEP	peak end-expiratory pressure
PEFR	peak expiratory flow rate
PEP	post-exposure prophylaxis
PEWS	paediatric early warning score
PGD	patient group direction
PICU	paediatric intensive care unit
PID	pelvic inflammatory disease
PIH	primary intracerebral haemorrhage
PIPJ	proximal interphalangeal joint
PMH	past medical history
PO_2	oxygen tension
POEC	progesterone-only emergency contraception
POP	plaster of Paris
PPE	personal protective equipment
ppm	paced pulses per minute
PR	per rectum
PT	prothrombin time
PUD	peptic ulcer disease
PV	per vagina; pulmonary vein
qds	four times daily
RA	right atrium
RBBB	right bundle branch block
RBC	red blood cell
RD	retinal detachment
Rh	rhesus

RIC	Risk Identification Checklist
RICE	rest, ice, compression, and elevation
RIF	right iliac fossa
RLQ	right lower quadrant (of abdomen)
ROM	range of motion
ROSC	return of spontaneous circulation
RR	respiratory rate
RSI	rapid sequence induction
RSV	respiratory syncytial virus
RTC	road traffic collision
RUQ	right upper quadrant (of abdomen)
RV	right ventricle
s	second
SA	sinoatrial
SAD	seasonal affective disorder
SaO_2	arterial oxygen saturation
SARC	Sexual Assault Referral Centre
SARS	severe acute respiratory syndrome
SC	subcutaneous
SCD	sudden cardiac death
SH	social history
SIADH	syndrome of inappropriate antidiuretic hormone
SIGN	Scottish Intercollegiate Guideline Network
SIRS	systemic inflammatory response syndrome
SL	sublingual
SLE	systemic lupus erythematosus
SLR	straight leg raising
SN-OD	Specialist Nurse for Organ Donation
SOB	shortness of breath
SP	spontaneous pneumothorax
SpO_2	oxygen saturation measured by pulse oximetry
SPT	superficial partial thickness
STEMI	ST elevation myocardial infarction
STI	sexually transmitted infection
SUFE	slipped upper femoral epiphysis
SVT	supraventricular tachycardia
T_3	triiodothyronine
T_4	thyroxine
TB	tuberculosis
TBI	traumatic brain injury

TBSA	total body surface area
TFT	thyroid function test
TIA	transient ischaemic attack
TM	tympanic membrane
TnI	troponin I
TnT	troponin T
TSE	transmissible spongiform encephalopathy
TSH	thyroid-stimulating hormone
TSS	toxic shock syndrome
TXA	tranexamic acid
U&E	urea and electrolytes
UK	United Kingdom
UPSI	unprotected sexual intercourse
URTI	upper respiratory tract infection
USS	ultrasound scan
UTI	urinary tract infection
UV	ultraviolet
VA	visual acuity
VBG	venous blood gas
VF	ventricular fibrillation
VHF	viral haemorrhagic fever
VLDL	very-low-density lipoprotein
Vt	tidal volume
VT	ventricular tachycardia
VTE	venous thromboembolism
WBC	white blood cell
WCC	white cell count
WNV	West Nile virus
wk	week
y	year

General principles of emergency nursing

Introduction

Emergency nursing is one of the most challenging specialties in nursing. It requires nurses to manage ambiguity and rapid changes in pace and intensity of work, and to have a knowledge of a significant number of clinical presentations, diseases, and conditions. The emergency nurse must also be able to relate to, and have an understanding of, all ages, from the very young child to the elderly. Emergency nursing is not for the faint-hearted!

Golden rules of emergency nursing

- An emergency is an emergency. It is only not an emergency in retrospect!
- There is no such thing as a 'minor' injury. Behind any so-called 'minor' presentation, there may be a 'major' one masquerading.
- Remember that what looks trivial to you may have significant ramifications for the patient.
- Do not forget the fundamentals—communication and observation.
- Always introduce yourself ('Hello, my name is … ').
- Monitors are an adjunct—nurse the patient, not the monitor.
- 'If you don't like the patient, spend twice as long with them'—that way you will minimize mistakes.[1]
- 'There is no such thing as a poor historian'—it is probably your inability to elicit the history.[1]
- A fall is only a fall after a collapse has been ruled out.
- Remember that what may be a common injury or illness to you may be a first for the patient and carers.
- Have a plan for the worst possible scenario—anything less is a bonus!
- Expect the unexpected.
- If the patient says they feel as if they are going to die, believe them and do something about it.
- Common things are common, but they can still kill you—you can bleed to death from your nose or from a large scalp laceration.
- The patient is not drunk until they have experienced the hangover—do not be misled by the smell of alcohol.
- In a woman of childbearing age with abdominal pain, actively rule out an ectopic pregnancy.
- In all unwell patients, *Don't Ever Forget Glucose* (DEFG).
- When caring for children, toys and distraction are essential tools.
- Do not attribute hyperventilation to hysteria until an underlying pathology has been ruled out.
- Do not dismiss or trivialize the frequent attender. They may have an underlying illness.
- Ensure that patients re-presenting with the same complaint are seen by someone senior.
- Make sure you are competent to use the equipment around you. You cannot always rely on someone else to troubleshoot.
- If you have a 'quiet' moment, use it to familiarize yourself with the latest guidelines and procedures.
- Enjoy what you do. Although it might not always feel like it, it is a privilege to be part of people's lives at a time of crisis.

Note

1 We wish to thank Mike Clancy for these contributions.

First principles

Never an average day!

Every day is different, but there are routine things you will do every day. One of the key skills necessary for emergency nursing is anticipation. This applies to the patients you are looking after, as well as to the team with whom you are working. For your patients, given that many will have undifferentiated and undiagnosed problems, anticipating the care, investigations, and treatment that they will need is an important component of your role. Emergency care is a team pursuit. Anticipating the needs and actions of the team around you, particularly in an emergency situation, is really important. The skill of anticipation is gained over time by exposure to many situations and recognizing the patterns that develop with similar patient presentations and disease/injury processes. Fundamental to this process is knowing the patient outcome; this feedback loop is important in building expertise. This requires discipline in following patients up, seeing how they are progressing, and establishing whether your identification of their problems was correct or not.

The patient's and relatives' experience of the emergency department (ED) can be shaped by you. How will you introduce yourself?

'Hello, my name is … '

General assessment of the ED patient

Initial assessment

Do a rapid head-to-toe visual scan of the patient. Look at:

- respiratory rate (RR) and effort;
- pallor;
- positioning;
- perfusion;
- haemorrhage—visible signs of blood loss;
- signs of distress—physical and psychological.

Do not forget the history—the clues to what is wrong with your patient will be in what has happened! Listen to those who have brought the patient to the ED.

Teamwork

Multidisciplinary teamwork is fundamental to successful emergency care. For effective teamwork, excellent communication and honesty are crucial. Particularly in emergency situations, where anticipation and proficiency are of utmost importance, training, learning, and rehearsing together for incidents can pay dividends in team performance. Clearly defined roles and responsibilities among the team can reduce ambiguity and duplication of effort, particularly in challenging clinical situations. In the resuscitation room, clear allocation of roles prior to the patient's arrival can help with effective resuscitation. The information provided by prehospital personnel is very important. If there are no immediate risks to the patient, the whole team should stop and listen to the handover. Important in developing effective teamworking is honest appraisal and feedback on performance within the team.

Inappropriate and frequent attenders at the emergency department

Inappropriate attenders

As health-care professionals, it is easy to make judgements about the reasons for, and legitimacy of, attendance. Pejorative judgements about patients and their attendance can influence their clinical assessment and ultimately their treatment.

Patients may seek care in an emergency care setting, because they have either been unable to contact, or are not satisfied with care from, other health-care providers. They may have sought advice from family or friends as to where they should receive care. Navigating through the health-care system, particularly during the 'out-of-hours' period, can be a challenge. The patient may have been referred to your service by another health-care provider such as 111. Expressing an opinion about the appropriateness of referral to the patient may undermine confidence in these services. It may well not be the individual who is an inappropriate attender, but rather it may be that the health-care system is providing an inappropriate service.

It is important to remember that, behind every so-called 'minor' presentation, there may be a problem with an undetected significant pathology. Be slow to judge the appropriateness of the attendance, and take time to explore the real reason for the presentation.

Frequent attenders

Every department or emergency service provider has regular attenders, callers, or service users. Many are known by name and are familiar to staff. Their reasons for attendance are often similar and may appear trivial. It is easy to see these individuals as nuisances or time wasters. However, they often have complex needs of a physical or psychological nature, compounded by challenging social circumstances. The 'regular attenders' are often high users of primary care services as well. They are a vulnerable and at-risk group, and require extra attention, not dismissal, when they attend services.

Among the seemingly trivial reasons for attendance may be significant pathology. Remember that, just because they are regular attenders, this does not mean that they are not sick or at risk of significant physical and psychological morbidity. One of the 'golden rules' (→ see Golden rules of emergency nursing, p. 3) applies here: 'If you don't like someone, you should spend twice as long with them'. Regular attenders should be seen as part of a vulnerable or at-risk group.

Emergency clinicians should work with individual patients and appropriate members of the multidisciplinary team to develop anticipatory care plans for high-impact service users. The team may include pain, liaison psychiatry, and emergency medicine consultants, relevant specialty consultants and/or nurses, the patient's general practitioner (GP), and other relevant health and social care staff. The provision of anticipatory care plans will optimize delivery of well-informed and consistent care in the ED.

Health promotion

This is an important part of emergency care. Patients and relatives are a captive audience. Consultations enable opportunistic health promotion opportunities. However, care must be taken not to be judgemental or to apportion blame for their attendance. Careful judgement of the individual's ability or willingness to accept health promotion information at the time of attendance is necessary. There is growing evidence for the use of 'brief interventions' and 'motivational interviewing' in bringing about behavioural change. A visit to the ED may include a teachable moment that could make a long-term difference to an individual.

Having written information that can be taken away is a useful way of providing health promotion. Appropriate information in different areas in the department should be considered for different age groups. It is important to consider access to written information for those whose first language is not English. Written information in the languages spoken by local communities is important.

Thematic displays of relevant health promotion advice and information can be used to good effect in emergency care settings. Patients or relatives may be inclined to seek information about general health and well-being, whilst waiting for care.

Injury prevention

The role of emergency care settings in surveillance of accident or incident hot spots has been under-recognized. Clear patterns may emerge for road traffic incidents or areas of particular violence or aggression in communities. Monitoring and recording of such incidents can provide useful data for preventing incidents in the future. Careful liaison with local authorities in sharing data can be useful in this respect. Emergency care staff have a key role to play in injury prevention, and should utilize every opportunity to provide education to prevent further incidents and create a culture that actively seeks to prevent accidents and incidents.

The College of Emergency Medicine recommends that EDs should routinely collect, electronically wherever possible, data about assault victims at registration.[1] These data should be shared with the local Community Safety Partnership and crime analysts in an anonymous and aggregate form. The information may be used to plan local authority and policing measures to reduce the incidence of violent crime.

Reference

1 College of Emergency Medicine (2009). *Guideline for information sharing to reduce community violence in EDs*. College of Emergency Medicine, London (revised May 2010 and August 2011).

Infection prevention

Preventing infection is everyone's responsibility. Each health-care profes-sional should have an understanding of infection control and be aware of how they can help to prevent hospital- or community-acquired infection. Key areas for concentration within the emergency setting are reduction of infections related to peripheral intravenous (IV) line insertion, reduction in urinary tract infections (UTIs) by reducing unnecessary urethral catheteriza-tion, and early isolation of patients with diarrhoea and vomiting. Emergency care personnel have a key role in surveillance—they may be the first to identify trends in disease or illness patterns such as seasonal flu or an ↑ incidence of similar types of presentations from the same source or area (e.g. an outbreak of food poisoning). In recent years, we have seen an ↑ in presentations of mumps and measles, which has been attributed to a poor uptake of immunization in the recent past. The emergency care system has an important part to play in identifying and reporting these diseases.

The use of personal protective equipment (PPE) is fundamental to pre-venting transfer of infection. In an emergency care setting, little is known about the patient's past medical history. Full protection precautions should be taken with bodily fluids. Given the nature of the working environment and the need to deal with a number of patients at any given time, care must be taken to change gloves and other protective items, and to clean the hands effectively between patients. The importance of hand hygiene cannot be overemphasized.

Notifiable diseases

Health-care professionals are required to notify a 'proper officer' of the local authority of suspected cases of certain infectious diseases. This is required under the Public Health (Infectious Diseases) 1988 Act and the Public Health (Control of Diseases) 1984 Act. This information is then passed in turn to Public Health England. Local information should be avail-able about to whom to report and the information required.

The following diseases are notifiable to Local Authority Proper Officers under the Health Protection (Notification) Regulations 2010:[2]

- acute encephalitis;
- acute infectious hepatitis;
- acute meningitis;
- acute poliomyelitis;
- anthrax;
- botulism;
- brucellosis;
- cholera;
- diphtheria;
- enteric fever (typhoid or paratyphoid fever);
- food poisoning;
- haemolytic uraemic syndrome (HUS);
- infectious bloody diarrhoea;
- invasive group A streptococcal disease;
- legionnaires' disease;
- leprosy;

- malaria;
- measles;
- meningococcal septicaemia;
- mumps;
- plague;
- rabies;
- rubella;
- severe acute respiratory syndrome (SARS);
- scarlet fever;
- smallpox;
- tetanus;
- tuberculosis (TB);
- typhus;
- viral haemorrhagic fever (VHF);
- whooping cough;
- yellow fever.

Reference

2 For further information, see Public Health England (2010). *Notifiable diseases and causative organisms: how to report.* Available at: ℘ https://www.gov.uk/guidance/notifiable-diseases-and-causative-organisms-how-to-report

Patients with learning disabilities

Recent evidence has identified that individuals with learning disability are at greater risk of health inequality and premature death than the general population.[3] Patients with learning disabilities require specific attention in the emergency care setting. This setting can cause considerable distress, exacerbating challenges to understanding and communication. Patients with learning disabilities are vulnerable. Staff should be trained to meet their needs and to be able to communicate effectively. Consideration should be given to the environment. The amount of stimulation from noise and human traffic can cause additional stress. Close links should be made with local learning disability specialists to facilitate early expert care.

Close involvement with relatives and carers in the assessment and management of those with learning disabilities is fundamental. Behavioural regression is not uncommon in emergency situations. Working with those who normally care for the individual will be invaluable in managing the situation. A high level of clinical care is required for this vulnerable client group, who are particularly at risk in an unfamiliar emergency environment.

Mencap has identified the following common factors that may have contributed to the premature death of people with learning disability:[4]

- lack of basic care;
- poor communication;
- delays in diagnosis and treatment;
- failure to recognize pain;
- inappropriate use of 'do not resuscitate' orders;
- flawed best-interests decision-making.

To improve care delivery, ED staff should:

- engage with the use of hospital passports;
- use appropriate communication aids (e.g. picture books);
- recognize that a change in behaviour may indicate pain or illness;
- provide a suitable environment for care delivery;
- make reasonable adjustments to meet the needs of people with learning disability;
- fully involve family members and carers in decision-making;
- involve specialist learning disability staff in care delivery;
- understand and utilize the provisions of the Mental Capacity Act (2005);
- undertake robust admission and discharge planning.

References

3 Department of Health (2013). *Confidential inquiry into premature deaths of people with learning disabilities.* For further information, see ℜ http://www.bris.ac.uk/cipold/.
4 Mencap (2012). *Death by indifference: 74 deaths and counting. A progress report 5 years on.* Mencap, London.

Models of unscheduled care delivery

A number of new models of service delivery are emerging. The exact configuration for service provision for the future is not clear. However, several key principles are evident. The principles are based on centralizing services to major emergency centres within an agreed network of providers. These new models of service delivery are driven by policy changes and clinical developments. The advent of thrombolysis for ischaemic stroke and the development of regional centres offering percutaneous coronary intervention (PCI) and the provision of an England-wide trauma system mean that service reconfigurations are needed. Changes in the commissioning of services are changing the shape of unscheduled care delivery. The new national 111 telephone service aims to provide a central point of navigation for patients and carers to direct them to services appropriate to their needs. The new models of urgent and emergency care will not only provide challenges, but also create opportunities for service delivery. However, many of the models in use have not been thoroughly clinically evaluated.

Fundamental to developing unscheduled services is the provision of consistent access with clear parameters of practice to ensure that the public knows where, when, and how to access unscheduled care. Given the current changes in service provision, it is likely that formal systems of unscheduled and emergency care will emerge such as the development of emergency care networks with centralization of a number of services.

Triage

Triage—that is, determining the urgency of care—is common in EDs in the United Kingdom (UK). The key processes are:
- rapid assessment;
- identifying life- or limb-threatening problems;
- initiation of investigations;
- providing analgesia;
- controlling patient flow.

A national consensus was reached between senior nurses and doctors from professional organizations in the UK in the 1990s about triage categories, times, and nomenclatures (➲ see Table 2.1).

See and treat

Many departments have changed their triage process in recent years to incorporate a 'See and treat' service. 'See and treat' works on the basis of bringing a senior decision-maker (an experienced emergency nurse practitioner or doctor) close to the triage area to identify patients who can be seen and treated almost as soon as they arrive. This process allows early management of some of the most straightforward presentations and removes them from the overall queue of patients waiting to be seen. Depending on the case mix of patients presenting, this has helped with managing demand in a number of departments.

Streaming

Many departments have also introduced the concept of streaming patients. This process involves allocating patients to streams of activity within the department or to other service providers from triage. An example of this may be identification of patients at triage who would be suitable for 'See and treat' and directing them to that stream or alternatively to a local walk-in centre from triage. The success of these initiatives relies on effective staffing and management of the streams to which patients are directed, to ensure that the patient's journey through the department is as smooth as possible.

Initial assessment

Departments have introduced an initial assessment process for patients arriving by ambulance. This is in response to the introduction of the Quality Indicators to replace the 4h time standard and focus on quality. The standard is for all patients who arrive by ambulance and should be achieved within 20min of arrival or handover by the ambulance crew. Initial assessment must include a pain score and physiological scoring. The aim is to reduce delays to assessment within the ED. This complements the focus on early ambulance crew handover of patient care (within 15min of arrival), facilitating early release of ambulances back into the community. A useful assessment framework for initial assessment is shown in Fig. 2.1.

Table 2.1 National triage scale

Category	Description	Time frame to be seen
1 Red	Immediate	Immediately
2 Orange	Very urgent	Within 10min of arrival
3 Yellow	Urgent	Within 1h of arrival
4 Green	Standard	Within 2h of arrival
5 Blue	Non-urgent	Within 4h of arrival

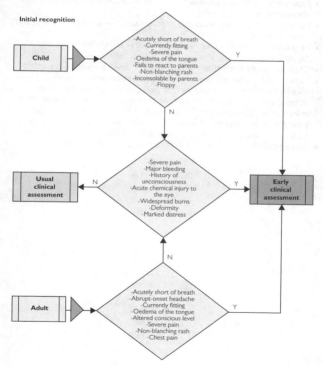

Fig. 2.1 Initial recognition.

(Reproduced with kind permission of the College of Emergency Medicine, from the 'Triage Position Statement', April 2011 (CEM, ENCA, FEN, RCN).)

Documentation

The gold standard for documentation is a contemporaneous record. When this is not possible, it is important to make it clear that the notes have been written retrospectively.

Key elements to document

- Time and date seen.
- Person giving the information (i.e. the patient, parent, relative, or carer).
- When using the patient's own words, use speech marks.
- Sign, time, and date every entry.
- Avoid using abbreviations.
- Develop a structured approach. This will act as an aide-memoire if you always use the same format.
- Record nursing assessments and interventions, personal care, drinks and meals given, etc.
- Handover of care to other nurses or health-care professionals should be recorded.
- Clear discharge instructions and plans for follow-up must be recorded.
- Increasingly, nurses are required to provide statements of events. These may be used in criminal, coroner, or negligence proceedings—your notes may be scrutinized in court. At the very least, you will need to refer to the patient record if you are asked to give evidence. Would your documentation stand up to this scrutiny? Remember that you may be asked to account years after the event and will only have your notes.
- Remember the old adage 'If it isn't recorded, it didn't happen!'

The handover of care

The handover of information from prehospital ambulance personnel to ED staff is crucial, particularly in emergency situations. Each ED should have an agreed process for this. On reception of the patient, the person(s) taking over the handover should be identified. Essential care of the patient should continue. Take the history and handover of care given en route. It is good practice to summarize the history and repeat it to the person handing over the patient, in order to ensure that the salient information is transferred. Wherever possible, handover should be given to the person taking ongoing responsibility for the patient—reducing the number of times that information is handed over will reduce the risk of inaccuracies or errors. A written record of prehospital care given is essential.

Pre-alerting EDs about patients who will require resuscitation or immediate intervention on arrival is good practice. The commonly used mnemonic 'ATMIST' by ambulance services ensures a concise method of delivering important information from the scene to facilitate correct preparation for trauma patients. This has been adapted to include aspects suitable for medical emergency presentations.

ATMIST

- *A*ge of patient.
- *T*ime of incident, injury, or onset of symptoms.
- *M*echanism of injury.
- *I*njuries or *I*llness (head to toe).
- *S*igns—vital signs.
- *T*reatments given and estimated time of arrival.

Interhospital or intrahospital/care setting handover

Information about the patient can be lost at any stage. Important information about the events that occurred preceding admission and during their treatment in the ED must be handed over to the next team providing care. Ideally, it should be the person who has cared for the patient who hands over care to the next team. If this is not possible, a careful briefing should be given. In some settings, a written handover of information is considered to be best practice. For critical care transfers, particular attention should be paid to preparation for transfer. Checking equipment for battery life, supplementary O_2, and resuscitation equipment are essential. Preparing for the worst possible scenario in transfer is good practice.

History taking

Obtaining a comprehensive history is fundamental in clinical practice, so spend time getting an accurate history. Vital information is gained from the patient, carers, parents (in the case of children), other family members, and community carers, including the GP and prehospital staff.

A general approach to history taking is as follows:
- Presenting complaint (PC)—why the patient has attended the department today (e.g. right wrist injury).
- History of presenting complaint (HPC):
  - what happened (e.g. fall on to outstretched hand);
  - how it happened (e.g. tripping over loose carpet);
  - when it happened (e.g. this morning at ~10 a.m.);
  - where it happened;
  - any additional information.
- In the case of illness:
  - recent events—any prodromal features, any recent foreign travel;
  - any other members of the family who are affected.
- Past medical history (PMH): information about previous injuries and/or illness. It is important to take time to ascertain information about PMH, as it may have a direct bearing on the PC. If, for instance, there is a history of postural hypotension, one might consider asking the patient if they had got up from a chair immediately before they fell.
- Medication ('meds'). What medication does the patient take? Ask about:
  - prescribed medications;
  - over-the-counter medications;
  - complementary medicines;
  - recreational drug use.

Consider:
  - medication as a cause of presentation, particularly polypharmacy in the older person;
  - how medications may affect different presentations (e.g. warfarin and head injury);
  - in the case of illness, immunization history, especially in children;
  - in the case of injury, remember to ask about tetanus status.
- Allergies—both pharmacological and non-pharmacological allergies are important. Medications can have a food base (e.g. eggs in some immunizations).
- Social history (SH):
  - alcohol consumption and recreational drug use;
  - smoking status;
  - for children—family structure (e.g. siblings, legal guardianships, school or college);
  - for adults—occupation, accommodation (particularly for the older person when considering mobility issues), hand dominance (important when considering arm and hand injuries).

Findings on examination (O/E)

- Inspection (look).
  - General appearance. Do they look unwell? Are they sweaty?
  - Note any deformity or discrepancy in contour, bruising, swelling, or bleeding. ▶ Compare with the unaffected side.
  - Note scars from previous surgery.
- Palpation (feel).
  - Note bony tenderness, crepitus, and deformity.
  - Check the circulation distal to the injury.
  - A full systematic systems examination may be required.
- Auscultation. Evaluation of lung fields, heart sounds, bruits, and bowel sounds as appropriate.
- Percussion. Chest and abdomen as appropriate.
- Movements. Test the range of movement, and describe it.
  - ▶ Compare with the unaffected side.
- Neurological. Test power, tone, and sensation of the affected area.
  - ▶ Compare with the other side.

Impression

A note of the impression formed after assessment is important. This can include a differential diagnosis (i.e. a number of diagnostic possibilities that can be either ruled in or excluded when the findings of any investigations are received). Although 'common things are common', it is important to consider rare presentations or conditions.

Plan

It is important to have a plan of investigations or plan of care for the patient. Careful documentation is important.

Final impression

A clear outline of what you believe to be the problem or diagnosis.

Final instructions

It is helpful to give the patient an outline of what to expect and/or the likely course of their illness or injury recovery. This is helpfully accompanied by instructions about where and when to seek further health-care assistance if there is a deviation from this predicted course. This is a safety net both for the patient and for you as the clinician.

For additional information about history taking and assessment in children and young adults, ➔ see Chapter 4, p. 74.

Careful documentation is part of good clinical practice.

Advanced practice

There are a number of advanced practice roles in emergency care. These roles commonly have an element of advanced practice using extended patient assessment skills and forming differential diagnoses. There is no formal regulation of advanced practice in the UK.

Emergency nurse practitioners

Emergency nurse practitioners (ENPs) were introduced in the UK in the 1980s. Most EDs now have ENPs as part of the clinical team. The role involves a more autonomous level of practice, including assessment, requesting and interpreting of investigations, differential diagnoses, patient management, and discharge. There is a developing evidence base of effectiveness of the role focused around minor injuries and illnesses. ↑ numbers of departments are now developing a 'major' nurse practitioner role.

There are no UK-wide agreements on scope of practice, educational preparation, or standards for testing or examining competence.

Advanced clinical practitioners

Advanced clinical practitioners (ACPs) are practitioners from different professional backgrounds such as nurses, paramedics, physiotherapists, and pharmacists. In some units where the workforce is entirely nursing, they are referred to as advanced nurse practitioners (ANPs). The ACP has a broader clinical role than the ENP. They practise at an advanced level in all areas of the ED, including the 'majors', the resuscitation room, minors, and paediatrics. The ACP is educated to Masters degree level.[5]

There is growing interest in this role. An England-wide competency framework, assessment, and credentialing process is being developed under the auspices of Health Education England.[6]

With the development of advanced roles and the changing medical workforce profile, many departments now have a multidisciplinary group of clinicians seeing and treating patients who, in the previous decade, would have been treated by doctors. There is a developing evidence base to support the use of ACPs.

Independent prescribing

Nurses who have undertaken a specific and recognized programme of education can now be registered as independent and/or supplementary prescribers, following a change in the law in 2001.[7] Since April 2012, qualified nurse independent prescribers have been able to prescribe any licensed medication for any medical condition within their competence. This includes controlled drugs (Schedules 2–5, with the exception of 3 named controlled drugs for the treatment of addiction (diamorphine, cocaine, and dipipanone)). Independent prescribing allows nurses to practise with a greater degree of autonomy and to expand the scope of their practice within a competency framework. Independent prescribing has been extended to other groups, including pharmacists and physiotherapists. Advanced and autonomous practice brings with it greater accountability and the potential for litigation.

References

5 Association of Advanced Practice Educators UK. Available at: ℘ http://www.aape.org.uk.
6 Health Education England (2013). *Emergency medicine: background to HEE proposals to address workforce shortages.* Health Education England, London.
7 Further information about independent and supplementary prescribing can be found in: Beckwith S and Franklin P (2011). *Oxford handbook of prescribing for nurses and allied health professionals.* Oxford University Press, Oxford.

Early warning scores

Early warning scores (EWS) and paediatric EWS (PEWS) are increasingly being recorded in emergency care areas as a means of identifying haemodynamic instability at an early stage. Evidence suggests that hospital staff are slow to recognize signs of early deterioration, and intervention is commonly delayed.[8] A National Early Warning Score (NEWS) has been agreed for use in adult patients and is now in common use in England.[9] There is no nationally agreed PEWS system, and there are a number of variations in use. A NEWS or PEWS score is calculated by adding together the scores attributed to various haemodynamic parameters. The sum total of each score gives an overall score, on which subsequent assessment, management, and escalation are based. An elevated NEWS or PEWS score requires intervention from senior staff to identify and treat the cause of the deranged physiology.

References

8 National Institute for Health and Care Excellence (2007). *Acute illness in adults in hospital: recognising and responding to deterioration.* Available at: ℘ https://www.nice.org.uk/guidance/cg50.

9 Royal College of Physicians (2012). *National Early Warning Score (NEWS). Standardising the assessment of acute-illness severity in the NHS.* Available at: ℘ http://www.rcplondon.ac.uk/resources/national-early-warning-score-news.

Major incidents and terrorism

A major incident can be described as a situation in which the demands imposed by the situation outstrip the resources available. A major incident can be called by an external agency such as the ambulance service or the internal organization. The type and nature of the major incident can vary widely. Consideration should be given to your local circumstances. For instance, if your department is near the coast or an airport, you could have a major incident related to a coastal event or an aircraft experiencing problems at landing or take-off. In more recent times, it has become necessary for heightened consideration to be given to chemical, biological, radiological, and nuclear emergencies (CBRN). Relevant training for dealing with major incidents is mandatory.

Each ED and National Health Service (NHS) trust must have an established major incident plan.

The notification of a major incident is often delivered using a structured format, known as METHANE:

- **M**ajor incident declared (or hospitals on standby);
- **E**xact location;
- **T**ype of incident—brief details of the type of incident, numbers of vehicles involved, buildings, aircraft, etc.;
- **H**azards—present and potential;
- **A**ccess and egress;
- **N**umbers and types of casualties;
- **E**mergency Services present and required.

In a mass casualty situation, it is fundamentally important that a structured approach is used. The CSCATTT principles are applied:

- **C**ommand;
- **S**afety;
- **C**ommunication;
- **A**ssessment;
- **T**riage;
- **T**reatment;
- **T**ransport.

Given the nature of a major incident, there are likely to be mass casualties. A different approach to triage is invoked. This is referred to as *triage* (*sieve and sort*).

The *triage sieve* is used to identify those who are most in need of immediate intervention. This is conducted at the scene. The *triage sort* takes place after this and is a more detailed assessment that is normally carried out at a casualty clearing station or receiving unit.

The triage categories used in a major incident are shown in Table 2.2.

It is essential that you are familiar with your local major incident plan.

Table 2.2 Mass casualty triage scale

Priority	Time frame	Colour
P1	Immediate—life-saving intervention	Red
P2	Urgent—intervention 2–4h	Orange
P3	Delayed—intervention >4h	Green
P4	Dead	Black or white

Terrorism

In recent years, the threat from terrorist attacks has ↑, and heightened awareness is therefore necessary. Any area of mass gathering is a potential target. When considering major incident planning, management of terrorist attacks should form part of the plan. Consideration should be given to the different types of injuries and illnesses that could be caused by such attacks, particularly when unfamiliar mechanisms or means are used to cause harm. Special consideration should be given to the preservation of evidence.

Prevent strategy

ED clinicians must ensure that they are aware of the UK Government's Prevent strategy, and of their role in identifying vulnerable patients who are at risk of becoming terrorists or supporting terrorism.

Three national objectives have been identified for the Prevent strategy:[10]
• Objective 1: respond to the ideological challenge of terrorism and the threat from those who promote it;
• Objective 2: prevent people from being drawn into terrorism, and ensure that they are given appropriate advice and support;
• Objective 3: work with sectors and institutions where there are risks of radicalization that need to be addressed.

The health sector contribution to the Prevent strategy focuses primarily on Objectives 2 and 3. In your work, you may notice unusual changes in the behaviour of patients and/or colleagues which are sufficient to cause concern. It is important that, if you have a cause for concern, you know how to raise it, as well as what will happen once you have done so.[10]

Guidance for health-care workers is provided by the Department of Health document *Building partnerships, staying safe: guidance for healthcare organizations.*[10]

Reference

10 Department of Health (2011). *Building partnerships, staying safe: guidance for healthcare organizations*. Department of Health, London.

Legal and ethical issues: consent, capacity, and confidentiality

Consent

Traditionally, emergency care practice has relied on the notion of implied consent. If the attendance is voluntary, the consent to examination and, to some extent, to treatment was assumed to be implied by the patient seeking assistance. However, given the increasingly litigious nature of society, implied consent is not sufficient. Emergency nurses must have an awareness of the legal framework for practice.

In many cases or procedures, such as the use of wound infiltration with local anaesthetic (LA) for exploration and/or closure or local nerve blocks, it is common to obtain verbal consent from the patient. However, a full explanation of the procedure, including the risks and benefits, should be given before proceeding. It is advisable that this process is witnessed. For procedures that require conscious sedation, such as the reduction of a fracture and dislocation, it is advisable to obtain written consent prior to the procedure. This would also apply to other procedures such as Bier's block.

Capacity

Decision-making capacity is the ability that an individual possesses to make decisions or to take actions that influence their life.[11] Under normal circumstances, every adult has the right to decide whether they will accept medical treatment, even if refusal may risk permanent damage to health. Competent adults may refuse treatment for reasons that are rational or irrational, or for no reason.

A person lacks capacity if, at the time when a decision needs to be made, they are unable to make or communicate their decision because of an impairment of, or disturbance in, the function of the mind or brain.[12] The impairment may be temporary (e.g. mental illness, reduced conscious level, intoxication) or long-term (e.g. dementia, learning disability, brain damage).

Capacity should be assessed in relation to each particular decision that has to be made, rather than by making a general assessment. The more serious the consequences of a decision, the greater the level of competence required to make that decision. If capacity is likely to improve, any interventions that are not urgent should be delayed until capacity has been recovered.

The Mental Capacity Act 2005 provides a statutory framework to empower and protect vulnerable people who are not able to make their own decisions.[12] It has five statutory principles:

- Principle 1: a person must be assumed to have capacity, unless it is established that they lack capacity;
- Principle 2: a person is not to be treated as unable to make a decision, unless all practicable steps to help them to do so have been taken without success;
- Principle 3: a person is not to be treated as unable to make a decision merely because they make an unwise decision;

- Principle 4: an act done, or decision made, under this Act or on behalf of a person who lacks capacity must be done, or made, in their best interests;
- Principle 5: before the act is done, or the decision is made, regard must be had as to whether the purpose for which it is needed can be as effectively achieved in a way that is less restrictive of the person's rights and freedom of action.

If staff have concerns about mental capacity, particularly if there is a high risk of treatment refusal and/or absconding, and a high risk of harm to self or others, mental capacity should be assessed and documented formally. A senior decision-maker should then be involved in formulating a management plan.

To assess capacity, clinicians should ask the following questions.
- Is there an impairment or disturbance of the person's mind or brain? This may be temporary or permanent.
- If the person has an impairment or disturbance of their mind or brain, are they (with support and assistance):
  - able to understand the information relevant to the question?
  - able to retain that information?
  - able to use or weigh up that information as part of the decision-making process?
  - able to communicate their decision?

In order to be robust in their documentation, clinicians should describe their method of assessment and why they reached their conclusion for each element of this process.

Confidentiality

ED clinicians should have access to a clear local information-sharing protocol to clarify how and when information may be shared with partner agencies.

Confidentiality is a right, except in exceptional circumstances. Consent from the patient to share information among members of the team should be sought. Relatives or friends may call to enquire whether a particular patient is in the department. Consent should be sought from the patient as to what information can be divulged and to whom. In situations where sharing this information outside of the team will have consequences for the patient, their consent must be sought.

If they withhold consent or are not able to give consent, information may only be shared where it can be justified as being in the public interest or if it is required by law or an order of court. In situations of safeguarding vulnerable adults and children, local policies and procedures must be followed. Further information can be found in the Nursing and Midwifery Code of Conduct.[13] You may need to defend your actions if you have breached confidentiality.

Emergency nurses should be aware of the General Medical Council (GMC) guidance about reporting gunshot and knife wounds.[14]

- In cases of alleged assault, considerable care should be taken when handling enquiries, as the assailant may want to find out where the alleged victim is being treated.
- The press are often interested in high-profile incidents or 'celebrity' attendees, and will often use a number of ruses or guises to obtain information. In sensitive cases, it may be appropriate to have a password that is shared among legitimate contacts to provide some degree of information security. Be aware, and brief your staff—reporters or journalists can be very persuasive, inventive, and persistent!
- Inadvertent breaches of confidentiality can occur during corridor conversations. No matter how interesting the case or presentation, the patient has a right to confidentiality.
- Hospital colleagues occasionally injure themselves and become sick. They too have a right to a confidential visit and consultation. It can be easy not to afford them the same rights when enquiries are received from concerned colleagues!

References

11 British Medical Association (2007). *The Mental Capacity Act 2005: guidance for health professionals*. British Medical Association, London. Available at: ℅ http://www.bma.org.uk.

12 Department of Health (2005). *Mental Capacity Act*. Department of Health, London.

13 Nursing and Midwifery Council (2008). *The code: standards of conduct, performance and ethics for nurses and midwives*. Available at: ℅ http://www.nmc.org.uk.

14 General Medical Council (2009). *Confidentiality: reporting gunshot and knife wounds*. General Medical Council, London.

Legal and ethical issues: assault and restraint

Assault and battery: supporting the victim

Within criminal law, assault and battery may be components of the same offence.

- Assault is an act that creates fear of imminent battery through intentional and unlawful threat to cause physical injury. No physical contact is involved.
- Battery is the intentional touching of a person against their will by another person, or by an object or substance used by that person, even if no physical injury is caused.

Careful record keeping during the clinical consultation, including body maps and/or clinical photography, may support any future legal proceedings. The patient should be asked whether the incident is part of ongoing victimization, such as domestic abuse or hate crime, and offered referral to the police and other partner agencies as appropriate. Acute stress reactions may occur as a result of assault and battery. These usually subside over a few days or weeks. If the experiences continue, worsen, or cause marked distress, the patient should be advised to contact their GP or local Victim Support team.

Treatment and restraint under the provision of the Mental Capacity Act 2005

No one can give consent on behalf of an incompetent adult. Treatment may be given under the Mental Capacity Act 2005 if it is necessary to save life or prevent deterioration, if the clinician has a duty of care to the patient, and if the intervention is in the patient's best interests. However, even if a person lacks capacity, they should still be enabled, as far as possible, to participate in the decision-making process.[15]

Restraint may only be used if the person using it believes it is necessary to prevent harm to the patient. The restraint used must be proportionate to the likelihood and seriousness of the harm. Restraint is defined as: (1) the use or threat of force when the patient is resisting, or (2) any restriction of liberty of movement, whether the patient resists or not.[16] Restraint may be applied via verbal, chemical (rapid tranquilization), or physical means. The minimum level of restraint necessary to protect the patient should be used, and physical intervention should only be considered as a last resort.

The National Institute for Health and Care Excellence (NICE) guideline *Violence: the short-term management of disturbed/violent behaviour in psychiatric in-patient settings and emergency departments* offers helpful guidance on the use of both rapid tranquillization and physical intervention.[17]

A local protocol that covers all aspects of rapid tranquillization and physical intervention should be made available to ED staff. These interventions should only be authorized by a senior clinician. Physical intervention should only be employed by an individual trained to do so. Restraint should be applied for no longer than 2–3min, and no direct pressure should be applied to the neck, thorax, abdomen, back, or pelvis. A clinician must remain responsible for monitoring patient safety and vital signs throughout the application of both rapid tranquillization and physical intervention.[17]

References

15 British Medical Association (2007). *The Mental Capacity Act 2005: guidance for health professionals.* British Medical Association, London. Available at: ℛ http://www.bma.org.uk.

16 Department of Health (2005). *Mental Capacity Act.* Department of Health, London.

17 National Institute for Health and Care Excellence (2005). *Violence: the short-term management of disturbed/violent behaviour in psychiatric in-patient settings and emergency departments.* Available at: ℛ http://www.rcpsych.ac.uk/PDF/NICE%20Guideline%202005.pdf.

Dealing with difficult situations: violence and aggression

Dealing with difficult situations

Challenging or difficult situations are not uncommon in emergency care. Consideration of, and planning for, some of the more predictable situations will be of benefit. Consideration must be given to the patient, their carers, and the staff dealing with these situations, as they may require considerable support.

Violence and aggression towards staff

Each department or setting must have clear guidelines and policies for managing violence and aggression. Patient and staff safety is paramount. Protection of staff is vital. This should include adequate provision for calling for assistance in the event of danger, as well as provision of training in de-escalation techniques and control and restraint.

Within any situation where violence or aggression occurs, the mental capacity of the aggressor should be assessed by a senior clinician, and the outcome of this assessment used to guide the response by the clinical and security team.

Key liaison with police and security staff is essential. Planning for, and rehearsing, responses to violent or aggressive incidents is a useful strategy.

Support frameworks and personnel should be provided for staff who have been involved in violent or aggressive incidents. This should include support from the employer to pursue legal redress against the assailant. Inadequate staff support following such an incident may lead to long-term problems for those involved.

Dealing with difficult situations: abuse

Domestic abuse

The Home Office revised the definition of domestic abuse in 2013 as follows:

> 'Any incident or pattern of incidents of controlling, coercive or threatening behaviour, violence or abuse between those aged 16 or over who are, or have been, intimate partners or family members regardless of gender or sexuality. The abuse can encompass, but is not limited to:
> - psychological
> - physical
> - sexual
> - financial
> - emotional.
>
> Controlling behaviour is a range of acts designed to make a person subordinate and/or dependent by isolating them from sources of support, exploiting their resources and capacities for personal gain, depriving them of the means needed for independence, resistance and escape and regulating their everyday behaviour.
>   Coercive behaviour is an act or a pattern of acts of assault, threats, humiliation and intimidation or other abuse that is used to harm, punish, or frighten their victim.'

Note that this definition includes so-called 'honour'-based violence, female genital mutilation (FGM), and forced marriage, and is clear that victims are not confined to one gender or ethnic group.

Health professionals are often the first point of contact for people who have experienced domestic abuse, and they should be trained to give an appropriate response. The use of routine enquiry about domestic abuse remains controversial. EDs should at least have a policy that promotes targeted screening within a safe, confidential, and supportive environment.

Following disclosure of domestic abuse, clinicians should reassure the individual and seek to make it easier for them to talk about their experiences by taking a non-judgemental stance. Assessment of risk to the patient and their children should be undertaken. The Coordinated Action Against Domestic Abuse (CAADA) Domestic Abuse, Stalking and Honour-Based Violence (DASH) Risk Identification Checklist (RIC) is a nationally recognized tool for assessing risk related to domestic abuse, including so-called 'honour'-based violence.

Staff should not encourage patients to leave their abusive partner, as only the individual will know when it is safe to do so. However, help should be given with safety planning, and clinicians can facilitate access to a refuge if the patient requests it. When domestic abuse is disclosed, clinicians should consider whether adult or child safeguarding factors exist and follow local Adult and Child Safeguarding policies as appropriate. Midwifery services should be advised of women who have been assaulted during pregnancy.

If the patient gives consent, referral to partner agencies, including the police and domestic abuse advocacy services, may help to reduce repeat victimization. Research has indicated a significant reduction in risk, following referral to an Independent Domestic Violence Advocate (IDVA).[18]

It is important that health staff contribute to local multi-agency partnerships to tackle domestic abuse such as the Multi-Agency Risk Assessment Conference (MARAC) and/or Multi-Agency Safeguarding Hub (MASH).

The government has published helpful guidance for professionals regarding information sharing in the context of domestic abuse.[19] Guidance regarding the care of victims of domestic abuse is also available.[18]

A vulnerable adult is someone 'who is or may be in need of community care services by reason of mental or other disability, age or illness; and who is or may be unable to take care of him or herself, or unable to protect him or herself against significant harm or exploitation'.[19]

Vulnerable adults are at risk of abuse which is often unrecognized and under-reported. The true extent of this abuse is not known. There should be as great a suspicion with vulnerable adults as there is with non-accidental injury (NAI) in children, particularly if the story or mechanism does not fit with the injury or illness or there are unexplained findings. There are many forms of abuse, including:

- physical—including hitting, misuse of medication, and restraint;
- sexual—including sexual assault and rape;
- psychological—including emotional abuse, humiliation, and threats to harm;
- financial or material—including fraud, theft, and misappropriation of benefits;
- acts of omission or neglect—including ignoring physical or medical needs, delays in seeking care, and failure to provide care or seek help;
- discrimination—including racist, sexual, or disability-based comments (➔ see Box 2.1).

Box 2.1 END ABUSE: a guide to intervention

- *Empowerment.* Enable people to know what their choices are—the choices need to be feasible and practical (information should be made available and known to staff in advance).
- *Neglect* is as much a form of abuse as a violent act. This may be the only sign; when identified, it requires action.
- *Documentation.* Careful documentation, if there is injury and/or illness, is essential for future reference if legal action is to be taken. Remember to document the patient's own words.
- *Advocacy.* In the case of a vulnerable elderly person who is either physically or mentally incapacitated and is unable to speak for themselves, you may have to act as their advocate.
- *Be aware* of the organizations that can assist and have to hand information that can be given to the victim (this may need to be done discreetly).
- *Understanding.* Part of the intervention is to help the victim understand that abuse is a crime, that they are a victim (it is not their fault), and that help is available.
- *Social services.* Early involvement of social services is essential when abuse is identified.
- *Education* of staff in the recognition of elder abuse and the sensitive steps to be taken when identified is fundamental.

Reproduced with kind permission from Crouch, R (2003) Emergency care of the older person. In *Emergency nursing care: principles and practice* (ed. G Jones, R Endacott, and R Crouch). Greenwich Medical Media, Cambridge University Press, London.

References

18 Department of Health (2005). *Responding to domestic abuse: a handbook for health professionals.* Department of Health, London.
19 Douglas N, Lilley SJ, Kooper L, and Diamond A (2004). *Safety and justice: sharing personal information in the context of domestic violence—an overview. Home Office Development and Practice Report No. 30.* Home Office, London.

Dealing with difficult situations: sexual assault

When caring for a patient who discloses sexual assault, clinicians should ascertain whether a vulnerable adult, child, or domestic abuse is a factor, and follow local adult and child safeguarding policy and/or domestic abuse guidelines, as appropriate.

Following sexual assault, victims have three main care needs: forensic, medical, and psychosocial.[20] Unless medical problems take precedence, forensic examination should be performed as early as possible, if consent has been given to do so.

- If the patient gives consent, they may be referred to the police, who will coordinate forensic and legal actions. Whether or not the police are involved, patients can be referred to a Sexual Assault Referral Centre (SARC), which will provide support and services (including forensic medical examination) following sexual assault.[21,22]
- If medical needs predominate, ED staff should optimize the preservation of forensic evidence during care provision. Helpful advice regarding preservation of forensic evidence may be gained from ℅ http://www.careandevidence.org.
- Urgent consultation with a specialist in genitourinary medicine (GUM) should be undertaken to discuss the risks associated with blood-borne viruses and other sexually acquired illness. Pregnancy testing and post-coital contraception should be offered where appropriate. Arrangements should be made for follow-up screening by GUM staff.
- Independent Sexual Violence Advisors (ISVAs) offer information, advice, and support to victims of sexual offences. ED clinicians should familiarize themselves with how to contact their local ISVA service.
- Referral for counselling via the patient's GP or a voluntary agency may be required. The Rape Crisis service provides face-to-face and telephone counselling by qualified and trained volunteers.

References

20 Cybulska B (2007). Sexual assault: key issues. *J R Soc Med* **100**, 321–4.
21 Department of Health and Home Office (2005). *National service guideline for developing sexual assault referral centres (SARCs)*. Department of Health, London.
22 Home Office (2006). *Tackling sexual violence: guidance for local partnerships*. Home Office, London.

Dealing with difficult situations: forensic issues

Patients may attend the ED as a result of an incident in which criminal proceedings may ensue. Preservation of evidence is of utmost importance. Care should be taken not to dispose of anything that could constitute evidence. Careful documentation of facts is important. Each department should have an agreed process for preservation of evidence and a sufficient supply of materials necessary for the storage of the evidence. A careful record of all personnel interacting or involved with the case should be kept. They may need to be contacted for witness statements at a later date.

Dealing with difficult situations: resuscitation, death, and communicating bad news

Witnessed resuscitation

In recent years, this has become commoner practice. Exposure to resuscitation scenes in television dramas appears to have had a role in preparing relatives for what they might witness. Some clinicians are still uncomfortable with the concept of relatives being present, whilst resuscitation is being carried out. Experience from practice suggests that relatives are focusing on their loved one, and not on what is going on around them. They often express gratitude and reassurance that it appears that all which could be done was done. Preparation and support of the relatives are fundamentally important. This should include the following:

• information about their loved one's appearance;
• a brief description and explanation of the equipment, lines, and tubes attached to the patient;
• brief information about the team;
• reassurance that they can leave the room at any time;
• an individual member of staff to stay with them and support them at all times.

The team also requires briefing and support before the relatives come in. It can be stressful and emotionally challenging to experience the raw grief that is often expressed in these circumstances. Senior experienced staff are essential in this situation for both the family and the team.

Bereavement care can be very demanding and time-consuming. Support mechanisms should be in place for staff who have been involved in bereavement support. The hospital chaplaincy team can provide support for relatives, loved ones, and staff involved in these situations.

Sudden death

Dealing with sudden death is common in the ED. It is a sad and traumatic event for the family and loved ones of those involved. Even in circumstances where the death was expected, when the actual death occurs, it can still seem sudden and traumatic. Nurses have a key role in breaking bad news and caring for the family and loved ones.

Breaking bad news

This is a key skill that requires preparation and experience. The person to break the bad news should be the person who has established the greatest rapport with the family or loved ones (and who has the greatest experience of breaking bad news). This could be either a nurse or a doctor. It is advisable to have two professional staff present who are able to break the news, provide comfort, and, where possible, answer questions. One person should be the link person and spend time with the family. Breaking bad news is not an exact science—every situation and circumstance is different, requiring rapid assessment and decision-making about the most appropriate approach and language to use.

The language used should be clear and unambiguous. Euphemisms, such as 'we lost him' or 'he has passed over' or 'he has gone to a better place', should not be used. Phrases, such as 'has died' or 'is dead', should be used. It is not uncommon to have to repeat these words in the first few sentences.

In situations where you are preparing relatives or loved ones for a poor outlook, again clear language should be used. It is better to be 'up front' with individuals and give the worst possible outcome, as well as the most optimistic one—but be realistic.

You should be prepared for a wide variety of reactions. These are also culturally dependent. Reactions can include anger, denial, crying, shouting, wailing, laughing, violent outbursts, self-flagellation, and collapse, to name just a few. In the case of sudden death in children, parents have been known to attempt to take their dead child home with them.

A checklist of information and key contacts can be useful in a bereavement situation. No matter how many times you have broken bad news, it is always stressful and emotionally challenging. The checklist should ensure that you have relevant contact numbers for follow-up, that correct documentation is given, and that the GP is informed. The necessary arrangements should be made to inform medical records, in order to ensure that inappropriate letters or appointments are not sent to the person who has recently died.

▶ Remember to offer the support of spiritual leaders from the patient's faith through either the family's contacts or the hospital chaplaincy team.

Keepsakes

It can be helpful to offer 'keepsakes' to relatives and loved ones. For adults, a lock of hair from the deceased, thoughtfully presented, can be offered. For children, a book of keepsakes can be provided, including foot and hand prints, locks of hair, and photographs (with the consent of the coroner).

Environment

Providing a quiet area for breaking bad news is important. The area should ideally be close to the resuscitation room, but with sufficient audio/visual separation. Making this area welcoming and comfortable is important.

The provision of a visiting room is highly desirable. The room should accommodate the deceased individual in comfortable surroundings without the equipment found in the clinical area. This area should allow the loved ones to spend time saying goodbye in an unhurried manner. Ideally, this room should be close to the relatives' room and the resuscitation room, but not in a busy thoroughfare.

Dealing with difficult situations: tissue and organ donation

There is a shortage of organs for donation in the UK. As a result, sadly, patients are dying, whilst waiting for a transplant. When faced with a sudden or imminent death, consideration should be given to raising the issue of organ or tissue donation (always check that there are no absolute contraindications first). Although staff are sometimes concerned about raising this issue at a time of major emotional crisis, evidence suggests that many relatives gain some comfort from knowing that others might benefit from the organs or tissues of their loved one. Recent awareness campaigns about the importance of organ donation have resulted in some families raising the subject of donation when bad news is broken, but this cannot be relied upon.

There are three different types of donation: donation after brainstem death (DBD), donation after circulatory death (DCD), and tissue donation. Local policies and procedures will determine how these processes are enacted.[23] NICE has issued a short clinical guideline on organ donation. This guideline applies to practice in England, Wales, and Northern Ireland, and recommends that hospital staff initiate discussions with a Specialist Nurse for Organ Donation (SN-OD) when one of the following criteria is met:

• an intention to use brainstem death tests to confirm death;
• an intention to withdraw life-sustaining treatment in patients with a life-threatening or life-limiting condition which will, or is expected to, result in circulatory death;
• admission of a patient with very severe brain injury (defined as a Glasgow Coma Scale (GCS) score of 3–4 with at least one absent brainstem reflex) that cannot be attributed to the effects of sedation.

Organs that may be retrieved from DBD donors include the heart and lungs, liver, kidneys, pancreas, and small bowel. DCD donors can donate the liver, kidneys, pancreas, lung, and tissue. Tissues that can be donated include eyes, heart valves, skin, and skeletal tissue (bone, tendon, and ligaments). Tissues can be donated up to 24–48h after death.

Absolute contraindications to organ donation are:

• age 85y or above;
• any cancer with evidence of spread outside the affected organ (including lymph nodes) within 3y of donation (however, localized prostate, thyroid, *in situ* cervical, and non-melanotic skin cancers are acceptable);
• melanoma (except completely excised Stage 1 cancers);
• choriocarcinoma;
• active haematological malignancy (myeloma, lymphoma, leukaemia);
• definite, probable, or possible cases of human transmissible spongiform encephalopathy (TSE), including Creutzfeldt–Jakob disease (CJD) and variant CJD, individuals whose blood relatives have had familial CJD, or other neurodegenerative diseases associated with infectious agents;
• TB—active and untreated;
• West Nile virus (WNV) infection;
• human immunodeficiency virus (HIV) disease (but not HIV infection).

Best practice is for the SN-OD to be involved in the approach with regard to organ donation, and therefore close liaison with the local SN-OD is necessary to support families and staff. The SN-OD team is also able to provide staff with information and knowledge to promote organ and tissue donation.

Reference

23 For further information, see ℘ http://webarchive.nationalarchives.gov.uk/+/www.dh.gov.uk/en/Healthcare/Secondarycare/Transplantation/index.htm.

Further reading

NHS Blood and Transplant. Organ donation. Available at: ℘ http://www.organdonation.nhs.uk/. Organ Donation and Transplantation. Available at: ℘ http://www.odt.nhs.uk/.

Investigations

Biochemical investigations: urea and electrolytes—urea

- Breakdown of protein produces urea.
- Around 90% is excreted by the kidneys.
- Urea levels in blood give an indication of kidney function.

Low urea

- Low-protein diet/malnutrition.
- In pregnancy due to blood volume.
- Liver disease.
- Very dilute urine.
- Lower levels can also be seen in infants and small children.

Raised urea (uraemia)

- Impaired renal function due to disease or poor blood flow to kidneys.
- Urinary tract obstruction.
- Dehydration.
- High-protein diet.
- Extensive tissue damage—necrosis or severe infection.
- Stress or shock due to ↑ release of adrenaline.
- Medication-induced (e.g. corticosteroids).

Biochemical investigations:
urea and electrolytes—calcium

- One of the most important minerals, and necessary for:
  - skeletal strength;
  - conduction of impulses from nerve endings for stimulation of muscle contraction;
  - blood clotting;
  - regulation of cell metabolism, including sodium (Na^+) shift;
  - cell wall structure and function.
- High Ca^{2+} level can cause muscle weakness and depress the nervous system.
- Low Ca^{2+} level can lead to overstimulation of muscles by nerve impulses. This is an important consideration for cardiac muscle.

Potential causes of hypercalcaemia

- Drug effects (e.g. thiazide diuretics, bendroflumethiazide).
- Renal problems affecting excretion of Ca^{2+}.
- Hyperparathyroidism.
- Neoplasms.
- High levels of vitamin D.
- Paget's disease.
- Sarcoidosis.

Potential causes of hypocalcaemia

- Reduced dietary Ca^{2+} intake.
- Hypoparathyroidism.
- Acute pancreatitis.
- Vitamin D deficiency.
- Renally related causes:
  - nephrotic syndrome (↓ levels of albumin lead to reduced transport)
  - chronic failure
  - stones.
- Septic shock.
- Drug-induced (e.g. cytotoxic therapy).
- Hypomagnesaemia.

Biochemical investigations:
urea and electrolytes—chloride

- Ingested in the diet.
- Function in electrolyte balance.
- Helps to maintain acid–base balance.
- Provides osmotic pressure—distribution of extracellular fluid.
- Abnormal chloride (Cl^-) levels could cause compensatory or abnormal movement of other electrolytes.

Possible causes of hyperchloraemia

- Na^+ retention.
- Dehydration.
- Metabolic acidosis.
- Respiratory alkalosis.
- Drug effect (e.g. corticosteroids).

Possible causes of hypochloraemia

- Significant loss of Na^+.
- Renal tubular damage leading to loss.
- Heat exhaustion.
- Hypokalaemic acidosis.
- Respiratory acidosis.
- Loss of Cl^- from the gastrointestinal (GI) tract through vomiting, intestinal obstruction, or nasogastric (NG) aspiration.
- Drug-induced, particularly by diuretics (e.g. furosemide, bendroflumethiazide).

Biochemical investigations:
urea and electrolytes—magnesium

- A mineral that is found in every cell of the body.
- Used for energy production, nerve function, and muscle contraction.
- Mg^{2+} in the body combines with Ca^{2+} and phosphorus to form bone.
- Only a small amount of magnesium (Mg^{2+}) in the body is found in blood.
- Intake of Mg^{2+} is mostly through diet.
- Regulation in the body involves a balance between absorption and excretion conservation through the kidneys.
- Mg^{2+} deficiencies cause (among other effects) cardiac arrhythmia, and ↑ irritability of the nervous system, with tetany.

Possible causes of hypermagnesaemia

- Renal failure.
- Ketoacidosis.
- Addison's disease.
- Medications containing Mg^{2+}.
- Hyperparathyroidism.
- Hypothyroidism.

Possible causes of hypomagnesaemia

- This is not equivalent to Mg^{2+} deficiency.
- Low dietary intake.
- Poor absorption due to GI disorders (e.g. Crohn's disease).
- Alcoholism.
- Long-term diuretic use.
- Chronic or prolonged diarrhoea.
- Severe burns.
- Hypoparathyroidism.

Biochemical investigations: urea and electrolytes—sodium

- Plays an important part in regulation of osmotic pressure and the distribution of water within the extracellular compartments of the body.
- Water and Na^+ balance is affected by dietary intake and renal excretion of both.
- Needed for fluid balance, muscle function, and acid–base balance.

Possible causes of hypernatraemia

- Dehydration 2° to lowered fluid intake, diarrhoea and/or vomiting, or polyuria.
- Pharmacological causes, due to the effects of steroids or antibiotics.

Possible causes of hyponatraemia

- Usually excessive loss, rather than dietary intake; can include loss from body surface as a result of sweating or burns.
- Renal disease (e.g. polycystic kidney disease).
- Metabolic disease (e.g. Addison's disease, hypothyroidism).
- ↑ circulatory water caused by excessive fluid intake or oedema.
- Pharmacological causes, due to the effects of diuretics.

Biochemical investigations: urea and electrolytes—potassium

- Present in all cells.
- Dietary intake (fruit, vegetables, and meat), absorbed through the intestinal mucosa.
- K^+ occurs in plasma, and intracellular and extracellular fluid.
- Distribution across cell membranes (i.e. intracellular versus extracellular) and balance between intake and excretion influence plasma K^+ concentration.
- K^+ concentration affects membrane excitability.
  - Hypokalaemia causes ↑ excitability, which can lead to atrial or ventricular arrhythmias. ECG changes: small or inverted T waves, prolonged PR interval, ST segment depression, prominent U wave after T.
  - Hyperkalaemia leads to ↓ excitability, with ECG changes, and can lead to heart block and asystole. ECG changes: tall tented T waves; wide QRS complex; small, broad, or absent P waves; atrioventricular (AV) dissociation or ventricular tachycardia (VT)/ventricular fibrillation (VF) (➲ see Fig. 3.1).

Possible causes of hyperkalaemia

- Dietary intake.
- Urinary output (renal failure).
- Aldosterone production.
- Excessive use of dietary supplements.
- Cell damage releasing K^+ (e.g. burns, trauma, sepsis).
- Chemotherapy.
- Metabolic acidosis.
- Insulin deficiency.
- K^+-sparing diuretics.

Possible causes of hypokalaemia

- Low intake.
- Dietary.
- Diuretics
- Prolonged ileus.
- Malabsorption.
- Loss from GI tract due to diarrhoea and/or vomiting.
- Rehydration during diabetic ketoacidosis (DKA) treatment.

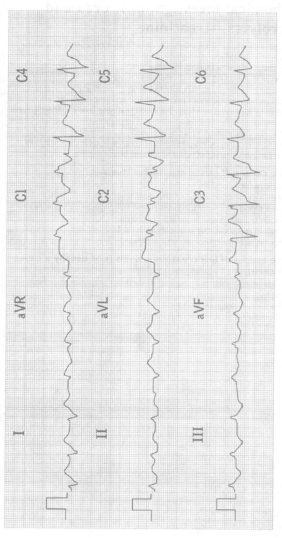

Fig. 3.1 Hyperkalaemia. Note the flattening of the P waves, prominent T waves, and widening of the QRS complex.
(Reproduced with permission from Longmore M. et al. (2014). *Oxford Handbook of Clinical Medicine*, 9th edn, p. 689. Oxford University Press, Oxford.)

Biochemical investigations: urea and electrolytes—creatinine

- Anaerobic skeletal muscle metabolism produces creatinine as a waste product.
- Normal values are related to muscle mass.
  - ↑ muscle mass → ↑ normal values of creatinine.
  - Creatinine values are normally higher in ♂ than ♀.
- Direct link between amount produced and amount excreted.
- Excreted by kidneys; therefore, ↑ blood creatinine levels suggest ↓ renal function.
- Muscle injury may also ↑ creatinine levels.
- Kidney function can be assessed with a creatinine clearance test, which includes a 24h urine collection and venous blood sample.

Possible causes of raised creatinine levels

- ↑ muscle mass.
- Renal disease or obstruction of the renal tract.
- Reduced blood supply to the kidneys due to congestive cardiac failure (CCF), dehydration, shock, or atherosclerosis.
- Diet high in red meat may cause short-lived ↑.
- Drugs causing impairment of renal function.

Possible causes of low creatinine levels (not usually a cause for concern)

- ↓ muscle mass—such as in the elderly or those with muscular dystrophy.
- Can be seen in pregnancy.
- Occasionally associated with advanced liver disease.

Biochemical investigations: liver function tests—albumin

- One of three main types of plasma protein and the one present in the greatest amount.
- Manufactured by the liver.
- Albumin levels give an indication of liver function.
- Sequential reduced albumin levels may indicate impaired hepatic function.
- Acts as a binding agent for transport of circulating substances such as hormones, bilirubin, and enzymes.
- Half-life is 20–26 days.
- Physical effects of a low albumin level are delayed.
- Albumin in capillaries provides osmotic pull.
- Lowered albumin levels will ↑ movement of water into tissues, resulting in oedema.
- Albumin may be reduced in:
  - liver disease;
  - nephrotic syndrome;
  - malnutrition;
  - marked inflammatory response;
  - Crohn's disease.
- Albumin may be elevated in:
  - dehydration;
  - inflammatory conditions (e.g. rheumatoid arthritis).

Biochemical investigations: liver function tests—alkaline phosphatase and bilirubin

Alkaline phosphatase

- A naturally occurring enzyme.
- Produced by cells in the bile duct (ductoles).
- Normally drains into the bile duct.
- In obstructive liver disease (cholestatic), the enzyme will build up in the liver and 'leak' into the circulatory system.
- Alkaline phosphatase (ALP) is also related to bone and placental growth (therefore can be ↑ in pregnancy) and can be produced by tumours.
- Can be ↑ with diseases of the gut (e.g. ulcerative colitis).
- Children can have higher ALP levels due to bone growth.
- Each of the tissues—liver, bone, placenta, and intestine—produces a slightly different ALP or isoenzyme.

Bilirubin

This is the major bile pigment. It is a by-product of haemolysis. Accumulation of bilirubin causes yellow discoloration of the sclerae, mucous membranes, and skin (jaundice).

- Destruction of red blood cells (RBCs) by the reticulo-endothelial system releases bilirubin into the blood.
- Bilirubin attaches to plasma proteins—unconjugated or indirect bilirubin. Passes through the liver where bilirubin conjugates with glucuronic acid to become conjugated or direct bilirubin.
- Conjugated bilirubin forms part of the bile and enters the digestive system; it is excreted partly in stools and partly in urine.

Possible causes of isolated increases in bilirubin levels

- Haemolysis.
- Ineffective erythropoiesis.
- Immature bilirubin metabolism (e.g. physiological neonatal jaundice); inherited defects in uptake or conjugation (e.g. Gilbert's syndrome).
- Modest elevation of serum bilirubin may be present with disorders such as vitamin B_{12} or folate deficiencies.

Possible causes of elevated conjugated bilirubin levels

- Inherited defects in excretion.
- Hepatocellular disease, post-hepatic disease, or cholestatic disease.
- Elevated faecal and urinary bilirubin can be present in haemolytic anaemias.

When there is an ↑ in bilirubin levels with other abnormal LFTs (gamma-glutamyl transferase (GGT), ALP, aspartate aminotransferase (AST), and alanine aminotransferase (ALT)), this can indicate:

- metastatic liver disease;
- cirrhosis;
- hepatitis;
- dilated common bile duct from gallstones;
- cancer of the pancreas.

Biochemical investigations: blood gases and 'cardiac enzymes'

Bicarbonate

- A measure of the total carbon dioxide (CO_2) in the body.
- Three forms:
  - carbonic acid (H_2CO_3);
  - CO_2;
  - bicarbonate (HCO_3^-).
- Main function: acid–base balance or pH.
- Works with K^+, Na^+, and Cl^- to maintain electrical neutrality.
- Test is part of routine urea and electrolytes (U&E) testing and also part of arterial blood gas (ABG) testing.

Abnormal findings
Elevated bicarbonate levels

- Imbalance of body pH through ↑ CO_2 levels or electrolyte imbalance, particularly K^+.
- Particularly with K^+ imbalance, consider diuretics as a cause.
- Can be associated with chronic obstructive pulmonary disease (COPD) and conditions or diseases that cause chronic metabolic alkalosis.

Low bicarbonate levels

- Can be associated with respiratory and/or metabolic acidosis, severe dehydration, and renal failure.

Creatine kinase

- Creatine kinase (CK) is an enzyme found in heart and skeletal muscles.
- Also found in brain.
- Three different forms:
  - CK-MB—mostly found in heart muscle;
  - CK-MM—found in heart and other muscles;
  - CK-BB—mostly found in brain and kidney (not usually found in blood).
- Elevated CK level indicates muscle damage. The type of CK enzyme isolated can indicate which muscles are damaged (e.g. heart or other muscle).
- In chest pain, CK-MB rises and falls over 72h, peaking at 24h. A rise can be seen at 4–6h, and this can be helpful in the diagnosis of myocardial infarction (MI).
- CK levels can also rise as a result of heavy or excessive exercise and other forms of muscle damage (from falls, crush injuries, etc.).
- Excess alcohol intake can lead to a small ↑ in CK levels.
- Afro-Caribbeans may have a higher CK than other ethnic groups.
- CK levels may fall in early pregnancy.

Cardiac troponin I (TnI) and troponin T (TnT)

- Complex of three regulating proteins integral to cardiac and skeletal muscle contraction.
- Cardiac-specific TnI and TnT (cTnI and cTnT).
- High-sensitivity cardiac-specific TnI (hs-cTnI) and TnT (hs-cTnT) are available at some centres.
- Cardiac troponin levels indicate cardiac cell death; the enzyme is released into the bloodstream on injury.
- Preferable to CK-MB—can be linked to skeletal muscle, whereas troponin is more specific to cardiac muscle.
- Used in the diagnosis of MI—can be elevated in unstable angina.
- Rises within 2–3h and can remain elevated for up to 10 days.
- TnT rises faster than TnI, 80% accurate at 6h, but a definitive result is obtained at 10–12h (follow local guidelines).
- Standard cTn—if not initially elevated and causing clinical suspicion, it should be repeated at 6–9h and 12h to rule out cardiac damage (follow local guidelines).
- hs-cTn—a second sample taken at 3h that demonstrates >20% rise confirms heart muscle damage; otherwise repeat after an additional 3h to rule out cardiac damage (follow local guidelines).

Note that not all laboratories use hs-cTn.

Biochemical investigations: lipids and other values

Lipid profile

- Lipids are fat or fat-like substances.
- Constituent of cells and sources of energy.
- Test conducted to assess risk of developing cardiovascular disease.
- In patients over 40y of age, perform a routine cardiovascular health check.
- Also tested if pancreatitis is suspected, looking particularly for elevated triglycerides.
- Two types of lipids—cholesterol and triglycerides—are transported by lipoproteins. Lipoproteins contain cholesterol, triglycerides, phospholipid molecules, and protein.
- Lipoproteins are classified according to density—high-density lipoproteins (HDLs), intermediate-density lipoproteins (IDLs), low-density lipoproteins (LDLs), and very-low-density lipoproteins (VLDLs). They are not all measured as part of the lipid profile.
- Total cholesterol.
- HDL-cholesterol (HDL-C) is the amount of cholesterol in HDL particles. HLD-C removes excess cholesterol and transports it to the liver.
- LDL-cholesterol (LDL-C) is the amount of cholesterol in LDL particles. Excess LDL is deposited in the walls of blood vessels and is a contributory factor in atherosclerosis. The amount of LDL is calculated using the results for total cholesterol, HDL-C, and triglycerides.
- Triglycerides measures all triglycerides, mostly found in VLDL, in the lipoprotein particles.
- 12h fasting is required, with the patient only able to drink water, before the sample is taken.

Glucose

- Simple sugar used as energy.
- Derived from breakdown of carbohydrate.
- Absorbed in the small intestine.
- Required by most cells.
- The brain and central nervous system (CNS) rely on glucose. Their functioning is susceptible to fluctuations in glucose levels.
- Insulin is required for uptake, metabolism, storage, and mobilization of glucose.
- Glucose is measured in the blood, and also tested for in urine.
- Raised blood glucose levels can lead to glucose excretion in the urine via the kidneys.
- Both hyper- and hypoglycaemia will affect brain function.

Possible causes of hyperglycaemia

- Impaired insulin production.
- Excessive food intake.
- Diabetes mellitus.

- Pancreatic insufficiency.
- Pancreatitis.
- Cushing's syndrome.
- Pregnancy/eclampsia.
- Hypertension.
- Obesity-induced type 2 diabetes.
- Chronic infection.
- Stress response (raised adrenaline levels):
  - trauma;
  - sudden illness;
  - seizures.
- Medication (e.g. corticosteroids).

Possible causes of hypoglycaemia
- Low dietary intake:
  - malnutrition;
  - vomiting.
- Exercise.
- Hypothermia.
- Excessive insulin:
  - overadministration;
  - overproduction—pancreatic tumour.
- Endocrine disorders:
  - Addison's disease;
  - hypothyroidism;
  - hypopituitarism.

Amylase

- An enzyme that is released into the digestive tract and used for breaking down starch.
- Found in large quantities in the pancreas, and smaller quantities in the salivary glands.
- Excreted by the kidneys, and therefore can be found in the urine.
- Usually requested as a test for patients presenting with abdominal pain.

Raised amylase (hyperamylasaemia) can be found with:
- acute pancreatitis (serum amylase usually ↑ 4-fold);
- DKA;
- hepatitis;
- peritonitis;
- renal failure;
- intestinal obstruction/perforation;
- burns;
- infections such as mumps;
- salivary trauma.

C-reactive protein ·

- This protein is made by the liver and secreted into the blood.
- Levels in blood become elevated within a few hours after infection or inflammation.
- This elevation may precede fever, pain, or other clinical conditions.
- There can be a significant ↑ in C-reactive protein (CRP) in response to inflammation, and then a rapid ↓ as the inflammation subsides.
- As CRP responds to both inflammation and infection, it is not specific to a particular disease or condition.
- Can be used to monitor reduction in infection or inflammation, as it falls quickly in the blood when infection or inflammation subsides.
- CRP levels are ↑ in bacterial infections and ↓ in viral infections.
- Erythrocyte sedimentation rate (ESR) is also used as an adjunct to CRP.

Possible causes of raised CRP

- Tissue injury or necrosis (e.g. pulmonary embolus (PE), MI, burns, necrosis).
- Inflammatory disorders (e.g. Crohn's disease, arthritis).
- Bacterial infections.
- Septic arthritis.
- Neoplastic disease.
- Tissue rejection.

Haematological investigations

Red blood cells

- Manufactured by the bone marrow.
- Responsible for the transport of O_2 and CO_2.
- RBCs act as an acid–base buffer, helping to maintain pH balance.
- Lower RBC counts are found in women.
- There is a ↓ in RBCs with age.
- Hypoxia stimulates the bone marrow to ↑ production of RBCs.
- The test counts the number of RBCs per litre of blood.
- Changes in RBC levels have to be interpreted in the context of other parameters such as haemoglobin (Hb) and haematocrit (Hct).
- RBC count is usually requested as part of a full blood count (FBC).
- If the RBC count shows a ↓ of >10% of the expected normal value, anaemia is diagnosed.
- If the RBC count is raised, polycythaemia is diagnosed.
- Lowered RBC count may indicate bleeding, anaemia (deficiency, pernicious, aplastic, or haemolytic), renal disease, bone marrow failure, or malnutrition.
  - *Fluid replacement after haemorrhage will reduce RBC volume.*
- Raised RBC count may indicate reduced circulatory volume (possible causes include dehydration, diarrhoea, and burns), bone marrow overproduction, and prolonged depletion of O_2 in the blood (e.g. in pulmonary disease, heart disease, and at high altitudes).

Haemoglobin

- Important in transportation of O_2.
- An iron-containing molecule found in RBCs.
- Hb picks up O_2, as it passes through pulmonary capillary blood vessels.
- O_2 is transported to cells across arterial capillary walls.
- Hb levels are adjusted for gender, age, and ethnic origin.

→ See Red blood cells above for causes of ↓ and ↑ Hb levels.

Coagulation screen

- Used to determine levels of different clotting factors (proteins).
- Test is requested when exploring any clotting derangement or potential derangement (i.e. in major haemorrhage).
- Nine coagulation factors are normally measured (factors I to XIV).
- Deficiencies can be inherited or acquired (→ see Chapter 17).
- Acquired deficiencies include overconsumption (e.g. due to haemorrhage, liver disease, some cancers, anticoagulation therapy, vitamin K deficiency, severe infections, etc.).

International normalized ratio

- The international normalized ratio (INR) is closely related to prothrombin time (PT).
- PT and measures such as prothrombin ratio and INR are measures of the extrinsic pathway of coagulation. The PT/INR are used to determine the clotting tendency of blood.

- The INR was introduced in an attempt to standardize PT.
- Using INR, the process and calculations are standardized internationally to provide consistency.
- The INR measures the effect of warfarin, a vitamin K antagonist, on clotting.
- It can also measure the effects of vitamin K deficiency.
- The INR is a ratio of the patient's PT to the normal control sample (this is adjusted using the International Sensitivity Index of the analytical system being used).
- The higher the INR, the less likely the patient's blood to clot is, and therefore more likely it is that bleeding will occur.
- The target INR for patients on warfarin is 2.0–3.0, although it may be higher in some circumstances, depending on the indication for anticoagulation.

Erythrocyte sedimentation rate

- Indirect measure of the degree of inflammation caused by disease.
- Not specific to any particular disease.
- Measures the rate of settlement (sedimentation) of unclotted blood in a tall, thin tube.
- The results are expressed as the number of millimetres of clear plasma present at the top of the column after 1h.
- A normal sample would have a little clear plasma at 1h.
- A rise in sedimentation rate occurs with ↑ red cell weight (↑ proteins, such as fibrinogen and immunoglobulins (Igs), as a result of inflammation through disease process ↑ weight) and causes RBCs to fall more rapidly.
- ESR is affected by age, gender, pregnancy, menstruation, and drugs.

Possible causes of raised ESR
- Inflammatory disorder or disease.
- Autoimmune disease.
- Recent trauma.
- MI (early response).
- Anaemia.

Possible causes of lowered ESR
- Sickle cell.
- CCF.
- Hypoproteinaemia.
- Hypofibrinogenaemia.
- Polycythaemia.

Although non-specific, ESR can be helpful for confirming two specific diagnoses—temporal arteritis and polymyalgia rheumatica.

White cell count

- Counts and quantifies each type of white blood cell (WBC) in the blood.
- Forms part of the FBC, showing total WCC and 5-part differential count.

- Raised WCC (leucocytosis) can indicate inflammation, bacterial infection, leukaemia (raised number of abnormal white cells), or trauma.
- Lowered WCC (leucopenia) can indicate autoimmune disease (e.g. lupus erythematosus), overwhelming bacterial infection, suppression of bone marrow, or vitamin B_{12} or folic acid deficiency.
- Stress, exercise, and pregnancy (last trimester) can ↑ WCC.
- Each type of white cell (leucocyte) is expressed as a percentage of the total count.

Differential white cell count
- Lymphocytes are formed in lymphoid tissue and bone marrow, and are needed for immunity. ↑ numbers of lymphocytes indicate stimulation of the immune response. They ↓ in viral infection.
- Eosinophils are related to allergic and parasitic conditions. They ↑ in asthma and allergic conditions.
- Neutrophils are related to defence against invading organisms. They act by phagocytosis, and their numbers ↑ during infection.
- Basophils are primarily related to an allergic response. Some defence against parasitic worms. Close relationship to mast cells.
- Monocytes mature into macrophages (in target tissue) in response to infection or inflammation. Macrophages work by phagocytosis, are involved in the generalized systemic reaction to inflammation, and pass information to lymphocytes to produce correct antibodies. Can also destroy tumour cells. Their numbers ↑ in chronic inflammatory disorders.

Other common investigations

Human chorionic gonadotrophin
- Human chorionic gonadotrophin (HCG) is a hormone associated with pregnancy, trophoblastic disease, or germ cell tumours.
- Can be detected in blood after implantation (i.e. before a missed menstrual period). At this stage, it may not be present in urine, leading to a false-positive result.
- HCG ↑ steadily during the first trimester of pregnancy.
- It peaks at around the tenth week after the last menstrual cycle.
- It levels off over the remainder of pregnancy.
- It is no longer detectable within a few weeks of the end of pregnancy.
- Measured either in urine (preferably an early-morning sample) or in blood.
- Urine HCG is reported as positive or negative—often point-of-care testing in the ED.
- False-negative and false-positive results are possible for urine HCG.
- The HCG level in blood, referred to as β-HCG, gives a quantitative value and is the gold standard test for establishing whether a woman is pregnant.

- If the results are questionable, consider a different mode of testing (i.e. ultrasound scan (USS)).
- ▶ Establishing pregnancy status in ♀ aged 12–55y attending the ED is important, as it is essential in the differential diagnosis of abdominal pain and GI disorders, imaging choices, and treatment.

HCG is also produced by some tumours such as germ cell tumours, trophoblastic disease, and teratoma. A positive result in ♂ can be associated with testicular cancer.

Urinalysis

Used for screening for infection, renal disease, and metabolic disorders. Although commonly performed, it is often done poorly! Inaccuracies can occur through early reading of screening sticks and the use of out-of-date sticks. Consideration should be given to the sensitivity and specificity of the tests in determining clinical decisions. Ideally, urinalysis should be conducted using a point-of-care machine, which gives more reliable results.

Routine urinalysis should be avoided—there should be a specific reason for testing urine.

Most testing strips will provide data on the following.

pH

Measures hydrogen ion concentration in the urine.

Possible causes of increased acidity
- Metabolic acidosis—diabetes mellitus, starvation.
- Respiratory acidosis.
- Alkaline loss through diarrhoea.
- Iatrogenic (e.g. ascorbic acid).
- Dietary—high meat content.

Possible causes of increased alkalinity
- Metabolic alkalosis.
- Respiratory alkalosis.
- Renal tube defects.
- Loss of acid through vomiting.
- UTI.
- Iatrogenic—sodium bicarbonate.
- Dietary—high vegetable content.

Specific gravity

Indicates the quantity of dissolved substances in the urine, which is not accurately measured with a dipstick.

Possible causes of raised specific gravity
- Reduced urine output (more concentrated), dehydration, etc.
- Elevated urea content.
- Elevated glucose content.
- Osmotic diuretics (e.g. mannitol).

Possible causes of lowered specific gravity
- ↓ urea content—low-protein diet.
- ↓ Na^+ concentration.
- ↑ urine output—overhydration, diabetes insipidus.
- Inability of kidneys to concentrate urine, particularly in the elderly.

Protein

Not normally found in urine. Possible causes of proteinuria (presence of protein in the urine) include the following:
- hypertension;
- heart failure;

- pyrexia;
- UTI;
- eclampsia.

Very dilute urine may produce false-negative results.

Glucose

Not normally found in urine. Possible causes of glycosuria (presence of glucose in the urine) include the following.

Hyperglycaemia (varying causes)
- Reduced renal threshold:
  - pregnancy;
  - eclampsia.
- Iatrogenic—corticosteroids, thiazide diuretics.

Ketones

Not normally found in urine. Possible causes of presence in urine are:
- dietary—reduced carbohydrate intake, high-fat/high-protein diet;
- metabolic—diabetes mellitus, ketoacidosis;
- ketones present in the urine signify metabolism of fat to produce energy, as insulin may not be available to metabolize glucose;
- pregnancy;
- eclampsia;
- rapid depletion of fat stores—rapid weight loss, ↑ metabolic rate, strenuous exercise;
- starvation or anorexia;
- hyperemesis;
- ↑ pituitary function;
- ↑ cortisone secretion.

Blood

Not normally found in urine.
- Macroscopic blood in the urine will alter its colour to rose/red.
- Microscopic blood may not be visualized.
- Reagent tests normally distinguish between haemolysed and non-haemolysed blood.
  - Haemolysed blood identifies free Hb/myoglobin released from breakdown or rupture of RBCs. May indicate that bleeding occurred in the higher urinary tract.
  - Non-haemolysed blood shows intact RBCs. May indicate that these undamaged RBCs originate from lower down the urinary tract.

Possible causes of haematuria (presence of RBCs)
- Renal disease or trauma.
- Renal calculi.
- Bladder neoplasm, stones.
- Cystitis.
- Prostate gland inflammation or neoplasm.

- Urethritis.
- Menstruation.
- Haemolysed blood external to the renal tract excreted through urine.

Nitrites and leucocytes

Should not be found in the urine.

- Nitrates and leucocytes can be indicative of urine infection.
- Most bacteria, but not all (those that do not have metabolic effects on nitrates), causing UTIs convert nitrates (normal waste product in the urine) to nitrites. UTIs cause an inflammatory response → ↑ presence of WBCs; ∴ ↑ leucocyte count.
- False-positive and false-negative results are possible.

Urinary chloride

- Cl^- excreted by kidneys (also lost through the skin in sweat).
- Urinary excretion is a function of balance, affected by pH, Na^+, and K^+ levels.
- Usually measured by 24h urine collection.

Forms of imaging

X-ray

This is a common investigation in the ED. It is commonly used to detect abnormalities of organs or tissues affected by injury, disease, or degeneration. It is also used to confirm or exclude suspicion of a fracture, dislocation, or certain foreign bodies (FBs), such as glass or metal in wounds, or ingested FBs such as coins.

The densities of the structures inside the body affect the penetration of X-rays, and therefore their appearance on the image. For example:

- air-filled spaces, such as the lungs or gas in the bowels, allow full passage of X-rays and appear black on the image;
- bones appear white, as they are dense and do not permit penetration of X-rays;
- organs and fat appear a darker grey, as they allow some penetration;
- fluid does not allow much penetration, so it appears white;
- specific dyes are used that are impenetrable to X-ray, and therefore appear white, allowing a contrast to the black image.

X-rays are not without risk, as long-term overexposure to radiation can lead to malignancy. Legislation governs the requesting, exposure, and evaluation of the images. Nurses and other allied health professionals are, under specific circumstances and local protocol, permitted to refer for a number of X-ray investigations. All referrers must be educated about, and conversant with, the Ionising Radiation (Medical Exposure) Regulations (IRMER) 2000 regulations.[1]

Computed tomography

This form of imaging is commonly used by ED clinicians as a diagnostic tool. In the computed tomography (CT) scanner, X-rays are used to form three-dimensional images of cross-sections of the body. Early CT scanning is now indicated for a number of conditions, including stroke.

CT images are often useful in diagnosis. However, the CT scanner is sometimes euphemistically referred to as the 'doughnut of death'! The patient must be adequately resuscitated before transfer to the scanner, in particular with regard to airway management and fluid resuscitation. An elective rapid sequence induction (RSI) of anaesthesia to protect the airway of a patient with a reduced GCS score in the resuscitation room is preferable to a flustered attempt with a vomiting patient in the CT scanner. Equally, if the patient is haemodynamically unstable, surgery to correct life-threatening haemorrhage may be indicated prior to definitive imaging. The ED nurse has a key role in raising questions about the safety and appropriateness of transfer of the unstable patient to the CT department. When critically ill patients are transferred to CT, they must be accompanied by experienced staff and emergency equipment.

Magnetic resonance imaging

The use of this form of imaging in the ED setting is ↑. Magnetic resonance imaging (MRI) uses magnetic and radio waves—there is no exposure to X-rays or other damaging radiation. As this form of imaging uses magnets, the referring clinician must take a history in order to determine whether the patient has metal implants, clips, or FBs that might be dislodged by the powerful magnets.

MRI can provide images of almost all tissues of the body and is able to make images of tissues that are surrounded by bone. It provides very detailed images, which is particularly useful when imaging the brain and cervical spine (C-spine). For example, MRI can identify ligamentous involvement in neck injury, which would not be detected on CT. The use of MRI is not limited to areas such as the brain and chest. Small-part MRI scanners are proving useful in the early definitive diagnosis of scaphoid fractures. As this imaging modality becomes commoner, early imaging of the wrists, knees, and ankles may well be a useful adjunct in the management of patients attending the ED with these injuries.

Ultrasound (sonography)

This investigation produces an image by the deflection of ultrasound waves from structures inside the body. It can be used to visualize muscle, tendons, and organs. 'Free fluid' within cavities can also be visualized.

Ultrasound can be used for diagnosis, as well as for guidance of procedures such as the visualization of the venous circulation before insertion of a central venous line.

In trauma, clinicians are being trained in focused assessment with sonography for trauma (FAST). The FAST scan is used, for example, to identify fluid in the pericardium, free fluid in the abdominal cavity, and the diameter of the aorta in the abdomen. It is a useful adjunctive scan and can assist in decision-making in both haemodynamically stable and unstable patients. Specific training courses in FAST scanning are available.[2]

ENPs may find ultrasound useful for the assessment of the Achilles tendon when injury is suspected, as well as for the identification of FBs that are not radio-opaque (e.g. wood). There is no legislative framework around referral for ultrasound. Referral will be dictated by local agreement.

References

1 For further information on the regulations, see Department of Health (2012). *Ionising Radiation (Medical Exposure) Regulations 2000 (IRMER)*. Available at: ℘ http://www.gov.uk/government/publications/the-ionising-radiation-medical-exposure-regulations-2000.
2 Further details can be found at Emergency Ultrasound UK. Available at: ℘ http://www.emergencyultrasound.org.uk/index.html.

Emergency care of the infant and child

Introduction

Many nurses working within the specialty of emergency care feel very anxious about looking after children. This can be for a variety of reasons: they are worried that children 'go off' quickly; they cannot relate to them; or they simply have had no exposure to children within their working career. However, caring for children and their families can be a very rewarding and gratifying experience.

When assessing children within the emergency setting, the nurse must take all of these aspects into account. On assessment, the nurse must rely on initial impressions and determine quickly whether the child is distressed or not. Often, when screening a child, it is the simple subtle clues, such as differing behaviours, non-feeding in infants, and no interest in surroundings, that are key. The ability to distinguish the unwell child from the well child is the key to paediatric emergency care and the principal objective of this chapter.

Top ten principles for assessing a child

- Make friends with the parents and the child.
- Never take the child away from the parents.
- Get down to the child's level.
- Babies are best examined on a couch, toddlers on the parent's lap.
- Be opportunistic.
- Always undress infants fully.
- Always weigh a child, and, if possible, assess a child's growth.
- Do not distress the child with unnecessary investigation.
- Take parental concerns into account.
- Always spend time watching the child, whilst taking a history.
- Written and verbal red flag/safety net advice should always be given before discharge.

Play and interaction

When caring for children, it is extremely important to remember that you also have to care for the family. Always take siblings into account, and be aware of the family dynamics and structure. Careful explanation of the child's condition must be given to the whole family, and the subsequent care planned with the family in partnership. Often the siblings get very distressed when their brother or sister is being treated, and time should be taken to explain the procedure to them as well as the patient.

Ten tips for play in the emergency department

- Provide a well-stocked playroom with toys and activities for children of all ages, not forgetting teenagers. Play is a normal and natural part of childhood—children will instinctively play. Encouraging children to play whilst waiting allows them (and their parents) to relax, which, in turn, will ↑ the likelihood of their cooperation. Remember, play is *fun*!
- All staff should take time to chat with children. Taking a moment to build a rapport with a child will ↑ that child's trust in the staff. If a child trusts the staff, they are less likely to resist examination and treatment.
- Children's greatest fear is often the fear of the unknown. The ED is an unfamiliar environment—with strange equipment and strange language. Therefore, take a few minutes to explain procedures to children in child-friendly language and to answer their questions. Remember to reassure parents also—children are receptive to their parents' anxieties, and a calmer parent will result in a calmer child. Play specialists can prepare children through play, using specially adapted dolls and teddies, as well as photo storybooks. Spending a few minutes preparing a child in this manner ↑ the child's cooperation with the procedure, which, in turn, saves valuable time and energy on the part of the staff, as well as making the experience more positive for the child and their parents.
- Distraction therapy offers children a coping mechanism for procedures. Play specialists employ a range of techniques, depending on the age and developmental level of the child, as well as the medical procedure being performed. Children do not have a choice over the procedure, so allowing them a choice over distraction technique empowers them to cope, as they feel a sense of control. Parents and siblings should also be involved with distraction—again, this encourages parents to stay calm, which helps the child stay calm and cooperative.
- There should be a definite 'finish' to the procedure that is clear to the child. This can be as simple as saying 'all finished' and should involve praise and some form of reward (stickers, certificates, and/or a small prize). 'Finishing' a procedure in such a manner allows everyone to relax.
- Post-procedural play should be offered when a procedure does not go well. Play specialists can talk through the experience with the child and their parents, and allow the child to play through emotions with medical play equipment. Allowing a child a few minutes in the playroom before they leave allows the child to de-stress. Follow-up visits can also be considered. All staff should reflect on such experiences, with the aim of avoiding such a situation in the future.

- Read children's body language. Children's 1° method of communication is through play. Watching a child at play and taking note of their body language can reveal much about how a child really feels about a procedure. Play specialists can spend time observing children at play, talking and playing with them, and reassuring them about procedures.
- Take time to position children comfortably before beginning a procedure. If the child is comfortable (often on a parent's knee), the child and parent will be more relaxed, increasing the likelihood of the child's cooperation with the procedure. Consider whether the child wants to watch the procedure and take positions accordingly. Remember to make space for the play specialist and distraction therapy.
- Staff must work together as a team. The child is the most important person, and staff should work with the child and their family to ensure the most positive experience in the best interests of the child.
- Play is a natural part of childhood. Children learn much through play and reach developmental milestones through play. Play specialists can observe children and assess their developmental level through play. Thus, developmental delay can be identified, allowing the child to receive appropriate interventions through referrals to outside agencies.

Further reading

Stephanie Lockwood, Play Specialist, Hospital for Sick Children GOSH.

The unwell child

One of the most frequent reasons that parents seek health-care advice is that the child or infant has fever or is hot to touch. Mostly, the causes are self-limiting viral infections. However, in young children, it can initially be very difficult to distinguish between a serious infection and a self-limiting one. Young infants and children are notoriously difficult to assess when they become unwell. Often the only sign you may get that the infant is unwell is a change in the infant's feeding patterns or the infant sleeping for prolonged periods. The parents know their child better than you, so statements 'that they just are not themselves' must be believed and taken seriously. Examine the infant fully, paying particular attention to the way they are behaving or handle (➲ see Fig. 4.1). All children <3y old presenting with a temperature over 38°C should be thoroughly examined, and a full infection screen considered. Most febrile illnesses in children will be caused by viruses, usually in the upper respiratory tract. It is important, however, to rule out other causes such as pneumonia, UTI, or septicaemia.

General rules

- Always carry out a full set of observations, including RR, pulse rate, temperature, and capillary refill (➲ see Vital signs in children, pp. 770–1).
- The younger the child, the lower the threshold for seeking senior advice and paediatric referral.
- Always take a urine sample. UTIs are a common cause of infection.
- Always take a blood sugar on children/infants who have a reduced level of consciousness or a history of a convulsion.
- Regular reassessment must be carried out if the child is not responding to simple measures such as antipyretics and fluids.
- A period of observation within the ED is always useful and should be encouraged.

▶ All children presenting to the ED or primary care centre must undergo a rapid assessment of ABCDE.

Assessment of ABCDE

(➲ see Vital signs in children, pp. 770–1.)
- Airway and breathing (AB). Assess:
  - work of breathing;
  - RR (➲ see Table 4.1 for normal values);
  - stridor, wheeze;
  - air entry on auscultation;
  - colour.
- Circulation (C). Assess:
  - heart rate (HR) (➲ see Table 4.1 for normal values);
  - pulse volume;
  - capillary refill time;
  - skin temperature;
  - urine output.
- Disability (D). Assess:
  - level of consciousness;
  - posture;

- pupils;
- blood sugar.
- Exposure (E). Assess:
  - rash;
  - skin temperature;
  - scars.

Table 4.1 Normal values of RR and pulse in children at different ages

Age (y)	RR (breaths/min)	Pulse (beats/min)	Systolic BP (mmHg)
Infant <1	30–40	110–160	70–90
Toddler 1–2	25–35	100–150	80–95
Preschool 3–4	25–30	95–140	80–100
School 5–11	20–25	80–120	90–110
Adolescent 12–16	15–20	60–100	100–120

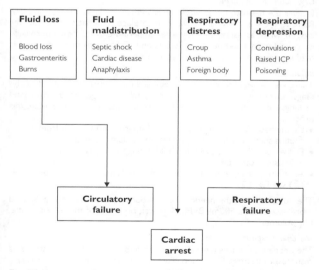

Fig. 4.1 Recognition of an acute unwell child.

(Adapted from Advanced Life Support Group (2016). *Advanced paediatric life support. The practical approach*, 6th edn. BMJ Books, London with the kind permission of Wiley–Blackwell Publishing.)

Resuscitation: introduction

Paediatric resuscitation is divided into that for the newborn, infant (<1y), and child (1y and puberty). International guidelines exist and should be followed.[1] Over the age of puberty, the adult resuscitation guidelines are used.

Resuscitation at birth

Deliveries in the ED or in the community—particularly if it is a concealed pregnancy—should be regarded as high risk, although typically such deliveries are incident-free.

Preparation

- Call paediatricians, midwife, and obstetric team.
- Stop obvious draught (e.g. window).
- Prepare resuscitation equipment. Either use a fully stocked resuscitaire (turn on overhead heater) or BVM (500mL), suction, and oxygen (O_2).
- Remember to start the timer at the outset of the resuscitation.

Neonatal resuscitation (➛ see Fig. 4.2) differs significantly from paediatric resuscitation, with the vast majority of neonates recovering following activity stimulus and/or inflation breaths. Very few neonates require compression/intubation/drugs.

Dry, warm, and stimulate

Deliver the neonate into a warm environment; wrap in a towel, and dry. Remove the wet towel and rewrap; then place on a flat surface. Deliver oxygen, whilst assessing the baby. The temperature of the newly born child is actively maintained between 36.5°C and 37.5°C, unless the decision is made to commence therapeutic hypothermia.

Inflation breaths

These are designed to open the alveoli and force amniotic fluid out of the lungs, as, during normal delivery, a baby takes a large breath to expand its lungs—if this has not happened, the resuscitator needs to replicate this process.

- Lie the baby flat, and open the airway—there is little benefit from routine suction of the airway (unless meconium is present).
- Deliver each breath slowly, and hold during the inspiration phase for 2–3s. Repeat five times.
- Assess response, crying, breathing, and HR. Resuscitate as per protocol (➛ see Fig. 4.2).

The sustained breaths needed for newborn resuscitation are produced more easily with a 500mL BVM. However, be aware of the risk of ↑ inflation volume.

Meconium aspiration

The neonate produces meconium (meconium is sterile faecal matter) as a response to distress. Fresh meconium is green in colour, and sticky aspiration of meconium leads to pulmonary damage.

- Immediately summon the paediatricians.
- Clean the face of meconium. There is no proven benefit from applying suction as the head is delivered.

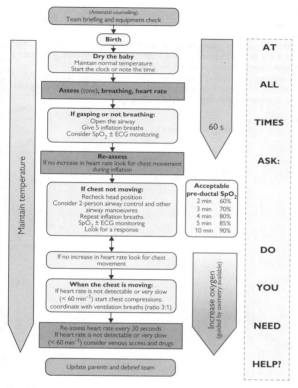

Fig. 4.2 Newborn life support.

(Reproduced with the kind permission of the Resuscitation Council (UK).)

- A vigorously breathing/crying baby has not aspirated.
- Floppy baby: suction the mouth and nose; attempt to remove all visible meconium.
- If no help has arrived and the baby is apnoeic, deliver inflation breaths.

Concerns over ventilating a baby with meconium are understandable, but if all obvious meconium has been removed, the baby remains floppy and apnoeic, and there is no help from an experienced advanced neonatal qualified resuscitator, ventilation becomes an immediate priority.

Compression and ventilation

Nasal continuous positive airway pressure (CPAP), rather than routine intubation, may be useful initially.

Set at 120/min in a compression:ventilation ratio of 3:1. The preferred method is to use two thumbs with the hands encircled around the neonate's chest, one fingerbreadth below the nipple line.

Two rescuers are required to do this effectively with an adequate RR. If only one rescuer is available, compressions using the tips of two fingers, one fingerbreadth below the nipple line, are acceptable.

Reference

1 For more information, visit ♪ http://www.resus.org.uk.

Paediatric basic life support

Children are split into infant and child, with the only difference in the basic life support (BLS) (➔ see Fig. 4.3) technique being used to provide compression.

- Base your assessment on a high index of suspicion, followed by confirmation of unresponsiveness, absence of effective breathing (beware of gasping ventilations), and no pulse (unreliable sign). If in doubt, start BLS.
- Get help as soon as you detect a problem, *but* note the next point.
- Once cardiac arrest is confirmed, early BLS may restore output. If on your own, delay going for help to deliver 1min of cardiopulmonary resuscitation (CPR) (five cycles).
- Significant numbers of critically ill children arrive by car. The triage nurse must instigate rapid assessment and should deliver the first five breaths immediately if a cardiac arrest is suspected—before moving to the resuscitation room.

Resuscitation

Open the airway (avoid hyperextension). Cover the mouth and nose (<1y), or cover the mouth and occlude the child's nose. Deliver five breaths: allow 1s per breath, and allow the child to exhale between breaths. Effective ventilation may reverse respiratory arrest with bradycardia.

Compressions should be instigated if no response to initial five breaths. If convinced that there is a pulse >60 beats per min (bpm), deliver 12–20 breaths/min. If in doubt, start compression, as the risk of significant injury is low.

Uninterrupted, high-quality chest compressions are vital.

- For a child <1y, use two fingertips, one fingerbreadth below the nipple line. The two-thumb method used for neonates (➔ see Compression and ventilation, p. 82) is more effective but becomes difficult to perform, as the child gets bigger.
- For a child >1y, use the heel of one hand or the adult two-hand approach in the centre of the child's chest. The aim is to depress the chest wall by 1/3 its diameter—in an infant or child, this equates to about 4cm and 5cm, respectively—at a rate of 100/min in a compression:ventilation ratio of 15:2, regardless of the child's age. If this proves difficult for a single rescuer to achieve, commence the adult 30:2 ratio, aiming to minimize the delays between breaths and compressions. The compression rate remains at 100–120/min.

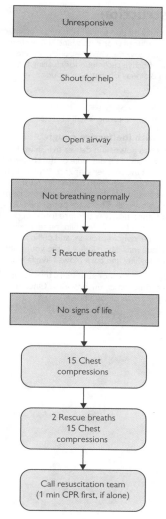

Fig. 4.3 Paediatric basic life support (health-care professionals with a duty to respond).

(Reproduced with the kind permission of the Resuscitation Council (UK). 2015 Guidelines.)

Airway obstruction

Airway obstruction may be due to an FB, trauma, or infection. FB obstruction tends to occur during play or eating, and is therefore rapidly identified. Treatment is based on how the child responds; an effective cough (➔ see Fig. 4.4) is the most effective technique for clearing the airway.

General signs of FB airway obstruction include:
- episode is witnessed;
- coughing/choking;
- sudden onset: no history of illness;
- history of playing with, or eating, small objects.

Conscious child with ineffective cough

- Back slaps. Place head down, and deliver five sharp blows to the back with the heel of the hand in the middle of the shoulder blades. If able, place the child across the rescuer's lap/arm, ensuring the child is head down. In older children, help them to lean forward.
- Chest thrusts and abdominal thrusts. In children <1y, perform chest thrusts once back blows fail. These are performed like cardiac compressions but done slowly with more force. In children >1y, use the abdominal thrust. Stand behind the child; place a clenched fist between the umbilicus and the xiphoid process, and pull backwards but upwards.
  - ⚠ This technique may cause injury in the young and should only be performed if coughing and back blows have failed.

Continue with back slaps/chest or abdominal thrusts, until either the airway is cleared or the child becomes unconscious. Once unconscious, instigate BLS, regardless of the presence of a pulse.

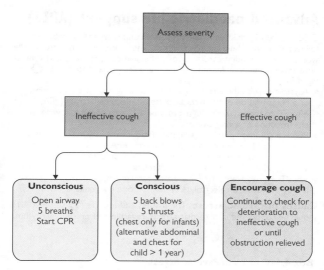

Fig. 4.4 Airway obstruction: immediate management.
(Reproduced with the kind permission of the Resuscitation Council (UK).)

Advanced paediatric life support (APLS)

Cardiac arrest in children is seldom sudden and is typically a deterioration following an overwhelming injury/illness. Therefore, outcomes are usually worse than in an adult cardiac arrest. Effective compressions and ventilations (avoid hyperventilation) are the principles of paediatric ALS (➔ see Fig. 4.5).

- Asystole may be the terminal rhythm, following prolonged downtime or a deterioration of bradycardic pulseless electrical activity (PEA; often 2° to hypoxia), although it may be a 1° arrhythmia following an electrocution or a drug overdose.
- PEA is a common presenting rhythm. Bradycardia may indicate hypoxia or end-stage hypovolaemia, and tachycardic PEA may indicate loss of circulating volume (sepsis, trauma, etc.). To treat loss of circulatory volume, administer a fluid bolus of 20mL/kg.
- VF/VT are relatively rare in paediatric cardiac arrest but may be due to a drug overdose, an electrolyte imbalance, or a congenital abnormality.

Causes of cardiac arrest The five Hs and four Ts (➔ see Box 4.1) should be considered in all cardiac arrests, regardless of presenting rhythm.

Box 4.1 Causes of cardiac arrest

5 Hs

- Hypoxaemia: common.
- Hypovolaemia: common. Not limited to trauma; can be 2° to dehydration, sepsis. Fluids and possibly blood will be required.
- Hyper-/hypokalaemia: may cause VF/VT or non-shockable rhythms.
- Hypothermia. Prolonged CPR may result in neurologically intact survivor.
- Hydrogen ions—acidosis.

4 Ts

- Tension pneumothorax: not limited to trauma. Consider in asthma. May be bilateral. PEA whilst on a ventilator or following CVP line placement.
- Tamponade. Traumatic tamponade = thoracotomy. Tamponade may be medical, e.g. in renal failure.
- Toxic/therapeutic cause. Should be considered in all paediatric arrests. It may affect treatment, e.g. role of adrenaline following solvent abuse.
- Thromboemboli: rare in young children, but possible in young adults.

Airway and ventilation

- Early supplementary O_2 before cardiac arrest is essential. Once cardiac arrest occurs, effective ventilation with a BVM is the priority—supplement with O_2 as soon as available, but do not delay ventilation if O_2 not immediately available.
- The use of oral and nasal airways will assist with effective ventilation. The process of measuring is the same as with an adult. Insert the oral airway with a laryngoscope/tongue depressor to immobilize the tongue. The airway is inserted the 'right way up'. Do not insert and rotate (➜ see Simple airway adjuncts, pp. 646–7).
- Suctioning is part of airway management. Use a soft suction catheter to clear the nose/mouth of fluid secretions; the ridged Yankauer suction catheter is more effective for vomit and blood. Use with a laryngoscope to minimize airway trauma.

Intubation

There is a significant variation in choice of endotracheal tubes (ETTs) for different age groups, but equipment must be checked and be available.

Equipment for paediatric intubation should include the following:

- Miller 0 and 1 laryngoscope blade with handle;
- Macintosh 2 and 3 laryngoscope blade with handle;
- Full range of ETTs cuffed and uncuffed (2.5–8.0mm, including half sizes);
- Catheter mount: adult and paediatric (make sure it fits ETTs);
- Elastoplast® tape and ETT tie tape;
- EtCO$_2$ monitor;
- Intubating stylet and paediatric bougies.

Drug administration in APLS

The two most effective routes for drug administration are IV or intraosseous (IO). Unless an IV access was established prior to loss of output, IO access should be the preferred drug route due to speed and ease of use.

- There are few contraindications to IO access (particularly during cardiac arrest), but infection, fracture above the chosen site, or multiple attempts (always move up the limb) are the main issues with IO access.
- Sites for insertion. The most commonly used site is the proximal tibia 2.5cm below the knee (or one fingerbreadth) on the flat anteromedial surface. Other sites include the calcaneum, distal tibia, distal femur, iliac crest, sternum, and clavicle (➔ see Intraosseous insertion, pp. 708–9).
- Drugs. The most commonly used resuscitation drugs are adrenaline (epinephrine), saline bolus, sodium bicarbonate, and 10% glucose. It is vital that the ED nurse is familiar with a drug dosage system (e.g. Broselow tape) for use during emergencies to minimize the risk of drug errors.

Adrenaline is administered every 3–5min at a dose of 10 micrograms/kg (0.1mL/kg of adrenaline 1:10 000) to improve coronary and cerebral perfusion. Although firm evidence for its effectiveness is still lacking, it is thought to stimulate spontaneous contractions and ↑ the intensity of VF, so increasing the likelihood of successful defibrillation.

Crystalloid bolus is frequently used during resuscitation. The initial dose is 20mL/kg, which represents 20–25% of a child's circulating volume. The choice of fluid is typically 0.9% saline/Hartmann's. After two boluses (40–50% of circulating volume), blood ± inotropic support should be considered. A bolus is used to achieve rapid administration. Therefore, the bolus should be administered under pressure via a 50 or 20mL syringe.

Sodium bicarbonate is used more often during paediatric resuscitation, as metabolic acidosis is usually an issue before cardiac arrest occurs. There is no evidence of clinical benefit. The dose is 1mmol/kg, which is 1mL/kg of 8.4% sodium bicarbonate. Also consider diluting it in equal parts of 5% dextrose.

Sodium bicarbonate should not be mixed with any other resuscitation drug, and the IV/IO line should be flushed prior to the administration of any other drug—use 0.9% saline.

Glucose 10% at a dose of 2mL/kg is the glucose concentration of choice during paediatric emergencies (50% glucose should never be used). During all paediatric emergencies obtain a capillary blood glucose (CBG) early to detect hypoglycaemia.

Amiodarone (5mg/kg) remains an option during VF/VT (but exclude drug overdose, if possible, first). Consider calcium chloride (10mL/10%) if K^+/Mg^{2+} are expected or following an overdose of a calcium channel blocker. These drugs have very limited roles during paediatric cardiac arrest.

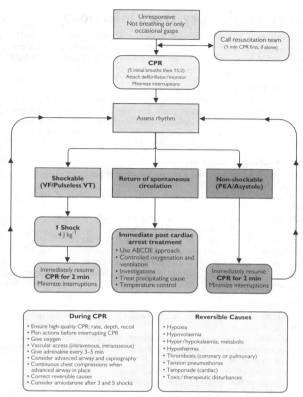

Fig. 4.5 Paediatric advanced life support.

(Reproduced with the kind permission of the Resuscitation Council (UK). 2015 Guidelines.)

Upper respiratory tract infections

Viruses cause ~ 90% of upper respiratory tract infections (URTIs). The upper respiratory tract comprises the ears, nose, throat, tonsils, pharynx, and sinuses. Whilst fever is common to all URTIs, remember that it can have many other causes (➡ see Box 4.2).

Acute nasopharyngitis

Most of the URTIs that occur in children can be classed as acute nasopharyngitis (common cold), of which there are over 200 viral types. However, the majority is caused by rhinoviruses. Children normally present with a low-grade fever, coryza, cough, and general malaise. Symptomatic management is all that is required and reassurance that it will be self-limiting.

Pharyngitis and tonsillitis

- Often children present with a painful throat, low-grade pyrexia, and difficulty in taking fluids.[2]
- This is commonly caused by a viral infection, but be aware of group A β-haemolytic *Streptococcus*.
- Children presenting with bacterial infections usually have a higher-grade fever, some lymphadenopathy, and severe pain.
- Various diagnostic tools have been developed to assist health professionals make their diagnosis (➡ see 'McIsaac score' in Box 4.3).
- Evidence produced by NICE suggests that products, such as benzydamine spray, can be useful in alleviating some of the pain, and thus encouraging the child to take more fluids.

Otitis media

- Children present with a fever and acute pain from the ear involved. They are often very distressed.
- Most inner ear infections are viral in nature, but some can be bacterial.
- On examination, a red, bulging tympanic membrane will be seen, with loss of light reflex.
- Ensure adequate fluid intake and reassurance.
- The tympanic membrane may perforate; this will produce a dramatic relief of the symptoms and will heal spontaneously.

Box 4.2 Causes of fever

- URTIs.
- Lower respiratory tract infections.
- Meningitis.
- Gastroenteritis.
- UTI.
- Acute abdomen.
- Tropical diseases.
- Leukaemia.
- Autoimmune disorders.
- Allergies.

Box 4.3 McIsaac score: sore throat or strep throat

This practical tool[3] will help primary care health professionals decide on the management of patients presenting with URTIs and sore throats.

Step 1 Determine the patient's total score by assigning points according to the following criteria

Criterion	Points
Temperature >38°C	1
No cough	1
Tender anterior cervical nodes	1
Tonsillar swelling or exudates	1
Age 3–14y	1
Age >45y	1

Step 2 Suggested management

Total score	Chance of strep infection (%)	Management
0	2–3	No antibiotics required
1	4–6	
2	10–12	Culture all: treat if culture positive
3	27–28	
4	38–63	Antibiotics and culture

McIsaac, W.J., Goel, V., Tot, T., and Low, D.E. (2000). The validity of the sore throat score in general practice. *Canadian Medical Association Journal* 163, 811–15.

Croup (viral laryngotracheobronchitis)

The commonest condition in the child presenting with stridor is viral croup. Most of the episodes are self-limiting, and the children get better with limited or no intervention. Clinical scoring systems are available for croup and may be useful in determining the severity of the croup and its clinical course.

- A full history and assessment must be carried out on the child to ensure that the right diagnosis is reached.
- Characteristically, the child presents with a barking cough, stridor, and low-grade pyrexia.
- Management depends on the symptoms.
  - Admit all children with respiratory distress, cyanosis, severe stridor, and fatigue.
  - There is very good evidence that oral dexamethasone 0.15mg/kg or nebulized budesonide 2mg is beneficial if stridor is present.[4]
  - In severe cases, adrenaline via a nebulizer can be beneficial.

- The main priority for the health professionals looking after this child is to try not to upset the child. This means that the child should be nursed in the parent's lap, and no attempt should be made to cannulate the child.
- If the stridor does not improve and the child is having some respiratory distress and is becoming exhausted, seek senior support and intensive care.

Acute epiglottitis

Acute bacterial epiglottitis is a rare life-threatening disorder caused almost exclusively by *Haemophilus influenzae* type b (Hib). It has become very rare since the introduction of the Hib immunization in the early 1990s. However, with a creeping ↑ of non-immunization, it is sadly on the ↑.

- The child presents with a history of a rapid-onset high fever and a painful throat. Classically, the children look shocked. They are unable to swallow; they often drool and have a soft inspiratory stridor.
- The treatment is supportive. Do not upset the child in any way, and allow them to find their own airways position.
- Do not attempt to cannulate them.
- You must seek senior anaesthetic, paediatric, and ear, nose, and throat (ENT) surgical help.
- The child will require intubation and IV antibiotics (third-generation cephalosporin, as per hospital antibiotic prescribing protocol) for up to 48h.
- Do not allow anyone to examine the child's throat, unless they are one of the senior specialists above.

References

2 Scottish Intercollegiate Guidelines Network (2004). *Management of sore throats and indications for tonsillectomy*. Royal College of Physicians, Edinburgh.
3 McIsaac WJ, Goel V, Tot T, and Low DE (2000). The validity of the sore throat score in general practice. *CMAJ* **163**, 811–15.
4 Westley CR, Cotton EK, and Brooks JG (1978). Nebulized racemic epinephrine by IPPB for the treatment of croup: a double-blind study. *Am J Dis Child* **132**, 484–7.

Lower respiratory tract infections

Pneumonia

Pneumonia is a term used to describe any infection of the lower respiratory tract, either viral or bacterial. Often it can be a very emotive term, and, if used, its full meaning must be explained to the child's parent.

- Most lower respiratory tract infections (LRTIs) in children are caused by viruses, the respiratory syncytial virus (RSV) being the most commonly known (associated with bronchiolitis). Parainfluenza virus, adenovirus, and the Coxsackie virus also cause LRTIs.
- Bacterial causes are *Streptococcus pneumoniae*, *Haemophilus influenzae*, *Mycoplasma pneumoniae*, and group B β haemolytic *Streptococcus* in the newborn.
- Acute presentation usually follows a history of an URTI, with the child having a worsening cough, fever, and shortness of breath. Infants are often heard to grunt.
- An X-ray should be performed, and blood cultures taken.
- Carry out regular observations, and look particularly for signs of ↑ respiratory distress and exhaustion. O_2 may be required to maintain SpO_2 >95%.
- Often infants and young children become quite dehydrated and require support with feeding or IV fluids for 24h.
- Administer antibiotics, as prescribed and in accordance with local policy.

Bronchiolitis

- RSV is the pathogen in 70–80% of cases; other causes include parainfluenza, influenza, adenoviruses and human metapneumovirus.
- It is a viral LRTI, generally affecting the under 12 months of age. After 12 months of age, consider overlap with viral-induced wheeze or asthma.
- Acute lower respiratory tract symptoms generally develop 2–3 days post-non-specific URTI. Characterized by a moist fruity cough, nasal discharge, fever, tachypnoea, tachycardia, subcostal and intercostal recession, head bobbing, and a widespread fine inspiratory crepitation with rhonchi and reduced O_2 saturations. Apnoea may be the presenting feature of RSV infection.

In healthy infants and young children, bronchiolitis is a self-limiting disease. Management in most cases is supportive, with little evidence for advocating alternative treatments other than to maintain oxygenation and hydration. (➔ see Table 4.2).

- Supplemental O_2: O_2 should be provided by nasal cannula, face mask, or head box to maintain saturations over 90–92%. Heated, humidified high-flow nasal cannula therapy is a non-invasive method of providing ventilatory support to infants with severe bronchiolitis. Studies have shown that the use of Optiflow™ has reduced the rates of babies requiring intubation and paediatric intensive care unit (PICU) admission. Flow rates of >6L/min appear to provide positive pressure throughout the respiratory cycle and optimize the respiratory support required.

Table 4.2 Bronchiolitis assessment and management

Severity	Signs	Management
Mild	Alert, pink on air	Manage at home
	Feeding well	Advise parents about course of disease and to return if concerned
	No underlying cardiorespiratory disease	
	SaO_2 >92%	Reduce quantity of feeds, but give often
		Review by GP 24/7
Moderate	Poor feeding	Admit
	Marked respiratory distress, underlying cardiorespiratory disease	Administer O_2 to maintain adequate saturations
	SaO_2 <92% or aged <6wk	Reduce quantity of feed, but give more frequently
		NG feed or IV fluid maintenance
		Regular observations
Severe	As for moderate with ↑ O_2 requirements	May require CPAP
	Obvious exhaustion	Involve senior paediatric staff
	CO_2 retention	Inform intensive care

Data from South, M. and Young, S. (2002). Emergency paediatric guidelines. Royal Children's Hospital, Melbourne.

- Bronchodilators: trials suggest that bronchodilators may be useful in infants and young children with moderate to severe bronchiolitis who are exhibiting signs of respiratory distress. Although a meta-analysis of randomized trials provides little evidence for the use of bronchodilators in bronchiolitis, the Scottish Intercollegiate Guideline Network (SIGN) and the American Academy of Pediatrics (AAP) suggest that they may be useful in a subset of patients during the early course of the disease. In addition, there is little evidence to suggest toxicity from the therapy. There is some evidence that, in severe bronchiolitis, adrenaline nebulizers may be useful.
- Hypertonic saline: hypertonic saline theoretically has the potential to reduce airway oedema and mucus plugging, and may be useful in the treatment of bronchiolitis. There is some evidence that it does shorten the length of hospital stay. A dose of 3mL of 3% saline via a nebulizer has been suggested.
- Hydration therapy: the fluid intake and output of the infant and child should be assessed regularly. Often the child will require NG feeding. Restricting fluids to two-thirds may be indicated due to the risk of plasma antidiuretic hormone levels rising and pulmonary congestion; however, this should be discussed with paediatrics. Occasionally, the child may require IV fluids if disease is severe.

Whooping cough (pertussis)

Pertussis more commonly is seen in children aged between 2 and 4y. Vaccination has reduced the incidence of pertussis within the western world. However, recent poor take-up of the vaccination has caused a resurgence in the numbers of children with whooping cough within the UK.

Whooping cough can last for 6–8wk. It consists of three stages: catarrhal, paroxysmal, and convalescent. Often the child presents with a paroxysm of coughing characterized by an inspiratory whoop. Mild fever and seizures are associated with the disease.

Management is mainly supportive. However, erythromycin can shorten the illness, if given within the early stages of the disease.

Asthma

Asthma is the commonest respiratory disorder requiring hospital admission in older children. In young children/toddlers, it can be very difficult to diagnose. A child with night-time spasmodic cough or a child with difficulty in breathing with no wheeze may indicate the diagnosis of asthma.

Assessment of the child presenting with asthma is extremely important, as the severity of the respiratory distress is not always easy to detect ($\ominus$ see Table 4.3). On initial assessment, if you are concerned about the child, senior help must be sought and treatment commenced.

Risk factors

- Parental smoking.
- Hospitalized for bronchiolitis.
- Preterm infant.
- Treatment of the acute attack.
- ♀.
- Family history.

Immediate management

- High-flow O_2 via a non-rebreathe mask.
- Bronchodilator therapy.
- If the child presents with mild to moderate asthma, salbutamol may be administered via a spacer, 2–10 puffs, depending upon the severity.
- If aged <2y, ipratropium bromide 125 micrograms via a nebulizer is sometimes effective. β-agonists rarely work in this age group, although it may be worth trying them and assessing their effects.
- >2y to <5y: nebulized salbutamol 2.5mg.
- >5y: nebulized salbutamol 5mg (1mL of nebulizer solution strength 1mg/mL with 2mL of normal saline), given by mouthpiece or face mask.
- Prednisolone 1–2mg/kg must be given.
  - ⚠ This tastes awful, and the child may vomit, so try to give it slowly and in the child's own time. Refer to the British Thoracic Society (BTS) guidelines for up-to-date drug dosages.

If life-threatening features are present

- Get senior support immediately.
- Prepare an IV infusion of salbutamol 15 micrograms/kg, followed by a continuous infusion 1–5 micrograms/kg/min (dilute to 200 micrograms/mL).
- Give hydrocortisone 4mg/kg.
- Consider the use of IV magnesium.
- Consider IV aminophylline 5mg/kg loading dose (omit if on oral theophylline), followed by an infusion 1mg/kg/h.
- Give nebulized $β_2$-agonist frequently back to back.
- Endeavour to maintain SpO_2 >92%.
- Watch for exhaustion.

Table 4.3 Assessment of asthma

Moderate	Acute severe	Life-threatening
• SaO$_2$ >92%	• Too breathless to feed or complete sentences	• Conscious level depressed or agitated
• No clinical features of severe or life-threatening attack	• RR >30/min (>5y) or >40/min (2–5y)	• Exhaustion
• Peak flow >50% best or predicted	• Pulse rate >125/min (>5y) or 134/min (2–5y)	• Poor respiratory effort
	• Peak flow <50%	• SaO$_2$ <92% on air
		• Silent chest
		• Peak flow <33%
		• Hypotension

Reproduced with kind permission from SIGN, QRG 141: British guideline on the management of asthma: (2014) ஃ http://www.brit-thoracic.org.uk/Portals/0/Guidelines/AsthmaGuidelines/sign101%20Jan%202012.pdf.

The child should be admitted if

- The attack is very severe when the child arrives at hospital. Initial SpO$_2$ level is <92% in air.
- There is little or no response to salbutamol after 30min, or there is response but then rapid deterioration.
- The child is discharged but returns within 4h.
- The child attends late in the evening or the parents are unable to cope. See Fig. 4.6 for the assessment and management of asthma in children.

The child is well enough to go home

- Make sure that the parents understand the instructions you have given about the treatment to be taken at home, and record your instructions in the notes.
- Ensure that the child is given a course of oral prednisolone, and ↑ the regular bronchodilator therapy for a couple of days.
- Contact the child's GP or the hospital respiratory team in order to ensure follow-up and further treatment.

Further reading

British Thoracic Society. *Asthma guideline*. Available at: ஃ https://www.brit-thoracic.org.uk/guidelines-and-quality-standards/asthma-guideline/.

(a)

MANAGEMENT OF ACUTE ASTHMA IN CHILDREN AGED 2 YEARS AND OVER

ACUTE SEVERE

SpO_2 <92% PEF 33–50% best or predicted

* Can't complete sentences in one breath or too breathless to talk or feed
* Heart rate >125 (>5 years) or >140 (2–5 years)
* Respiratory rate >30 breaths/min (>5 years) or >40 (2–5 years)

LIFE-THREATENING

SpO_2 <92% PEF <33% best or predicted

* Silent chest
* Cyanosis
* Poor respiratory effort
* Hypotension
* Exhaustion
* Confusion

CRITERIA FOR ADMISSION

✓	Increase β_2 agonist dose by giving one puff every 30–60 seconds, according to response, up to a maximum of ten puffs.
✓	Parents/carers of children with an acute asthma attack at home and symptoms not controlled by up to 10 puffs of salbutamol via pMDI and spacer, should seek urgent medical attention.
✓	If symptoms are severe additional doses of bronchodilator should be given as needed whilst awaiting medical attention.
✓	Paramedics attending to children with an acute asthma attack should administer nebulized salbutamol, using a nebulizer driven by oxygen if symptoms are severe, whilst transferring the child to the emergency department.
✓	Children with severe or life-threatening asthma should be transferred to hospital urgently.
B	Consider intensive inpatient treatment of children with SpO_2 <92% in air after initial bronchodilator treatment.

The following clinical signs should be recorded:

* Pulse rate – increasing tachycardia generally denotes worsening asthma; a fall in heart rate in life-threatening asthma is a pre-terminal event
* Respiratory rate and degree of breathlessness – i.e. too breathless to complete sentences in one breath or to feed
* Use of accessory muscles of respiration – best noted by palpation of neck muscles
* Amount of wheezing – which might become biphasic or less apparent with increasing airways obstruction
* Degree of agitation and conscious level – always give calm reassurance

NB. Clinical signs correlate poorly with the severity of airways obstruction. Some children with acute severe asthma do not appear distressed.

INITIAL TREATMENT OF ACUTE ASTHMA

OXYGEN

✓	Children with life-threatening asthma or SpO_2 <94% should receive high flow oxygen via a tight fitting face mask or nasal cannula at sufficient flow rates to achieve normal saturations of 94–98%.

Fig. 4.6a Assessment and management of asthma in children.

(Reproduced from *Thorax*, British Thoracic Society Scottish Intercollegiate Guidelines Network, 69, p.15–16, 2014, with permission from BMJ Publishing Group Ltd.)

(b)

MANAGEMENT OF ACUTE ASTHMA IN CHILDREN AGED 2 YEARS AND OVER

BRONCHODILATORS

A Inhaled β_2 agonists are the first line treatment for acute asthma.

A A pMDI + spacer is the preferred option in children with mild to moderate asthma.

B Individualize drug dosing according to severity and adjust according to the patient's response.

A If symptoms are refractory to initial β_2 agonist treatment, add ipratropium bromide (250 micrograms/dose mixed with the nebulized β_2 agonist solution).

✓ Repeated doses of ipratropium bromide should be given early to treat children who are poorly responsive to β_2 agonists.

C Consider adding 150 mg magnesium sulfate to each nebulized salbutamol and ipratropium in the first hour in children with a short duration of acute severe asthma symptoms presenting with an oxygen saturation less than 92%.

✓ Discontinue long-acting β_2 agonists when short-acting β_2 agonists are required more often than four hourly.

STEROID THERAPY

A Give oral steroids early in the treatment of acute asthma attacks.

- Use a dose of 20 mg prednisolone for children aged 2–5 years and a dose of 30–40 mg for children >5 years. Those already receiving maintenance steroid tablets should receive 2 mg/kg prednisolone up to a maximum dose of 60 mg.
- Repeat the dose of prednisolone in children who vomit and consider intravenous steroids in those who are unable to retain orally ingested medication.
- Treatment for up to three days is usually sufficient, but the length of course should be tailored to the number of days necessary to bring about recovery. Tapering is unnecessary unless the course of steroids exceeds 14 days.

SECOND LINE TREATMENT OF ACUTE ASTHMA

B Consider early addition of a single bolus dose of intravenous salbutamol (15 micrograms/kg over 10 minutes) **in a severe asthma attack where the patient has not responded to initial inhaled therapy.**

A Aminophylline is not recommended in children with mild to moderate acute asthma.

B Consider aminophylline for children with severe or life-threatening asthma unresponsive to maximal doses of bronchodilators and steroids.

IV magnesium sulfate is a safe treatment for acute asthma although its place in management is not yet established.

Fig. 4.6b (contd.).

The child with fever

The NICE (2013) feverish child clinical guidelines (CG160) were intended for health-care professionals for the assessment and initial management of infants and young children under the age of 5 with feverish illness. The guidelines were developed to ensure that patients were adequately assessed and cared for, before a definitive diagnosis was made. In essence, the guidelines have been developed to ensure that health professionals do not undertreat those children requiring aggressive management or overtreat those that do.

The conditions to which the fever guidelines give special attention are those that could potentially be life- or limb-threatening to an unwell child and could be spotted by systematic assessment and careful regard to the signs and symptoms of the presenting child:

- meningococcal disease;
- bacterial meningitis;
- herpes simplex encephalitis;
- pneumonia;
- UTI;
- septic arthritis;
- Kawasaki disease.

Assessment is based on the traffic light system, as detailed in Table 4.4.

Table 4.4 Traffic light system for assessment of the feverish child

Children considered at high risk for serious illness (RED)

- Pale
- No response to social cues
- Appearing ill to health-care professional
- Does not wake or, if roused, does not stay awake
- Weak, high-pitched, or continuous cry
- Grunting
- RR >60 breaths/min
- Moderate or severe chest indrawing
- Reduced skin turgor
- Bulging fontanelle

Children considered at intermediate risk for serious illness (ORANGE)

- Pallor of skin
- Not responding normally
- No smile
- Wakes only with prolonged stimulation
- ↓ activity
- Dry mucous membranes
- Poor feeding in infants
- Reduced urine output
- Rigors

Children considered to be at low risk for serious illness (GREEN)

- Normal colour of skin, lips, and tongue
- Responds normally to social cues
- Content/smiles
- Stays awake or awakens quickly
- Moist mucous membranes
- Strong, normal cry or not crying
- Normal skin and eyes

Reproduced with permission from the National Institute for Health and Care Excellence (2013) *Feverish illness in children: Assessment and initial management in children younger than five years.* NICE CG160.

Meningococcal septicaemia

Meningococcal disease presents in two different ways: meningitis and septicaemia. Early recognition and aggressive management can greatly improve the prognosis. Diagnosis in the early stages of the disease is often problematic. Children present with non-specific febrile illness, indistinguishable from a viral URTI or influenza. Health professionals therefore need to be very diligent with their clinical examination and history taking. If children are sent home, following a febrile illness, parents should be advised about what signs and symptoms to look for and told to return immediately if worried.

There are four clinical indicators that health professionals must look out for and manage accordingly.

- Rash. In the early stages, the rash may be blanching and maculopapular. It then develops into a non-blanching purpuric rash. Often the rash is a very small, subtle rash found in the skin crease. It is very important to undress the patient and to search the skin fully. A rapidly evolving petechial rash is a very worrying sign.
- Shock. Cold hands and feet, fast irregular breathing, tachycardia, and poor capillary refill are all signs of septicaemia (➔ see Box 4.4).
- ↓ level of consciousness. Often subtle signs, such as irritability, not feeding, and drowsiness, can be indicative of severe sepsis.
- Neck stiffness. This is very difficult to assess in young children but must be taken seriously when present.

Any child presenting with any of the above symptoms must be very carefully observed. Senior clinical support must be obtained at an early stage, and the child cared for in a high dependency area. Early and aggressive intervention is the key to management of any kind of sepsis (➔ see Box 4.5). In symptomatic infants and children, lumbar punctures are contraindicated and must not be carried out.

Box 4.4 Signs of early compensated shock

- Tachycardia.
- Cool peripheries.
- Delayed capillary refill.
- Reduced level of consciousness.
- Tachypnoea.
- Poor urine output.
- Hypotension.

Box 4.5 Management of severe sepsis and septic shock in infants and children

- Recognize ↓ mental status and perfusion.
  - Begin high-flow O_2.
  - Establish IV/IO access.
  - Urgent bloods sent for venous blood gases (VBG), U&E, FBC, CRP, PCR, Ca^{2+}, and Mg^{2+} (do not forget to check blood glucose or lactate).
- Push boluses of 10–20mL/kg of isotonic saline, up to 60mL/kg, with reassessment in between each bolus—until perfusion improves, or hepatomegaly or crackles develop.
  - Correct hypoglycaemia and hypocalcaemia.
  - Start antibiotics; IV cefotaxime 50mg/kg.
- Fluid-refractory shock: start dopamine up to 10 micrograms/kg/min.
- Intubate, and gain central access.
  - For cold shock: add in central adrenaline if dopamine-resistant.
  - For warm shock: add in central noradrenaline.
- NG tube and urinary catheter.
  - Transfer to PICU.

Adapted from the American College of Critical Care Medicine (2007). Clinical practice parameters for hemodynamic support of pediatric & neonatal septic shock, *Crit Care Med* 2009 Vol **37**.No2.

Kawasaki disease

Kawasaki disease is an autoimmune disease that is seen predominantly in the under 5s. This is a relatively rare disease but, if left untreated, can be fatal due to coronary artery aneurysm (~1% of children with the disease). The pathogen that causes the disease remains unknown and could be linked to a pre-existing viral infection.

Criteria for diagnosis of Kawasaki disease

- Fever of ≥5 days' duration, associated with at least four of the following five changes:
  - bilateral non-suppurative conjunctivitis;
  - one or more changes of the mucous membranes of the upper respiratory tract, including throat redness, dry cracked lips, red lips, and 'strawberry' tongue;
  - one or more changes of the arms and legs, including redness, swelling, skin peeling around the nails, and generalized peeling;
  - polymorphous rash, primarily truncal;
  - large lymph nodes in the neck (>1.5cm in size).
- Disease cannot be explained by some other known disease process.
- A diagnosis of Kawasaki disease can be made if fever and only three changes are present, if coronary artery disease is documented by two-dimensional echocardiography or coronary angiography.

If suspected, routine bloods should be taken (U&E, CRP, LFTs, FBC, including ESR); urine should be collected, as well as an electrocardiogram (ECG) recorded and an echocardiography requested. The child should be referred to paediatrics for admission and subsequent management.

Management of the disease includes high-dose IV immunoglobulin (IVIG) (2g/kg), aspirin for 6wk, and occasionally steroids.

Further reading

National Institute for Health and Care Excellence (2013). *Feverish illness in children: assessment and initial management in children younger than five years.* CG160. National Institute for Health and Care Excellence, London.

Herpes simplex encephalitis

Herpes simplex encephalitis (HSE) is rare; however, if missed, it can have severe consequences, with a 70% mortality rate if left untreated. Children will present to the ED with ↓ level of consciousness or fitting, a history of fever, and often a vesicular rash. If HSE is suspected, senior paediatric support must be called for immediately.

The child should be treated with IV aciclovir and, if *in extremis*, requires intubation, ventilatory support, and careful fluid management.

Rashes

One of the commonest reasons for parents to seek health-care advice is because their child has developed a rash or skin lesions. More often than not, these rashes are self-limiting and tend to be innocuous. With all of these lesions, it is important to treat the child, and not the rash (➔ see Table 4.5). There are many causes of a rash or skin lesion:

- infection;
- irritation;
- injury;
- infestation;
- iatrogenic;
- dermatological disease.

The history that should be taken includes the following:

- Is the child well or febrile?
- Is the rash itchy?
- Are there any predisposing factors or associated symptoms?
- PMH.

The rash should be described, focusing on characteristics, distribution, and the presence of enanthem (➔ see Table 4.5).

Treatment is dependent on the cause and severity of the rash. Often simple management is indicated, but be careful not to miss the telltale signs of sepsis and other life-threatening illness. Be concerned about non-blanching rashes that are evolving and severe staphylococcal infections such as scalded skin syndrome. Signs for toxic shock must be picked up and acted on immediately.

Table 4.5 Rashes in children

Type of lesion	Description	Example
Macular rash	Flat lesion <1cm, pink or red in colour	Rubella
Papular	Raised lesion >1cm in diameter	Insect bite
Maculopapular	Mixture of above	Iatrogenic
		Measles
Vesicles	<1cm, fluid-filled	Chickenpox
Wheals	Raised lesions, erythematous, irregular shape	Urticaria
Desquamatous	Scaly eruption	Kawasaki disease
Purpura	Non-blanching, red/purple, >0.5cm	Henoch–Schönlein purpura
		Meningococcaemia
Petechiae	Non-blanching, red/purple, <0.5cm	ITP
		Leukaemia
		Meningococcaemia

Urinary tract infections

All unwell infants and children presenting to the ED should be tested for a UTI. Although UTIs are relatively common in young infants and toddlers, they can be hard to detect on symptoms alone. Classical symptoms, such as dysuria, frequency, fever, and enuresis, may not be present. Often infants present with irritability, not feeding, vomiting, diarrhoea, and failure to thrive.

- The commonest organism causing a UTI in children is *Escherichia coli*. However, other organisms, such as *Proteus, Pseudomonas*, and *Klebsiella*, may also be detected.
- UTIs are often caused by vesicoureteric reflux where there is a backflow of urine from the bladder up the ureter.
- Diagnosis is dependent on the urine culture, but a urine dipstick test should be the initial screening test.
  - ⚠ Dipstick tests have poor sensitivity and limited specificity for detecting UTIs. Do *not* rely upon them as the sole means of diagnosis.
  - Where available, urgent urine must be obtained to aid with diagnosis.
  - Urine collection in children can be problematic.
- In infants, a suprapubic aspirate can be a very useful way of obtaining a urine sample. This should be carried out by an experienced clinician, using ultrasound as a guide.
- Obtain clean-catch urines by sitting the infant or young child on the parent's lap without a nappy, whilst feeding with a sterile collecting utensil. It is very important the child's perineum and genitalia have been cleaned properly to reduce the chance of sample contamination.
- Urine-collecting pads can be used in accordance with the manufacturer's recommendations. The use of gauze, cotton wool, or sanitary towels is contraindicated and should be avoided.

Management

- Any child <3 months of age (this is dependent on local guidelines) or who is systemically unwell should be admitted under the paediatricians for IV antibiotics and further investigations and management.
- Discharge older children on co-trimoxazole for 3 days if they have a lower UTI or cystitis (refer to *Children's BNF* for guidance about dosages and further advice). They will require follow-up and further investigations. Give advice to parents about encouraging fluids, personal cleansing, and appropriate underwear.
- Refer to the NICE guidelines for the treatment of UTIs.[5]

Reference

5 National Institute for Health and Care Excellence (2007). *Urinary tract infection: diagnosis, treatment and long-term management of urinary tract infection in children*. CG54. National Institute for Health and Care Excellence, London.

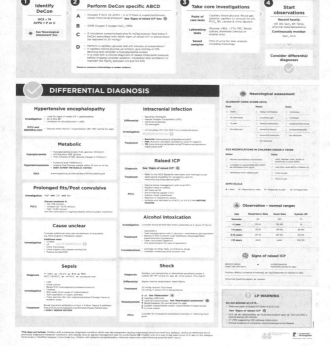

Fig. 4.7 Algorithm for the management of a child aged 0–18y with a decreased conscious level.

(Reproduced from *The management of children and young people with an acute decrease in conscious level*, 2015 update, with permission of Royal College of Paediatrics and Child Health. Available at: http://www.rcpch.ac.uk/improving-child-health/clinical-guidelines-and-standards/published-rcpch/management-children-and-you)

The fitting child

Children commonly present to the ED with seizures or episodes of altered consciousness associated with abnormal posturing, movement, or behaviours. There can be many causes of these seizures or syncopal occurrences (➔ see Box 4.6). A clear history and description of the events and episode can be very useful in establishing the cause.

Box 4.6 Causes of syncope in children

- Epilepsy.
- Febrile convulsion.
- Hypoglycaemia.
- Vasovagal episode.
- Lyme disease.
- Breath-holding attacks.
- Gastro-oesophageal reflux.
- Congenital heart condition.
- Migraines.
- Panic attacks.
- Meningitis.
- Electrolyte disturbances.
- Trauma.
- Poisoning.

Key history points

- Previous history of convulsions.
- How long has the seizure lasted?
- Obtain an accurate description of the seizure itself. Was it focal or generalized?
- Were they well or unwell prior to the seizure?
- Did any incident precede the event?
- Any family history or developmental abnormalities?

These events can be very frightening to the child's parents or carers. Often, because of the dramatic nature of the episode, they are concerned that the child may be critically ill or die. The parents and carers need constant reassurance and care.

Management

(➔ See Fig. 4.8.)

- The immediate management of the fitting child must be to maintain the child's airway and support their breathing with an airway adjunct and high-flow O_2.
- Use anticonvulsants to stop the seizure, and check the child's blood sugar. Administer 2mL/kg of 10% glucose if the CBG is <3mmol/L.

- Insert an IV cannula, and take bloods for FBC, U&E, Ca²⁺, and Mg²⁺.
- If the child has a temperature >38°C, administer rectal paracetamol.
- A senior clinician must be involved in the child's care.
- Refer all infants presenting with their first fit to the paediatricians for admission or follow local first fit pathway.
- Children can present with a ↓ conscious level from many causes. The algorithm presented in Fig. 4.7 presents a useful evidence-based guideline for the initial management of children who present to hospital with a reduced level of consciousness.

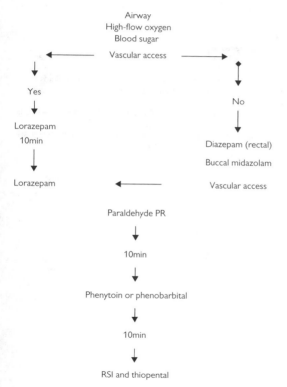

Fig. 4.8 Management of fitting in children.

(Reproduced with kind permission of Wiley–Blackwell Publishing from Advanced Life Support Group (2011). *Advanced paediatric life support. The practical approach*, 5th edn. BMJ Books, London.)

Diabetic ketoacidosis

This is defined as uncontrolled catabolism associated with insulin deficiency seen in patients with type 1 diabetes resulting in hyperglycaemia, ketosis that causes metabolic acidosis, and osmotic diuresis resulting in profound dehydration.

Clinical features include:
- hyperventilation;
- dehydration;
- nausea and vomiting;
- drowsiness and coma;
- can present as severe abdominal pain and is often mistaken for an acute abdomen.

Management
- Resuscitation as necessary.
- Venous or capillary blood gas, including glucose, pH, bicarbonate, and lactate.
- Cautious fluid management replacing deficit and maintenance fluids over 48h, along with correction of electrolyte imbalance. Repeat U&E regularly.
- Insulin should be commenced 1h after the fluids have been commenced. Blood sugars should be reduced slowly at <5mmol/L/h.
- Watch for signs of raised intracranial pressure (ICP) caused by cerebral oedema. If suspected, seek senior help urgently.

Apparent life-threatening episode (ALTE)

Children <1y who present to the ED, following an episode involving one or more of the following symptoms, should be admitted under the paediatricians for investigation and observation. On assessment, they may be perfectly well, and your examination may not reveal any underlying condition. In some cases, there is an obvious diagnosis. Manage children who are obviously unwell, as their condition dictates:

- apnoea (stopping breathing);
- colour change (cyanosis or pallor);
- choking (except straightforward choking on a feed);
- unresponsiveness;
- hypertonia (stiffening of limbs or neck);
- floppiness.

It is essential to take a detailed history from all observers.

▶ Ask who was taking care of the infant at the time of the incident.

Examination

- Fully undress the baby, and examine thoroughly, including a careful look for bruises, petechiae, rash, and injury.
- Examine the ears and eyes; the optic fundi should be examined for haemorrhages.

Gastroenteritis

Diarrhoea and vomiting are very common in infants and young children. They are most often caused by viruses such as the rotavirus. However, they can be of bacterial origin, e.g. caused by *Campylobacter*, *Shigella*, *Escherichia coli*, and *Salmonella*, among others. Key distinguishing factors pointing to a bacterial infection are fever, severe abdominal pain, and blood or mucus in the stool. It is very important to note that there are other causes of diarrhoea and vomiting in infants and children, and these must be considered (➔ see Box 4.7). If the vomit is bile-stained, senior clinical advice must be obtained and a surgical opinion sought.

- Most children who have gastroenteritis have a self-limiting condition lasting no longer than 48h.
- They can be simply managed by reducing their milk feed for a small amount of time and encouraging oral dehydration solutions such as Dioralyte®.
- It is important to note that early refeeding reduces the duration of the gastroenteritis and therefore should be encouraged.
- Babies who are breastfed should be encouraged to carry on. However, the parents should be encouraged to observe the infant's weight to ensure that they do not become too dehydrated.

Box 4.7 Causes of diarrhoea and vomiting

- Gastroenteritis.
- UTI.
- Febrile illness.
- Tonsillitis.
- Irritable bowel syndrome.
- Gastro-oesophageal reflux.
- Small bowel obstruction.
- Constipation.
- Pyloric stenosis.
- Intussusception.
- Acute appendicitis.
- Sepsis.
- Food intolerance.
- Metabolic disorders.

Dehydration

Dehydration is the major concern in children presenting with gastroenteritis. Assessment should be made as to the degree of dehydration (➔ see Table 4.6).

The most useful assessment of hydration is the comparison of weights. However, this is not always available.

- Mild dehydration (<5%) can be treated at home, using oral rehydration therapy, but the parents must be advised that, if vomiting persists, they must return. In pre-weaned children, milk feeds or breastfeeding should be continued.
- Moderate to severe dehydration requires hospital admission. Infants may require IV fluids to correct any electrolyte imbalance.
- Too rapid rehydration can lead to large shifts in fluids and hyponatraemia. Most infants and young children can be fed via an NG tube, which negates the need for IV fluids, and thus the risks associated with them. Keep careful documentation of the child's fluid balance, as well as of the vital signs and weight.

Table 4.6 Assessment of dehydration

	Mild	Moderate	Severe
Mucous membranes	Dry	Dry	Dry
Urine output	Normal	Reduced	None for 12h
Mental state	Normal	Lethargic	Coma
Pulse rate	Normal	Tachycardia	Tachycardia
BP	Normal	Normal	Low
Capillary refill	Normal	Delayed	More delayed
Skin and eye turgor	Normal	Reduced	More reduced
Fontanelle	Normal	Sunken	Very much sunken
Dehydration (%)	<5	5–10	>10

Reproduced from Advanced Life Support Group (2011). *Advanced paediatric life support. The practical approach*, 5th edn. BMJ Books, London, with kind permission of Wiley–Blackwell Publishing.

Management of the injured child

Management of the seriously injured child can be extremely challenging, but principles of treatment priorities are identical to those for an adult. Preparation is often the key. Working out the child's treatment variables before arrival speeds up care and reduces much of the stress. The weight of the child is the priority for this. Although there has been much clinical debate regarding the approximation of a child's weight, a reasonably accurate way to do this is by calculating the age of the child + 4 × 2 = approximate weight in kilogram (up to age of 10y).

The team should be prepared with PPE, and roles should be assigned.

Primary survey
- C (Catastrophic haemorrhage).
  - Any massive haemorrhage must be controlled, using appropriate wound dressings, tourniquets, or splintage, along with direct pressure.
- A (Airway).
  - Assess; clear and secure the airway, whilst maintaining control of the C-spine.
  - Maintain in-line C-spine immobilization. (Do not immobilize combative patients.)
- B (Breathing).
  - Assess breathing and oxygenation. Give O_2. Prepare to manage any life-threatening chest injury.
- C (Circulation).
  - Assess circulation, and control haemorrhage.
  - Insert two large-gauge IV cannulae.
  - If evidence of hypovolaemic shock, give a bolus of normal saline in 10mL/kg, and reassess early.
  - Think about the need for blood early; initiate the Massive Transfusion Policy, but be aware of overtransfusion: Rapid infusion devices can be harmful to young children; use with caution. Initially 5mL/kg of RBCs and 5mL/kg of FFP warmed; up to 15mL/kg should be given.
  - Direct pressure to external bleeding sites; appropriate early splintage is important—protect the pelvis!
  - Tranexamic acid 15mg/kg should be prescribed and given.
  - Consider the use of platelets 5mL/kg, cryoprecipitate 5mL/kg, and $CaCl_2$ 10% 2mL/kg.
  - Manage the lethal triad of hypothermia, coagulopathy, and electrolyte abnormalities (lactate). Aim for fibrinogen >1.5g/L, platelets >100 × 10^9/L, Ca^{2+} >1mmol/L, Hct >0.3.
- D (Disability). Carry out a simple neurological assessment using:
  - level of response (AVPU: A, alert; V, responds to vocal stimuli; P, responds to painful stimuli; U, unresponsive);
  - pupil reaction and equality;
  - do not ever forget to take CBG.
- E (Exposure).

Undress the patient completely, taking care to protect the whole of the spine. Remember children lose heat very quickly, so they should always be covered and warmed, if hypothermic. All fluids should be warmed.

Once ABC is stabilized, proceed to the secondary survey.

Remember to manage hypothermia, electrolyte imbalances, and haemolysis.

Secondary survey

It is very important to manage the child's pain effectively and ensure the child is comforted throughout. Allow the child's parents to be in attendance at all times. Carry out a full set of observations, and monitor the patient accordingly. Take the child off the spinal board as soon as possible, and carry out a full assessment for other injuries.

Examine the whole patient systematically

A suggested system is:
- head and face, neck;
- chest;
- abdomen;
- pelvis and perineum;
- back and spine; minimal patient handling if pelvic fracture is suspected;
- extremities;
- neurological status;
- pupil reaction;
- GCS score;
- any lateralizing signs.

Paediatric head injury

Head injuries are the commonest cause of traumatic death in children aged 1–15y. They are most often caused by falls, road traffic collisions (RTCs), sporting injuries, and non-accidental injury (NAI).

The first priority is to perform a primary survey, assessing the child's airway and C-spine. Make sure that breathing and circulation are secure and stabilized.

History and examination

Perform an assessment of the child, looking specifically at the following.
• Neck and C-spine. Deformity, tenderness, muscle spasm.
• Head. Scalp bruising, lacerations, swelling, tenderness, bruising behind the ear (Battle sign).
• Eyes. Pupil size, equality, and reactivity; fundoscopy.
• Ears. Blood behind the eardrum, CSF leak.
• Nose. Deformity, swelling, bleeding, CSF leak.
• Mouth. Dental trauma, soft tissue injuries.
• Facial fractures.
• Motor function. Examine the limbs for the presence of reflexes and any lateralizing weaknesses.
• Perform a full children's coma score. Beware that children can have raised ICP with a normal GCS; look for signs of a low pulse, coupled with a high blood pressure (BP) (Cushing's sign). Always report abnormal findings to a senior clinician immediately.
• Consider the possibility of NAI.
• Other injuries.

Additional information
• Time, mechanism, and circumstances of injury.
• Loss or impairment of consciousness and duration.
• Nausea and vomiting.
• Clinical course prior to consultation: stable, deteriorating, improving.
• Other injuries sustained.

Management

Minor head injury
• No loss of consciousness.
• One or no episodes of vomiting.
• Stable, alert, conscious state.
• May have scalp bruising or laceration.
• Normal examination otherwise.

These children may be discharged from the ED into the care of their parents. Ensure that the child and parents have clear instructions regarding the management of the child at home—especially when they should return to hospital immediately. (A written advice sheet must be provided.)[6]

▶ If there is any doubt as to whether there has been loss of consciousness, assume there has been, and treat as a moderate head injury.

Moderate head injury
- Brief loss of consciousness at time of injury.
- Currently alert or responds to voice.
- May be drowsy.
- One or more persistent episodes of vomiting.
- Persistent headaches.
- May have a large scalp bruise, haematoma, or laceration.
- Normal examination otherwise.

Assess the child, and admit for observations as per local protocol.
- The child may be discharged home if there is improvement to normal conscious levels and no further vomiting. It is important that the child has been observed playing normally during this period of observation and has tolerated fluids and diet.
- Persistent headaches, a large haematoma, or a possible penetrating wound may need further investigation. If the child is still drowsy or vomiting after a period of observation or there is any deterioration during this time, discuss with a senior as a matter of priority. Consider further investigations, and admit the child under the inpatient team caring for children with head injuries (➔ see Box 4.8).

Remember the term 'head injury' is very alarming for parents and carers; it is therefore imperative to offer reassurance and give sound advice, which is reiterated in a written advice leaflet.[6]

Box 4.8 Guidelines for admission of children following head injury

- Patients with new, clinically significant abnormalities on imaging.
- Patients who have not returned to GCS 15 after imaging, regardless of the imaging results.
- Continuing worrying signs (e.g. persistent vomiting and severe headaches) of concern to the clinician.
- Persistence of symptoms >4h after the event.
- Suspected NAI.
- Social. Home situation suspected of being unsuitable for adequate observation.
- Mechanism of injury indicative of more severe trauma, e.g. falling from height.
- Other medical conditions that may involve a risk of intracranial complications, e.g. haemophilia, ITP, etc.
- Re-attendance with head injury if there are persisting signs or symptoms.
- Bleeding from the ear and nose.

Criteria for immediate request for CT scan of the head, which must be performed within 1h of the risk factors being identified

- Suspicion of NAI.
- Post-traumatic seizure, but no history of epilepsy.
- On initial assessment within the ED, GCS <14; or for children under the age of 1y, GCS <15.
- At 2h after injury, GCS <15.
- Suspected open or depressed skull fracture or tense fontanelle.
- Any signs of basal skull fracture.
- Focal neurological deficit.
- For children under 1y: presence of bruise, swelling, or laceration of >5cm on the head.
- For children who have sustained a head injury and have >1 of the following risk factors:
  - loss of consciousness lasting >5min (witnessed);
  - abnormal drowsiness;
  - three or more discrete episodes of vomiting;
  - dangerous mechanism;
  - amnesia lasting >5min.

Reference

6 National Institute for Health and Care Excellence (2007; updated 2014). *Head injury: assessment and early management*. CG176. National Institute for Health and Care Excellence, London. Available at: ℞ http://www.nice.org.uk/cg176.

Children's fractures

A fracture is a disruption or a break in the cortex of a bone. Children with fractures often present with swelling, pain, and regional tenderness, lack of movement, angulation, and deformity. However, due to the cartilaginous properties of developing bone, signs and symptoms in young children can be very subtle. Often toddlers will present with symptoms such as not using their arm or crying inconsolably. Children will often find it hard to localize specific areas of pain, and this can lead to needless X-rays and investigations. It is important that the nurse or clinician spends time examining the limb appropriately and determining from where the child's pain is coming, rather than resorting to excessive X-rays. The growth and development of bones in children vary with age and sex (➔ see Table 4.7).

General guidelines
• All fractures are painful. Give the child regular analgesia.
• All fractures are generally more comfortable immobilized.
• Refer fractures that look clinically deformed to the orthopaedic team.
• Full arm plasters are required on all babies, as backslabs tend to slip off.
• All children with grossly deformed limbs require regular neurovascular observations.
• Be alert for children <2y who present with fractures. Take a very careful history, and be mindful of NAI.

Greenstick fractures

Greenstick fractures of the forearm are the commonest fractures seen in children in the ED. A greenstick fracture (➔ see Fig. 4.9) is an incomplete fracture where the cortex of the bone is only disrupted on one side and buckled on the other. Place these fractures in a backslab for support, and send to the fracture clinic for further follow-up. Treat greenstick fractures of the proximal end of the radius with an above-elbow backslab, as there is significant evidence to suggest that they are unstable and become more angulated over time.

Buckle fractures Buckle/torus fractures (➔ see Fig. 4.10) are minimally impacted fractures within an intact periosteum. These occur at the metaphysis. Treat buckle/torus fractures conservatively with splintage. These fractures tend to heal in 2–4wk. Follow-up should be arranged as per local guidelines.

Open/compound fractures

Suspect a compound fracture in a child if there is any overlying wound to the fracture.
• These fractures must be properly assessed by an orthopaedic surgeon.
• They require thorough surgical clean and anti-staphylococcal antibiotic.
• It is appropriate for these wounds to be cleaned and dressed.
• A Polaroid™ or digital picture may be taken of the wound to reduce multiple exposure of the wound.
• Be aware that children may lose a large amount of blood from these injuries. Haemodynamic monitoring is therefore essential.

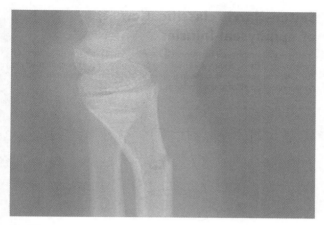

Fig. 4.9 X-ray of a greenstick fracture.

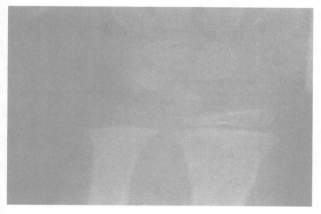

Fig. 4.10 X-ray of a buckle fracture.

Salter–Harris classification of epiphyseal injuries

Epiphyseal/metaphyseal fractures (➔ see Fig. 4.11) are fractures through the growth plate or epiphysis. These can be of particular importance, as any disruption of the growth plate in a growing child can have serious implications. Follow up all of these fractures.

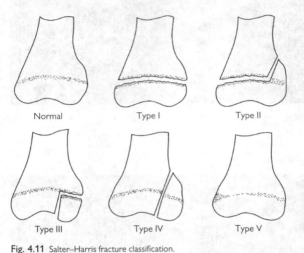

Normal　　　Type I　　　Type II

Type III　　　Type IV　　　Type V

Fig. 4.11 Salter–Harris fracture classification.
(Reproduced with permission from Wyatt, J. et al. (2012). *Oxford Handbook of Emergency Medicine*, 4th edn, fig 15.19, p. 719. Oxford University Press, Oxford.)

Table 4.7 Common fracture sites related to age

Toddler	Distal tibia Distal radius Clavicle	Clavicle fracture common in children that fall down stairs
School age	Clavicle, proximal humerus, supracondylar, radius/ulna, phalanges, midshaft femur	
Teenager	Epiphysis fracture, distal humerus, proximal humerus, clavicle, midshaft radius and ulna, distal radius and ulna, fifth metacarpal, midshaft tibia and fibula, distal tibial epiphysis	

Upper limb fractures

Clavicle fractures

Most clavicle fractures in children can be treated conservatively. Often they only require simple analgesia, an arm sling, and review in a fracture clinic. Occasionally, when there is severe angulation or tenting of the skin, orthopaedic intervention may be required.

Shoulder injuries

Dislocation of the shoulder in children is extremely rare and often requires a great deal of force. However, some children have some degree of laxity within their rotator cuff and dislocate reasonably easily. As in adults, anterior dislocation is commoner than posterior.

- Give children with a dislocated shoulder analgesia, and encourage them to relax.
- Numerous techniques are available for the reduction of dislocated shoulders; you are advised to follow local guidance and practised techniques.
- There is evidence to suggest that immobilization of the limb in a collar and cuff for 3wk is beneficial.
- Refer the patient to the orthopaedic outpatient clinic for follow-up.

Humeral shaft fractures

- Assess the integrity of the radial nerve. If any deficit or displacement is found, refer the child to the orthopaedic team.
- If the fracture is minimally displaced and there is no neurological deficit, place in a collar and cuff, and refer to the fracture clinic.
- Be suspicious of all spiral fractures in children, and investigate for NAI.

Elbow injuries

Supracondylar humeral fracture

This is a relatively common fracture in children, often resulting from a fall on to an outstretched hand. The child normally presents holding the arm rested on their abdomen, with a swollen and tender elbow.

- Assess the neurovascular status of the limb. The integrity of the radial and median nerves, as well as of the brachial artery, must be given special consideration. Maintain frequent monitoring of the radial pulse.
- On initial assessment, administer analgesia; place the child in a comfortable position, and request an X-ray.

Management

- Refer patients for manipulation under anaesthetic (MUA) immediately if:
  - neurovascular deficit is present;
  - >50% displacement;
  - >20° angulation of the distal part posteriorly;
  - >10° medial or lateral angulation.
- Admit patients with a large amount of swelling and pain for analgesia and observation.

- If there is no swelling or angulation, give the child analgesia; place in a collar and cuff, and refer to the next fracture clinic.
  - The arm must be placed at 90° in the collar and cuff and kept inside the clothes.
- If the elbow is very painful, use an above-elbow back slab for immobilization.
- Angulation of the elbow: seek senior advice.

Lateral epicondylar epiphyseal injuries Often require orthopaedic intervention. Always seek advice, if unsure. Children require analgesia and careful positioning. Always assess the neurovascular status. If the fracture is undisplaced, treat in an above-elbow back slab, and collar and cuff at 90°; ensure analgesia is given, and arrange fracture clinic for the next day.

Medial epicondylar epiphyseal injury Treat in a collar and cuff at 90°, with analgesia and fracture clinic follow-up. Seek orthopaedic opinion if any suggestion of ulnar nerve involvement or excessive displacement of the fracture site.

Elbow injury without obvious fracture Children sometimes present with no obvious fracture on the X-ray, but with fat pad signs of injury, i.e. a raised anterior fat pad and the presence of a posterior fat pad (effusion into the elbow joint). Treat in a collar and cuff; give analgesia, and follow up in the fracture clinic.

Radial head fractures Treat in a collar and cuff or broad arm sling; give analgesia, and follow up in the fracture clinic. If significant angulation, seek orthopaedic opinion.

Subluxation of the radial head/pulled elbow Often results from a sudden pulling of the forearm and only occurs in children <4y. The child presents holding the affected arm on one side and not using it. If a good history of a pull and no trauma, no X-ray is necessary. Reduce by flexing the arm to 90°, and then place gentle traction onto the forearm, supinating the limb at the same time. Often a subtle click is felt when it has been successfully reduced. The child will start using the arm again after 10–20min.

Radial/ulnar shaft fractures Children often present with significant deformity or angulation to their forearm. These children require immediate assessment and analgesia.
- Place the child in a comfortable position, and refer to X-ray.
- Refer these children to an orthopaedic surgeon.
- Always ensure that X-rays are taken of the whole forearm, so as not to miss Monteggia and Galeazzi fractures.

Distal radius and ulna fractures
Fractures of the distal radius and ulna are relatively common in children. They are characterized by pain, swelling, and deformity. Often you can feel the haematoma.
- Give the child analgesia and a broad arm sling before sending them to X-ray.
- Treat simple torus/buckle fractures using a torus splint or plaster of Paris (POP) back slab. Follow-up should be arranged as per local

guidelines. The nurse should discuss analgesia with the parents and point out that the fracture site often takes at least 2–4wk to heal.
- In fractures where there is moderate or severe displacement, seek a senior opinion.
- If the wrist is clinically deformed, the child may require an MUA.

Scaphoid fractures

Rare in children under the age of 12; this is because the bone only calcifies after the age of 8. A scaphoid fracture should be suspected in children who have fallen on to outstretched hands and are tender over the anatomical snuffbox. Treat these patients according to the adult protocol (➔ see Wrist injuries, pp. 304–5).

Hand injuries Treat as per adult protocols (➔ see Hand injuries, pp. 306–8).

Lower limb injuries

Hip injuries
(➋ See The limping child, pp. 134–5.)

Femoral shaft fractures
Femoral shaft fractures in children are relatively common and are usually the result of a motor vehicle accident. Be mindful that a significant force is needed to fracture a femur, so it is important to assess the child for other injuries. Children can lose up to 40% of the circulating blood volume from the fracture site and thus require a full assessment and ongoing observation.
- If the child is cardiovascularly unstable, give 10mL/kg of normal saline and re-evaluate.
- Ensure analgesia, either intranasal diamorphine or IV morphine, is given as prescribed. A femoral nerve block may also be considered.
- Place the child in a traction splint as soon as possible.
- Seek orthopaedic opinion without delay.

Knee injuries
- Most knee injuries in children are due to twisting, whilst playing sport, and often consist of a sprain.
- Serious ligamentous injury is rare, due to the laxity of children's ligaments.
- Serious fractures in the knee are very rare, but tibial plateau fractures can occur. Refer all fractures within the knee to the orthopaedic team.
- Otherwise, treat knee injuries with a knee brace, crutches, analgesia, and physiotherapy.

Dislocated patella
A reasonably common presentation, especially in teenage girls. The knee will be held in flexion with lateral displacement of the patella, and the patient will be in a great deal of pain.
- Reduction is usually achieved using Entonox®.
- Occasionally IV sedation and analgesia are required (➋ see Knee injuries, pp. 314–16).
- Once the knee has been reduced, obtain an X-ray, and immobilize the knee in a knee brace or cylinder POP. Arrange orthopaedic follow-up.

Tibial shaft fractures
Treat all tibial shaft fractures, as you would those in an adult. Always be aware of the potential for compartment syndrome. If you are at all concerned, seek a senior opinion.
- These children need analgesia, an above-knee back slab, and regular neurovascular observations.
- Compound fractures should be treated with IV antibiotics.
- Displaced or angulated fractures require orthopaedic intervention, often an MUA.

Toddler fractures

These fractures are seen in children <4y, usually caused by a twisting injury and associated with learning to walk. Often the child presents with a reluctance to place their foot on the floor. On examination, there is often no swelling or bruising. However, when the foot is twisted, pain is elicited.

- An X-ray should be taken. These can be difficult to interpret, as the fracture can be very subtle.
- If at all concerned, refer for a senior opinion.
- Place the child in a below-knee back slab; give analgesia, and refer for an orthopaedic appointment.

Ankle injuries

- Treat ankle injuries as in an adult: analgesia, ice, elevation, and rest. A recent study suggests that the Ottawa ankle rules are valid in children >8y.
- Avulsion Salter–Harris 1 fractures of the distal tibia or fibula may be diagnosed. Give these children a below-knee back slab, analgesia, and crutches, and arrange follow-up.
- Nurses must ensure that good advice is given on using crutches, as children often find them difficult to use.
- Be aware that, in older children, venous thromboembolism (VTE) guidance must be followed.

Foot injuries Treat as for those in an adult (➲ see Calcaneal fractures, p. 327).

The limping child

This is one of the commonest reasons for children to attend the ED. For many, the causes are obvious from the history, e.g. sprained ankle, FB in the foot, broken toe, etc. For others, the cause is less obvious, because:
- the child is too young to say where it hurts;
- the child is too young to say what happened and no one witnessed it, e.g. an accident;
- poor localization of pain, e.g. hip/thigh/knee;
- pain may be referred from elsewhere, e.g. young children will often complain of knee pain when their hip is the problem.

Toddlers will often continue to limp and play on a tibia that has sustained a greenstick or hairline fracture (toddler fracture). There is often no definable swelling or bruising and apparently no tenderness—only a vague history of the toddler not using that limb or the limb being slightly warmer to touch.

Causes of limp in a child
- Trauma.
- Sepsis: septic arthritis.
- A bleed into a joint due to an underlying haematological problem.
- Perthe's disease.
- Slipped femoral epiphysis.
- Viral illness, including rubella.
- Bacterial infection, e.g. meningococcal disease.
- Allergy.
- Recent immunization.
- Rheumatological conditions.
- Leukaemia.

History and examination
In most of these cases, it is possible to localize the problem. Look for:
- visible signs, e.g. swelling, bruising, redness;
- the style of the limp;
- local warmth;
- muscle wasting or tenderness;
- pain on movement (but be careful that only one joint is moved).

Investigations
- X-rays only if able to identify where the problem may be.
- FBC, CRP, ESR if the child is systemically unwell or has a raised temperature.

Treatment
If you cannot make a diagnosis and the child is well, it may be appropriate to review the child the following day. By this time, the cause may be obvious, or the child may be getting better. Send the child home with appropriate analgesia and advice.

Perthe's disease is a degenerative disorder of the hip joint. It causes avascular necrosis of the upper femoral epiphysis. Mainly affects children aged 2–12y (majority 4–8y). Characterized by pain and limping. Interference with vascularity of the femoral head, but the cause of this is still unknown. X-ray appearances are of progressive irregularity, flattening, and ↑ density of the femoral head; also changes visible in the adjacent metaphysis. Detecting Perthe's is important to ensure the femoral head is correctly contained within the acetabulum, as it reforms with time. This is usually achieved with rest, analgesia, and regular follow-up by the orthopaedic surgeons. If Perthe's is suspected, refer to the orthopaedic team. Occasionally, surgical intervention is required.

Slipped upper femoral epiphysis (SUFE) occurs around puberty (8–15y). It is thought to be due to hormonal changes that weaken the epiphyseal plate. It may be gradual in onset (chronic) or sudden (acute), e.g. during a game of netball. Limp or pain predominates, depending on chronic or acute history. Pain is often experienced in the knee. Classically, the affected limb is short-ened and the hip is externally rotated, or attempts to flex the hip result in external rotation. Have a high index of suspicion in teenage girls and over-weight children. Detection of a slipped femoral epiphysis is important to allow pinning of the epiphysis before further slip occurs. Delay may result in a functionally worse joint position or in an ↑ risk of avascular necrosis of the femoral head. A frog lateral X-ray of the hips is therefore needed in 8–16y olds with hip pain. Examination of the contralateral hip is also important, as bilateral SUFE is not uncommon.

Irritable hip—transient synovitis, observation hip
- Infective, traumatic, and allergic causes have been suggested.
- Pain caused by inflammation of the synovial lining of the hip joint, leading to an effusion and distension of the capsule. Often bilateral, but one side may start a day or two before the other.
- Some children have a lot of pain and are comfortable only when lying down with the affected hip flexed to 30° or 40°. Others may be up and about, but limping a little.
- Recent or current URTIs are common associations. There may have been previous episodes or a family history of irritable hip.
- Look for associated systemic signs such as pyrexia, rash, lymphadenopathy, URTI, etc.

Investigation of the painful hip
- X-ray at presentation if: any significant trauma; any fixed deformity, shortening, or functional deformity; child >8y old (look for SUFE).
- FBC, ESR, and CRP if the child is systemically unwell, in severe pain, or, on examination, there are signs of infection.
- USS. Many consider this examination of choice. Seek senior opinion.

Management
- Ensure appropriate analgesia to children diagnosed with septic arthritis, hip fracture, Perthe's disease, or slipped femoral epiphysis. Refer to the orthopaedic team on call. Patients with septic arthritis must commence IV antibiotics as soon as possible.
- Manage children with transient synovitis with simple analgesia and rest. Arrange follow-up within 3 days to ensure they are recovering appropriately and other diagnoses have not been missed.

Surgical emergencies

The assessment of a child presenting to the ED with abdominal pain depends upon the clinician taking an accurate history and carrying out a detailed examination. Often the history given can be very confused and misleading. Clinical findings can mimic other disorders such as gastroenteritis. If unsure, always seek senior help.

- Consider appendicitis in all children presenting to the ED with abdominal pain until adequately ruled out.
- Treat any infant or child who presents with bile-stained vomit as a surgical emergency until proven otherwise.

General principles for management of surgical emergencies

- Administer adequate analgesia.
- Administer IV fluids if required.
- Consider taking bloods for U&E, FBC, amylase, and sending for C&S urine.
- Always check the child's blood sugar.
- NG tube insertion if bowel obstruction is suspected.
- Keep the child fasted, and seek senior surgical opinion.
- Carry out any specific treatments, depending on the condition and diagnosis.

Appendicitis

Appendicitis can occur at any age; however, it is very rare in infants. It occurs either when the appendix becomes obstructed or by lymphatic hyperplasia. Box 4.9 lists the general principles for detecting appendicitis.

- The clinical features associated with appendicitis are: mild fever, anorexia, nausea, vomiting, tachycardia, and right iliac fossa pain. Children <5y often present with atypical features, as they are unable to localize the pain.
- Diagnosis is usually made clinically. FBC and CRP may be useful to identify inflammatory markers. However, they can be poor prognostically and should not to be relied upon for diagnosis. Ultrasound can be very useful in diagnosis if carried out by a skilled practitioner. Where there is uncertainty about the diagnosis, the child should be seen by a senior clinician and admitted for observation. Usually the diagnosis becomes clear over time.

Box 4.9 Tips for not missing appendicitis

- Consider the diagnosis in every patient with an appendix and abdominal pain.
- Symptoms can progress rapidly over a few hours or slowly over days.
- Smaller children are unable to localize pain.
- Antibiotics may mask the signs.
- Appendicitis may mimic gastroenteritis.
- Overweight children mask it.
- Children with communication problems and learning difficulties are a high-risk group.
- If in doubt, get an ultrasound.

Management of a suspected appendicitis
- Regular examination.
- Regular analgesia.
- Regular observations of temperature and pulse.
- Chart intake/output.
- IV fluids (if required).
- Ultrasound can be useful in the diagnosis.
- Appendectomy, if required.

Intussusception

In intussusception, one segment of the bowel telescopes into another. Typically seen in children aged 6–12 months.
- Clinical features include vomiting, colicky abdominal pain, and redcurrant jelly stools. Often a sausage-shaped mass can be felt in the abdomen.
- Signs of severe obstruction and shock can develop over 24–48h. Often the child presents as very unwell.
- All children with a suspected intussusception must be referred to a paediatric surgical team for early management.

Pyloric stenosis

Pyloric stenosis is caused by hypertrophy of the pylorus muscle. It usually develops in the first 6wk of life.
- Clinical features include projectile vomiting after every feed, weight loss, dehydration, and a hungry cry. Often a walnut-shaped hard mass can be felt in the epigastric area.
- U&E may be helpful, as the prolonged vomiting will result in low serum K^+, Cl^-, and Na^+.
- Management includes the correction of any dehydration and electrolyte imbalance, and then surgery.

Volvulus is associated with the malrotation of the midgut. Infants present with signs of severe bowel obstruction, bile-stained vomiting, and shock. Refer these infants to the paediatric surgical team immediately for surgical management and resuscitation.

Torsion of the testicle The peak age range for presentation with testicular torsion is 15–30y. Clinical features include sudden-onset testicular pain, inability to walk upright, and nausea often associated with right iliac fossa pain. On examination, the testis is riding high, extremely tender, and non-mobile. Refer all patients with a suspected torsion of the testicle to the urology team immediately. Give analgesia as a supportive measure.

Paraphimosis The foreskin gets retracted, then, due to the swelling, it is unable to be replaced. Try to replace the foreskin using a lubrication gel; application of an ice pack can be useful prior to this procedure. Often application of direct pressure to the oedematous area can ease the replacement of the foreskin; this is often helped by a dose of Entonox®. If unable to replace manually, the patient may require operative release.

Ear and nose foreign bodies

➲ See Nasal foreign bodies, p. 483 and Ear (auricular) foreign bodies, p. 484.

Safeguarding children

There are national guidelines regarding the management of NAI, highlighting the need for health, police, and social services to work collaboratively together, both within the hospital and the community, in identifying and protecting children appropriately. There have been a number of reports that demonstrate failures in this process; therefore, it is vital that, if you suspect that a child has suffered from some form of abuse, your suspicions must be reported and acted upon.

Types of child abuse

- Physical abuse.
- Sexual abuse.
- Emotional abuse.
- Neglect.
- Fabricated illness.

Suspicion arising from history

Aspects of the history may alert the nurse/health-care professional to the possibility of child abuse:

- frequent attendances;
- delay in seeking health care;
- injuries inconsistent with developmental stages;
- injuries inconsistent with history;
- third party attendance;
- vague or poor history;
- changing, inconsistent history;
- abnormal parental attitudes;
- distant relationship between the child and parents;
- the child may disclose abuse;
- the child may be abnormally affectionate to strangers.

Physical signs of abuse

- Abnormal bruising.
- Torn frenulum of the upper lip.
- Multiple bruising of differing ages.
- Finger imprinting or wounds that may have been caused by a cigarette.
- Long bone fracture in children <3y, especially humerus and femur.
- Human bite marks.
- Petechiae associated with smothering.
- Scalds in the stocking/glove distribution.
- Perineal wounds or burns.
- Skull fractures.
- Subdural haematoma in an infant or toddler.
- Failure to put on weight.
- Unkempt and dirty (be careful—do not be too judgemental!).

Signs of sexual abuse

- Injuries to the genitalia or anus.
- Inappropriate sexual behaviour.
- Perineal discharge or bleeding.
- Behavioural disturbances, enuresis, encopresis.
- Disclosure of sexual abuse.

If abuse is suspected

Unless you are a specialist in safeguarding children, your role in suspected child abuse cases is restricted to the detection and referral of children who you suspect may have been abused. If you suspect a child or sibling under your care has been abused:

- Notify a senior early, preferably a consultant paediatrician with a remit for safeguarding children.
- Take a detailed history, including direct quotes. Include family and social history.
- Arrange for the child to be fully examined by a senior clinician; if necessary, a forensic physician should be involved to minimize the number of examinations.
- The child must be treated clinically, and all relevant investigations and treatments carried out.
- Child protection teams from the police and social services must be notified and involved in the child's care.
- Immediate protection for the child must be considered, and a place of safety organized and discussed.
- A Laming checklist must be completed and placed in the notes.

If the child is discharged after examination by the paediatrician, ensure the health visitor is aware of the child's attendance to the ED to ensure follow-up. If you still have concerns about the child being discharged, make these concerns known to a senior member of the team before the child leaves the department. The importance of valuing the views of all team members, however junior, as an essential factor in protecting the child was highlighted by the Laming Report.[7] Accurate record-keeping is essential. However, emergency treatment and clinical management of the presenting complaint should not be delayed.

Reference

7 Lord Laming (2003). Report of the Inquiry into the death of Victoria Climbié, London: Department of Health. Available at: ℞ https://www.gov.uk/government/uploads/system/uploads/attachment_data/file/273183/5730.pdf.

Self-harm

Self-harm among young people is becoming increasingly common. A survey of young people aged 15–16y estimated that >10% of girls and 3–5% of boys had self-harmed in the previous year. A wide range of mental health issues, such as depression, dependence on alcohol or drugs, borderline personality disorders, schizophrenia, and bipolar disorder, are associated with self-harm.

Self-harm refers to any act of self-poisoning or self-injury carried out by an individual, irrespective of the motive.

All young people who self-harm must be treated with dignity and compassion, and their needs catered for sensitively in a non-judgemental environment.

To improve the care given to young people who have self-harmed and to eradicate the stigma surrounding the vulnerable young people who self-harm, NICE guidance CG16 (2004) and CG133 (2011) have been published which have now become a quality standard to which all trusts must adhere.

- *Respect, understanding, and choice.* Young people who have self-harmed should be treated with the same care and respect as any other patient.
- *Staff training.* Staff caring for young people who self-harm should be trained to understand and care for their needs appropriately.
- *Activated charcoal.* Ambulance and ED services whose staff may be involved in the care of people who have self-harmed by poisoning should ensure that activated charcoal is immediately available to staff within the appropriate time frame.
- *Triage.* All people who have self-harmed should be offered a preliminary psychosocial assessment at triage (or at the initial assessment in primary or community settings), following an act of self-harm.
- *Environment.* If a person who has self-harmed has to wait for treatment, he or she should be offered an environment that is safe and supportive and minimizes any distress. For many patients, this may be a separate quiet room, with supervision and regular contact with a named member of staff to ensure safety.
- *Treatment.* People who have self-harmed should be offered treatment for the physical consequences of self-harm, regardless of their willingness to accept psychosocial assessment or psychiatric treatment.
  - Adequate anaesthesia and/or analgesia should be offered to people who have self-injured throughout the process of suturing or other painful treatments.
  - Staff should provide full information about the treatment options and make all efforts necessary to ensure that someone who has self-harmed can give, and has the opportunity to give, meaningful and informed consent before any and each procedure or treatment is initiated.
- *Assessment of needs.* All people who have self-harmed should be offered an assessment of needs, which should be comprehensive and include evaluation of the social, psychological, and motivational factors specific to the act of self-harm, current suicidal intent, and hopelessness, as well as a full mental health and social needs assessment.

- *Assessment of risk.* All people who have self-harmed should be assessed for risk. This assessment should include identification of the main clinical and demographic features known to be associated with risk of further self-harm and/or suicide, and identification of the key psychological characteristics associated with risk, in particular depression, hopelessness, and continuing suicidal intent.
- *Psychological, psychosocial, and pharmacological interventions.* Following psychosocial assessment for people who have self-harmed, the decision about referral for further treatment and help should be based upon a comprehensive psychiatric, psychological, and social assessment.

Further reading

British Psychological Society and Royal College of Psychiatrists (2004). *Self-harm. The short-term physical and psychological management and secondary prevention of self-harm in primary and secondary care.* National Clinical Practice Guideline Number 16. British Psychological Society, Leicester, and Royal College of Psychiatrists, London.

Obstetric emergencies

Overview

Pregnancy is a natural condition, but complications do arise, and pregnant patients may attend the ED with medical problems associated with pregnancy or with what the patient perceives as a problem related to pregnancy. Women may also attend in labour. It should be borne in mind that some patients suffering from trauma may also be pregnant.

Most emergency nurses are not qualified midwives. They should therefore always refer to specialist staff in the event of an obstetric emergency, and not undertake any procedure if they are not competent or qualified to do so. The role of the emergency nurse in obstetric terms is to maintain the safety of the mother and her unborn baby until expert help arrives, and also to identify pregnant patients who are vulnerable and potentially at risk. It is therefore important that nurses working in emergency care have a rudimentary knowledge of obstetrics, in order to ensure the safety of a pregnant patient and speedy access to specialist care.

This chapter will focus on the conditions of pregnancy that most frequently present as an emergency. It is also important that emergency nurses have an awareness of the patients who are most vulnerable in pregnancy due to either health or socio-economic reasons. The *Eighth Report of the Confidential Enquiries into Maternal Deaths* in the UK[1] shows that there has been a significant reduction in the overall maternal death rate, from 13.95 per 100 000 maternities in the previous triennium to 11.39 per 100 000 maternities in this 2006–2008 triennium.

However, the report also highlights that, whilst some clinical causes of maternal death, particularly thrombosis, have fallen sharply, new problems are emerging as major contributors to maternal mortality, namely obesity, sepsis, and the emergent threat from influenza A (H1N1/2009).

Those considered to be at risk include:
- socially disadvantaged, poor communities;
- some ethnic minorities;
- asylum seekers;
- black African women;
- women who booked late and whose attendance at antenatal clinics was poor;
- obese women;
- victims of domestic violence;
- substance abusers.

ED nurses are familiar with these vulnerable groups, but it is imperative that they are especially aware of the added vulnerability of pregnant women who are also socially disadvantaged. Ensuring optimum outcomes calls for collaborative working practices between health and social care agencies.

Reference

1 Centre for Maternal and Child Enquiries (CMACE) (2011). Saving Mothers' Lives: reviewing maternal deaths to make motherhood safer: 2006–08. The Eighth Report on Confidential Enquiries into Maternal Deaths in the United Kingdom. *BJOG* **118**(Suppl. 1), 1–203.

The pregnant patient

The physiological, anatomical, and biochemical changes that occur in pregnancy are both systemic and local. Most of these changes revert to normal 6wk after birth.

Cardiac output

- To provide the developing fetus and placenta with a greater blood flow, cardiac output (CO) ↑ in the first trimester of pregnancy by 30–50%. This remains elevated until about the 30th week, after which it may ↓ as the enlarging uterus obstructs the vena cava.
- CO causes an ↑ in HR from the normal 70bpm to 80–90bpm, whilst BP falls slightly.
- Circulating volume ↑ proportionally with CO, but the ↑ in plasma is greater initially than RBC mass. This may produce a dilutional anaemia until the 28th week, when the ↑ in RBCs matches the plasma volume ↑.
- WBCs ↑ from about 9000 to 12 000/microlitre.
- Clotting factors are altered during pregnancy. It is essential to understand this and respond with alacrity to patients presenting with more serious complications such as haemorrhage or clotting disorders. Changes in the coagulation and fibrinolytic systems occur in pregnancy. These changes include an ↑ in a number of clotting factors (I, II, VII, VIII, IX, and XII), a ↓ in protein S levels, and inhibition of fibrinolysis.
- As pregnancy progresses, the activity of activated protein C, an important anticoagulant, ↓. These physiological changes are important for minimizing intrapartum haemorrhage, but they also ↑ the risk of thromboembolism during pregnancy and the post-partum period.

Respiratory changes

Changes in lung function during pregnancy are attributed to the effects of progesterone and to pressure on the diaphragm from an enlarging uterus.
- Tidal volume (Vt), RR, plasma pH, and O_2 consumption ↑.
- The ↑ Vt causes a ↓ in plasma $PaCO_2$, but vital capacity and plasma PaO_2 remain unchanged.

Renal changes

- Glomerular filtration rate (GFR) ↑ by about 50% during pregnancy, although the volume of urine passed each day is not ↑.
- The renal plasma flow rate also ↑ by 25–50%.
- Glycosuria in pregnancy may be attributed to ↑ GFR and impaired reabsorption of filtered glucose. Although this may not be considered abnormal, ↑ glycosuria may predispose the pregnant woman to UTIs.
- Relaxation of ureters due to ↑ progesterone may lead to urinary stasis and subsequent infection.
- Proteinuria should not be present during pregnancy, so any significant rise in proteinuria should raise suspicion of a disease process.
- Pressure on the bladder from the enlarging uterus may cause frequency of micturition.

Gastrointestinal changes

- Gastric motility in pregnancy is reduced, due to the elevated levels of progesterone.
- Gastric reflux and heartburn are common, due to the slower emptying time of the stomach and the relaxation of the cardiac sphincter.
- Constipation is also common, due to compression of bowel segments and ↓ gastric motility.

Nursing assessment of the pregnant patient

Pregnant patients presenting with any health problem will understandably be anxious and need reassurance.

- From an emergency perspective, patients presenting in the first trimester are regarded as gynaecological patients and managed in the ED or in an early pregnancy unit.
- In most hospitals, patients who are >20wk pregnant are usually assessed in the labour ward, unless delivery is imminent and there is no time to transfer, or the patient's condition is too unstable for transfer.
- If childbirth is imminent and there is no time to transfer the patient, call the paediatrician, as well as the obstetrician. Inform the labour ward, and have a neonatal incubator/Resuscitaire® ready.

Remember that there are two lives to be considered. Do not delay in calling for specialist help.

History taking

History from a pregnant patient should include:

- last menstrual period (LMP);
- pregnancy test and result;
- number of times pregnant (gravida);
- first pregnancy (primigravida);
- number of viable births (para);
- method of delivery (vaginal or Caesarean);
- number of miscarriages and stillbirths (miscarriage is fetal death before 24wk gestation; stillbirth is fetal death after 24wk gestation).

Additional signs and symptoms that must be recorded include any history of the following.

Vaginal bleeding

Bleeding in the first trimester of pregnancy may suggest an ectopic pregnancy or a threatened miscarriage. In the second and third trimesters, it may be associated with placenta praevia, placental abruption, traumatic injury, or the onset of labour.

Abdominal pain

In the first trimester, abdominal pain may be associated with ectopic pregnancy, especially if the pain radiates to the shoulder. Cramping abdominal pain may also indicate miscarriage. Abdominal pain in the third trimester of pregnancy may be associated with placental abruption or impending labour. It is important to consider other causes of abdominal pain such as UTI, pelvic inflammatory disease (PID), or appendicitis.

Nausea and vomiting

Nausea and vomiting of varying severity is common (>50% in the first trimester). Persistent vomiting (hyperemesis gravidarum) can lead to dehydration and weight loss, with the patient needing urgent fluid replacement. This can also predispose the patient to greater risk of serious complications such as deep vein thrombosis (DVT).

Headaches, visual disturbance, or swelling in the limbs

These are features that may be associated with pre-eclampsia, which usually manifests after 20wk gestation. Signs of pre-eclampsia include oedema, proteinuria, and elevated BP.

Trauma

Any recent injury should be recorded. (Nurses should bear in mind that pregnant women are at ↑ risk of domestic violence.)

Fetal movements

A ↓ or change in the normal pattern of fetal movements may be a sign of fetal distress.

Other signs and symptoms

As with any other history taking, the patient's PMH, current medication, and any known allergies must be recorded.

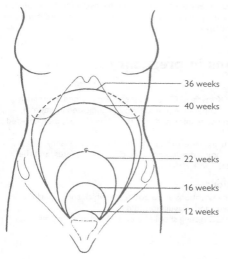

Fig. 5.1 Uterine size in pregnancy.

(Reproduced with permission from Wyatt, J. et al. (2012). *Oxford Handbook of Emergency Medicine*, 4th edn, fig 13.1, p. 577. Oxford University Press, Oxford.)

Physical assessment in pregnancy

Physical assessment
Physical assessment of the pregnant patient includes inspection, palpation, and auscultation.

Inspection
- Observe the colour and amount of vaginal loss, and inspect any clots or products that have been passed.
- Observe the external genitalia for any sign of imminent delivery such as crowning of the head.
- Observe for any cord protrusion from the vagina; this calls for immediate intervention.

In all cases of imminent childbirth, get expert help without delay.

Palpation
Palpate the abdomen for uterine size and position (➡ see Fig. 5.1).

Auscultation
Listen to the fetal heartbeat with a Doppler probe or a Pinard stethoscope. The fetal HR should be 110–160bpm. Where there is any anxiety about the well-being of the fetus or any uncertainty about hearing a fetal heartbeat, a midwife or obstetrician should be called without delay to ensure optimum care for mother and baby.

Investigations in pregnancy

Imaging
- As far as possible, X-rays and CT scans should be avoided in pregnancy. If an X-ray or CT is imperative (e.g. CT may be indicated in trauma), the radiographer must be informed, and the patient's abdomen covered with a lead apron.
- Ultrasound is useful for determining the location of pregnancy (intrauterine or ectopic), the size and well-being of the fetus, and the site of the placenta.

Other investigations
- The commonest investigations are blood tests, which should include FBC, group and save, and coagulation studies.
- Urinalysis and β-HCG testing should be performed in early pregnancy.

Nursing interventions

Recording of vital signs and monitoring

This should include BP, pulse rate, pulse oximetry, RR, blood sugar level, temperature, and fetal HR, where indicated. Urinalysis should also be performed. CBG levels should be recorded in patients who are diabetic and when gestational diabetes is suspected.

Care should be taken when interpreting observations, especially BP, as even slight ↑ may suggest pre-eclampsia. Refer, if possible, to a validated obstetric EWS.

Venous access

Establish venous access for fluid replacement as a priority, particularly if the patient is bleeding. Insert a wide-bore cannula, and infuse normal saline or Hartmann's solution, as prescribed. In cases of major haemorrhage, two wide-bore cannulae should be sited. Blood should be obtained at the same time for laboratory investigation. Ensure that samples are correctly labelled and sent to the laboratory as a matter of urgency.

Pain management

Ensure that the patient receives effective and timely analgesia. Entonox® (50% nitrous oxide, 50% O_2) can be safely administered to the pregnant patient. The medication prescribed will depend on the presenting condition. Always evaluate the effectiveness of the analgesia given.

Caution: Always check prescribed medications in the *BNF* for any pregnancy contraindication.

Pelvic examination

Prepare and assist with vaginal examination, ensuring privacy and dignity during the procedure, and subsequent comfort.

Psychological support

Unforeseen medical problems relating to a pregnancy are likely to cause fear and anxiety for the patient and her family. It is important for staff to understand and acknowledge such distress and offer support and empathy. As far as is reasonable, the patient's partner should be allowed to stay with her, and the nursing staff should involve them both in all decision-making.

Female genital mutilation

FGM (sometimes referred to as female circumcision) refers to procedures that intentionally alter or cause injury to the ♀ genital organs for non-medical reasons. This traditional practice is widespread in sub-Saharan Africa and parts of the Middle East, and, although illegal in the UK, it has been estimated that over 20 000 girls under the age of 15y are at risk of FGM in the UK each year, and that 66 000 women in the UK are living with the long-term consequences of FGM, which include complications in pregnancy and childbirth. These patients who are high-risk must be treated with empathy and compassion, and referred to midwifery and obstetric services without delay.

There has been greater recognition of FGM in recent years, and the Safeguarding Children Team must be informed of patients under 18y of age who are thought to be at risk.

Emergency delivery: labour

Childbirth is a natural event that is best managed by midwives and obstetricians. It is not uncommon, however, for a patient to present in the ED in advanced labour.

In such situations, it is vital to summon specialist help immediately.

Stages of labour

- The first stage of labour is characterized by the onset of regular painful contractions and dilatation of the cervix >3cm. There may be a 'show' (mucus and blood discharge from the vagina), or the membranes may have ruptured.
- The second stage extends from full dilatation of the cervix until the baby is born.
- The third stage extends from the birth of the baby and the delivery of the placenta until the retraction of the uterus.

Assessing the patient in labour

- Record maternal vital signs, particularly pulse and BP.
- Palpate the abdomen, and listen for fetal HR using a Doppler probe or Pinard stethoscope.
- Observe the rate of contractions.
- Check the perineum and vulva. If the head is crowning or the mother says she wants to push or says 'the baby is coming', summon help urgently (an obstetrician, paediatrician, or midwife), and prepare to assist delivery. Inform the labour ward, and arrange to have a neonatal incubator/Resuscitaire® ready.
- If there is time, transfer the patient to the labour ward.

Assisting delivery

(➔ See Fig. 5.2.)

The delivery process must be controlled to avoid trauma to the baby from a precipitate birth or tearing of the perineum.

- Sit the mother upright, and continue to reassure her and her partner (if present).
- Offer Entonox® as pain relief.
- Put on sterile gloves to assist delivery from the patient's right side.
- If the head is crowning, instruct the mother to pant and not bear down.
- As the head emerges, spread the fingers of the left hand over the baby's head, applying gentle pressure to prevent rapid expulsion of the head.
- The baby's head will then turn to the side, and their shoulders will rotate into an anterior/posterior position.
- Firmly, but gently, guide the head downwards, and deliver the anterior shoulder. Give oxytocin 10IU, as prescribed, with the birth of the anterior shoulder.
  - *Oxytocin must be prescribed and should not be given by an unqualified or inexperienced person. It is safer to give nothing, and keep the cord intact until expert help arrives.*
- Then guide the head upwards, and deliver the posterior shoulder.
- The rest of the baby will then deliver immediately.
- Dry and wrap the baby, and place them on the mother's abdomen or alongside her to facilitate skin-to-skin contact.

- Clamp the cord in two places, and cut between the clamps when the cord has stopped pulsating.
- Use a Hollister crushing clamp 1–2cm from the umbilicus.

Delivery of the placenta

- Soon after the infant is delivered, the uterus will contract again to detach and expel the placenta. The cord will lengthen, and there may be a gush of blood from the vagina.
- Apply gentle downward traction on the cord, whilst exerting upward pressure on the abdomen.
- Examine the placenta, and check that it is complete. Record the findings, and retain the placenta for further examination by a midwife or obstetrician or as per hospital protocol.

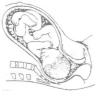

(1)
1st stage of labour. The cervix dilates. After full dilatation the head flexes further and descends further into the pelvis.

(2)
During the early second stage the head rotates at the level of the ischial spine so the occiput lies in the anterior part of pelvis. In late second stage the head broaches the vulval ring (crowning) and the perineum stretches over the head.

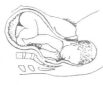

(3)
The head is born. The shoulders still lie transversely in the midpelvis.

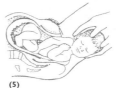

(4)
Birth of the anterior shoulder. The shoulders rotate to lie in the anteroposterior diameter of the pelvic outlet. The head rotates externally. Downward and backward traction of the head by the birth attendant aids delivery of the anterior shoulder.

(5)
Birth of the posterior shoulder is aided by lifting the head upwards whilst maintaining traction.

Fig. 5.2 Stages of labour.
(Reproduced with permission from Wyatt, J. et al. (2012). *Oxford Handbook of Emergency Medicine*, 4th edn, fig 13.2, p. 579. Oxford University Press, Oxford.)

Documenting the birth and post-natal nursing interventions

Documentation

- Record the exact time of birth.
- Calculate the American Pediatric Gross Assessment Record (APGAR) score.
- Ensure that both mother and baby have identity bracelets.
- The baby's identity bracelet should include:
  - the mother's name and hospital number;
  - the gender of the baby;
  - the date, time, and type of delivery;
  - the ward, and other information in accordance with local policy.
- Administer vitamin K orally or intramuscularly (IM) to the newborn, as prescribed.

APGAR score

This is an internationally recognized scoring system (➔ see Table 5.1) that is used to assess the condition of the infant. A score is given for each sign at 1min and 5min after birth. If there are problems with the baby, an additional score is given at 10min.

- A score of 7–10 is considered normal.
- A score of 4–7 may require some resuscitative measures.
- Babies with a score of ≤3 require immediate resuscitation.

Immediate post-natal nursing interventions

- Record vital signs, particularly pulse and BP.
- Encourage and assist the mother to breastfeed the infant.
- If indicated, prepare for repair of episiotomy.
- Assist the patient with washing, and make them comfortable.
- Ensure that the baby is wrapped up and kept warm. Transfer the mother and child to the post-natal ward.

Table 5.1 The APGAR scoring system

		Score		
		2	1	0
A	Activity (muscle tone)	Active movement	Arms and legs flexed	No movement; floppy tone
P	Pulse	Normal	<100	Absent
G	Grimace (reflex irritability)	Sneeze, cough, pulls away	Facial movement only; grimace	Absent; no response to stimulation
A	Appearance (skin colour)	Normal over entire body	Normal, except for extremities	Blue-grey, pale all over
R	Respiration	Normal rate and effort; crying	Slow, irregular	Absent; no breathing

Childbirth complications

It is expected that specialist help will be available for an emergency delivery in the ED, but, in the event of delivery taking place in another setting, such as a walk-in centre, it is important that nurses can respond in a safe and professional way.

Prolapsed cord

Prolapsed cord occurs after rupture of the membranes. It is associated with prematurity, malpresentation, fetal abnormality, and multiparity. Once the cord is out of the uterus, the fetal blood supply may become obstructed. Emergency Caesarean section is usually indicated.

- Whilst preparations are being made for the Caesarean delivery, the cord should be pushed back into the vagina and kept in place by a pack or, if necessary, by hand.
- Positioning the mother and raising the foot of the bed may help to further reduce cord compression.
- Supplemental O_2 should be given to the mother.

This is a serious complication, and under no circumstances should the patient be left alone.

Breech presentation

This occurs when the baby's legs or bottom present first. It is commoner with premature labour and is much riskier for the mother and baby.

Encourage the mother to pant, rather than push, and summon specialist help immediately.

Post-partum haemorrhage

Blood loss during childbirth is normally about 250–300mL. Greater loss than this is cause for concern. Post-partum haemorrhage may be due to retained placental tissue, laceration to the vagina or perineum, uterine atony, or inversion. These are all obstetric emergencies that must be managed by a specialist.

The nurse's role in these situations is as follows.
- Ensure IV access, and collect blood for cross-matching/transfusion.
- Commence IV infusion, as prescribed.
- Maintain meticulous recording of vital signs. Support the mother and her partner.
- Assist the obstetrician or midwife in controlling the bleeding.
- If the bleeding is due to a tear, apply a sterile dressing and direct pressure, whilst the obstetrician or midwife prepares to suture.
- If it is due to uterine atony, the nurse should massage the fundus of the uterus to stimulate a contraction, or encourage the mother to breastfeed her infant, as this will also stimulate contractions.
- If the bleeding is not quickly controlled, operative intervention in theatre may be indicated.
- Prepare the patient for theatre.

Vaginal bleeding in pregnancy

Vaginal bleeding in pregnancy is a common presentation in the ED. It is also very worrying for the patient and, in some cases, represents a serious threat to the well-being of the mother and baby. It is also important to remember that patients may present with vaginal bleeding and may either deny pregnancy or not be aware that they are pregnant. Early accurate assessment, intervention, and continuous monitoring are essential.

Causes of vaginal bleeding

Causes of bleeding relate to the gestational stage.

First trimester causes
- Spontaneous abortion (miscarriage).
- Ectopic pregnancy.
- Trophoblastic disease.

Second trimester causes
- Spontaneous abortion.
- Placenta praevia.
- Placental abruption.
- Trophoblastic disease.
- Cervical erosion, polyp, or malignancy.

Third trimester causes
- Placenta praevia.
- Placental abruption.
- Early labour 'show'.

Terminology

Spontaneous abortion

To the lay person, the term 'abortion' implies intention to terminate a pregnancy, and therefore seems an inappropriate and insensitive term to a patient who is experiencing a spontaneous abortion. 'Miscarriage' is a more acceptable and more widely understood term, and therefore more appropriate to use when caring for patients in the ED.

Miscarriage

This refers to loss of the pregnancy before 24wk gestation. There are several different types of miscarriage.
- Threatened abortion—vaginal bleeding, but the cervical os is closed. Pregnancy may be viable.
- Inevitable abortion—vaginal bleeding; the cervical os is open, and there is crampy abdominal pain. Pregnancy cannot continue.
- Incomplete abortion—the cervical os is open, and tissue is visible in the vagina. Pregnancy is not viable.
- Complete abortion—the cervical os is closed, and tissue has passed. Pregnancy has ended.

Missed abortion

The cervical os is open; no products have been passed, and the fetus is not viable. On rare occasions, patients may present in the ED long after fetal death and be unaware of what has happened.

Septic abortion

Infection may complicate abortion, once the cervix starts to dilate or instruments are introduced into the uterine cavity. Sepsis may follow spontaneous or surgical abortion, particularly an illegal abortion.

- There is vaginal bleeding and an offensive discharge.
- The cervical os is open. Tissue may have been passed or is in the cervix or vagina.
- Temperature is elevated, and BP is lowered.
- There is abdominal and vaginal tenderness on examination.
- The patient is generally very unwell.

Trophoblastic disease

This occurs when the fertilized ovum forms abnormal trophoblastic tissue but no fetus. The abnormality ranges from benign hydatidiform mole to invasive choriocarcinoma requiring chemotherapy.

Choriocarcinoma is a rare occurrence (1 in 50 000 pregnancies) but is nonetheless devastating for the patient. The patient may present with vaginal bleeding at 12–16wk gestation. They may also present with abdominal pain and hyperemesis gravidarum, which may be due to very high HCG levels. Diagnosis is by ultrasound and serum HCG measurement. These patients require very skilled psychological, as well as physical, care.

Patient assessment

Signs and symptoms will depend on the type of miscarriage. Assessment follows the principles outlined in this chapter (➋ see Physical assessment in pregnancy, p. 150; Investigations in pregnancy, p. 150). Treatment is directed at managing pain, controlling blood loss to prevent shock, and, in septic abortion, treating infection.

- Observe for signs of shock. Record vital signs, especially pulse, BP, RR, and temperature.
- Undress the patient, and assess blood loss (how long the patient has been bleeding, whether any clots have been passed, and how many pads are being used).
- Assess pain, and offer analgesia as prescribed.

Investigations

These include blood tests, FBC, coagulation studies, cross-matching, and USS. If septic abortion is suspected, blood cultures and vaginal swabs should be taken before commencing antibiotic therapy.

Nursing interventions

Ensure early assessment of the patient.

- Reassure and comfort the patient and her partner.
- Regularly record vital signs, fluid balance, and blood loss.
- Establish venous access using wide-bore cannulae if blood loss is moderate or severe.
- Send blood samples urgently for FBC, clotting screen, and group and save.
- Administer appropriate pain relief, and evaluate its effectiveness.
- Initiate infusion of normal saline or Hartmann's solution, as prescribed.

- Enquire about the need for anti-D Ig if the mother is rhesus (Rh)-negative and miscarriage has occurred or is inevitable.
- Assist with gynaecological examination. Keep the patient nil by mouth (NBM), in case emergency surgery is indicated.
- Accompany the patient to the scanning room. Prepare them for theatre, if this is indicated.

Do not leave the patient unattended or alone—they can deteriorate rapidly and will also be very anxious and frightened. Document all interventions.

Discharge

If miscarriage is threatened or complete, and the patient is allowed to go home from the ED, give follow-up advice.

- The patient should rest, avoid sexual intercourse, and use sanitary towels and not tampons.
- The patient should see her own doctor or return to the ED if the condition or bleeding does not settle, or if she develops crampy abdominal pain.

Sensitive disposal of fetal tissue and products of conception

In the event of miscarriage in the ED, fetal tissue and products of conception must be handled in a dignified and very sensitive manner.[2]

This is an extremely distressing event for the patient and her partner, and nurses need to be well informed about the correct procedures, so that they do not compound the distress. Be mindful that the patient may want to see and hold the fetus—this must be facilitated in a compassionate way.

No fetuses or fetal tissue should be disposed of as clinical waste. The fetus or products of conception should be placed in a container with a sealed watertight lid.

Ensure that a Certificate of Medical Practitioner or Midwife in Respect of Fetal Remains is completed, to include the following:

- name of patient;
- hospital number;
- date of delivery;
- gestational age;
- signature of the doctor who examines the products of the pregnancy.

Follow local policy.

Reference

2 Royal College of Nursing (2001). *Sensitive disposal of all fetal remains: guidance for nurses and midwives*. Royal College of Nursing, London.

Ectopic pregnancy

Ectopic pregnancy has ↑ in recent years to about 1 in 100 pregnancies. It occurs when the products of conception implant outside the uterine cavity, most commonly in the Fallopian tube. Risk factors include:
- previous history of salpingitis or PID;
- previous ectopic pregnancy;
- intrauterine contraceptive devices (IUCDs);
- abnormal tubal structure or tubal surgery;
- fertility treatment.

An ectopic pregnancy is a gynaecological emergency. Rupture will lead to profound hypovolaemic shock and can be fatal if not diagnosed and treated swiftly. Treatment is aimed at preventing shock, terminating the pregnancy, and preserving the Fallopian tube where possible.

If there is any suspicion of an ectopic pregnancy, close monitoring and early assessment by the gynaecologist are essential.

Patient assessment

Patients with an ectopic pregnancy may not be aware that they are pregnant or may deny pregnancy. For this reason, an ectopic pregnancy must always be considered as a possible diagnosis in any ♀ patient of childbearing age with abdominal pain or vaginal bleeding, or in young women who collapse for no obvious reason.

Presenting symptoms

These may include:
- abdominal pain;
- pain referred to the shoulder;
- possible vaginal bleeding (there may also be no bleeding);
- one or two missed menstrual periods;
- feeling dizzy, weak, or faint;
- diarrhoea and vomiting (atypical symptoms).

Signs
- Observe for signs of shock.
- Vaginal examination may be painful, and blood may be visible around the cervix.
- Positive pregnancy test.
- Pain in the abdomen may range from mild discomfort to severe pain with rebound tenderness and peritonism.

Investigations
- Recording and monitoring of vital signs, especially BP and pulse, are imperative from the time of arrival in the ED.
- Record CBG.
- Urinalysis is important to exclude urinary infection as a cause of abdominal pain.
- Pregnancy test is usually positive, but serum β-HCG may be below normal.

- Blood samples must be taken for FBC, coagulation studies, and group and save. Cross-match ~6 units of blood.
- A transvaginal USS is usually performed to confirm an ectopic pregnancy.

Nursing interventions

- Commence regular monitoring and documentation of vital signs.

Do not be lulled into a sense of false security by normal vital signs on initial assessment, although it is likely that the patient will have a tachycardia.

- *Remember that these patients are otherwise healthy young women who will initially compensate, despite shock, and then rapidly deteriorate.*
- Give O$_2$.
- Establish venous access as a priority, and obtain blood samples.
- Ensure that samples are sent to the laboratory without delay.
- Initiate infusion of normal saline or Hartmann's solution, as prescribed.
- Administer appropriate analgesia, as prescribed, and monitor the effects.
- Assist with pelvic examination.
- Prepare the patient for theatre.
- Give anti-D Ig, if prescribed.

Antepartum haemorrhage

Antepartum haemorrhage is bleeding from the genital tract after the 24th week of pregnancy and before the birth. Causes include placental abruption and placenta praevia.

Placental abruption

Abruptio placentae is a premature separation of the placenta from the uterine wall before the delivery of the fetus. It usually occurs after 20wk gestation. Risk factors include multiparity, diabetes, smoking, pre-eclampsia, and trauma.

Fetal distress and death may occur, and maternal haemorrhage may lead to disseminated intravascular coagulation (DIC).

Placenta praevia

Placenta praevia occurs when the placenta is implanted low in the uterus, either partially or completely covering the os. The patient may present during the second or third trimester with fresh painless vaginal bleeding. As the uterus grows, the placenta praevia may move upwards away from the cervix, and bleeding ceases. If this does not happen, bleeding will ↑ in the third trimester, particularly when the cervix begins to dilate in labour. If placenta praevia is suspected, a vaginal examination with a speculum should be avoided.

Nursing interventions

Antepartum haemorrhage is an obstetric emergency that threatens the well-being of the mother and baby. It is a terrifying experience for the patient and their partner. It is therefore essential that the emergency nurse (who may be the first person to assess the patient) acts swiftly, whilst also maintaining a sense of calm.

- Call for an obstetrician and paediatrician immediately.
- Commence regular monitoring and documentation of vital signs.
- Monitor fetal HR.
- Give O_2.
- Establish venous access as a priority, using wide-bore cannulae, and obtain blood samples for FBC, U&E, glucose levels, clotting screen, group and save, cross-match, and Rh and antibody status.
- Ensure that samples are sent to the laboratory without delay.
- Initiate infusion of normal saline or Hartmann's solution, as prescribed.
- Administer appropriate analgesia, as prescribed, and monitor the effects.
- Prepare the patient for an emergency Caesarean section.

Other causes of abdominal pain in pregnancy

Any abdominal pain may be a chance happening and unrelated to pregnancy, but nonetheless it is very frightening for the patient. It is therefore advisable to involve the obstetrician from the outset.

Urinary tract infection

The main causes are stasis of the urine and ↑ susceptibility to ascending infection.

Gallstones

Biliary colic may present for the first time in pregnancy. Treatment is usually conservative.

Appendicitis

In early pregnancy, appendicitis may be difficult to differentiate from an ectopic pregnancy. In later pregnancy, the pain may be located in the right hypochondrium.

Assessment

Nurses should follow the same assessment guidelines as for pregnant patients, being mindful that there are two lives to be considered.
- Call for specialist help early on.
- Referral to the surgeons, as well as the obstetrician, may be indicated.
- Check that any prescribed medications are not contraindicated in pregnancy.

Medical problems in pregnancy

Pregnancy will affect established, and otherwise stable, diabetes and may also precipitate impaired glucose tolerance in non-diabetic patients. Hyperglycaemia is a common presentation in pregnancy. Diabetic patients often find their condition more difficult to manage, as their insulin requirement ↑, and DKA may occur more frequently. Early collaboration between the physician and obstetrician is essential for optimum outcomes.

It is good practice to record a CBG reading on any patient presenting in the second or third trimester of pregnancy, and at any stage in established diabetic patients.

Pre-eclampsia and eclampsia

Pre-eclampsia is a disease of the second half of pregnancy. It is characterized by proteinuria, hypertension, and oedema. It occurs in 7% of primigravid pregnancies. In previously well patients, it is regarded as 'primary' pre-eclampsia. In patients with pre-existing hypertension or renal disease, it is regarded as secondary pre-eclampsia.

- Pre-eclampsia is diagnosed when the patient exhibits two or more of the following:
  - hypertension (BP >140/90mmHg);
  - proteinuria;
  - oedema.
- Pre-eclampsia causes an alteration in the placental circulation that may adversely affect the fetus.
- Risk factors for pre-eclampsia include diabetes, multiple pregnancies, pre-existing renal disease, and substance misuse.

Eclampsia and HELLP syndrome

Pre-eclampsia is a disease of signs but no symptoms. If it is not detected, it can escalate to eclampsia, which is an obstetric emergency where the patient may complain of the following:

- headache;
- visual disturbance;
- abdominal pain.

The patient may appear restless, agitated, or hyper-reflexive. Other symptoms include:

- raised BP;
- tremor;
- confusion;
- an epileptic-type seizure may occur.

A related variant of pre-eclampsia is HELLP syndrome (haemolysis, elevated liver enzymes, and low platelet count). Immediate treatment is crucial to prevent DIC. Eclampsia and HELLP, although relatively rare (incidence of <1 in 1000), are dangerous complications of pregnancy.

- Maternal mortality from eclampsia is 2%.
- Perinatal mortality is 15%.
- *Nurses must be aware of these signs and symptoms in a pregnant patient, and summon help urgently.*

Vomiting in pregnancy

Nausea and vomiting are common in pregnancy, affecting around 70–85% of pregnant women. Initial management should be conservative and may include reassurance, dietary recommendations, and support. Alternative therapies may include acupressure and hypnosis.

Hyperemesis gravidarum, or pernicious vomiting of pregnancy, is a rarer complication of pregnancy that is characterized by:
- continuous severe nausea and retching;
- dehydration caused by vomiting;
- weight loss;
- ketosis;
- hypotension;
- a risk of DVT due to dehydration.

These patients will require IV fluid resuscitation and admission to provide symptomic relief and correct electrolyte imbalances, as untreated hyperemesis can have adverse effects on the fetus.

Asthma in pregnancy

Asthma is a serious health problem worldwide, and it is the commonest chronic condition in pregnancy. The RR and vital capacity do not change in pregnancy, but the Vt, minute ventilation (40%), and minute O_2 uptake (20%) ↑, with a resultant ↓ in functional residual capacity and residual volume of air, due to the elevated diaphragm. In addition, airway conductance is ↑, and total pulmonary resistance is reduced, possibly due to the influence of progesterone.

A hyperventilatory picture is normal in the latter half of pregnancy, so a normal pCO_2 in a pregnant patient may be a sign of distress and impending respiratory failure. Nurses must be aware that changes in respiratory status occur more rapidly in pregnant patients than in those who are not pregnant.

ABG results often show a ↓ in PaO_2. The physiological changes that occur in the pulmonary system during pregnancy slightly alter normal ABG values, such that pH is 7.4–7.45, pO_2 is 95–105mmHg, pCO_2 is 28–32mmHg, and HCO_3^- is 18–31mEq/L.

Almost all anti-asthma drugs are safe to use in pregnancy and during breastfeeding. In fact, under-treatment of the pregnant patient is a frequent occurrence, because these patients are worried about the effects of medication on the fetus.

β-adrenergic agonists remain the mainstay of treating exacerbations and handling mild forms of asthma. For moderate to persistent asthma, a β-adrenergic agonist, combined with an inhaled anti-inflammatory agent or inhaled corticosteroid, is recommended for treatment. In severe asthma, oral corticosteroids and β-agonists are recommended.

Corticosteroids can be used in the acute phase and have been shown to be relatively safe in pregnancy. The IV, IM, and oral preparations can be used for acute exacerbations, whereas the inhaled preparations are reserved for outpatient maintenance therapy.

Carpal tunnel syndrome in pregnancy

Carpal tunnel syndrome (CTS) is a relatively common condition that causes pain, numbness, and a tingling sensation in the hands, especially the fingers. It is a common condition in pregnancy, affecting up to 50% of pregnant women. It is caused by compression of the median nerve that controls sensation and movement in the hands. Fluid retention during pregnancy can narrow the carpal tunnel, putting pressure on the nerves, which causes pain or numbness in the fingers. Symptoms include:

- numbness in the hands;
- tingling and pain in the thumb and fingers of one or both hands, usually worse at night;
- occasionally, there is reduced manual dexterity.

Treatment is usually aimed at giving reassurance and relieving the symptoms. Paracetamol may reduce the symptoms, and a wrist splint used at night can also help to alleviate the symptoms.

Overdose in pregnancy

The use of alcohol, cigarettes, and street drugs (e.g. cocaine, marijuana, heroin) is considered unsafe during pregnancy.

The physiological changes that occur during pregnancy alter drug metabolism, making some drugs even more harmful. The growing fetus is unable to metabolize drugs and cannot eliminate them effectively, which can result in permanent damage. Mothers who are substance abusers are more likely to overdose and are also more susceptible to certain diseases, especially if they share needles. In addition, they are more vulnerable to domestic violence and accidents. ED nurses need to be aware of the risks for these patients and ensure that they are referred appropriately to both obstetric and mental health services.

Paracetamol overdose

Paracetamol is the most commonly used substance in self-poisoning in the UK. Paracetamol overdose during pregnancy should be treated with either oral or IV acetylcysteine. This should be started within 10h after ingestion, in order to prevent maternal, and potentially fetal, toxicity. Paracetamol overdose does not appear to ↑ the risk of adverse pregnancy outcome, unless there is severe maternal toxicity.

Iron overdose

Acute iron toxicity in pregnancy is a medical emergency, and maternal resuscitation must be the 1° objective. High maternal serum iron loads do not affect the developing fetus but can result in maternal multisystem organ failure, which can lead to spontaneous abortion, preterm delivery, or even maternal death.

Treatment may include whole-bowel irrigation using polyethylene glycol electrolyte lavage, desferrioxamine treatment, and supportive care. Desferrioxamine is not thought to cross the placental barrier and is therefore considered to be safe for use during pregnancy.

Neurological emergencies

Overview

Altered consciousness and coma are common reasons for presentation to the ED. Coma (which is derived from the Greek word for deep sleep) is defined as a prolonged period of unconsciousness. This is an acute life-threatening situation, and early recognition and *rapid intervention by nursing and medical staff is* essential, in order to prevent or minimize further neurological damage. Active resuscitation may be indicated, in order to maintain and support the cardiovascular and respiratory systems. Coma is caused by bilateral hemisphere damage, failure of the reticular activating system, or both.

An impaired level of consciousness may be due to:

- haemorrhage or structural lesions that compromise the CNS (e.g. stroke, subdural or subarachnoid haemorrhage, fits, infection, or space-occupying lesions (tumours));
- ↓ supply of O_2 or glucose to the brain (e.g. hypoxia due to respiratory conditions, hypoglycaemia as a symptom of diabetes);
- ingestion of, or exposure to, substances that adversely affect the CNS such as drugs or alcohol (increasingly common);
- psychogenic causes such as psychiatric disorders (very rare).

Some knowledge of functional anatomy will aid the nurse in making an informed assessment.

- Lesions in the left hemisphere of the brain will cause right sensory and motor deficits.
- Lesions in the right hemisphere will produce left sensory and motor deficits.
- Occipital lobe injury will affect visual interpretation and interpretation of written language.
- Parietal lobe injury will affect sensation and recognition of body parts.
- Frontal lobe injury will affect personality, humour, motor movement, spatial awareness, and perceptual information.
- Temporal lobe injury will affect hearing, long-term memory, and understanding of speech and written language.

The role of intracranial pressure

The brain, spinal cord, and CSF are encased in a rigid bony enclosure. The volume of blood, CSF, and brain in the cranium must remain constant, in order to maintain a normal ICP of 7–15mmHg (Monro–Kellie hypothesis). Thus, any ↑ in volume due to swelling or a haematoma results in a rise in the ICP. As the ICP ↑, cerebral perfusion pressure ↓, as:

Cerebral perfusion pressure = mean arterial pressure − ICP

Once the cerebral perfusion pressure falls to below 70mmHg, significant 2° brain injury may occur. ↑ in the ICP leads to a reflex ↑ in systemic arterial BP and an associated bradycardia.

▶ It is imperative that nurses caring for patients with any neurological injury understand this process.

Neurological assessment

The assessment of a patient with an actual or potential neurological deficit should follow the same format, irrespective of the cause. The aim of assessment is to:
- establish baseline vital signs;
- identify any deviations from the baseline;
- recognize significant neurological changes.

A quick and simple tool for use in initial assessment is AVPU:
- *A*lert;
- responsive to *V*oice;
- responsive only to *P*ain;
- *U*nresponsive.

▶ Any patient who is not alert on AVPU assessment requires senior intervention.

History taking

In cases of altered level of consciousness, a history obtained from the patient can be unreliable. A history is more likely to be obtained from a family member, friend, carer, or paramedic. In most emergency situations, history taking and initial management occur simultaneously. Where a history can be obtained, questions must be asked about any trauma, any exposure to environmental hazards, and chemical or substance misuse, as well as routine questions about the PC and PMH. It is important to establish whether there is any history of seizures or psychiatric illness.

Physical examination

This should focus on determining the depth of coma or any obvious signs that may give a clue to the cause of altered consciousness.

Evaluate the patient using the GCS to assess the level of consciousness (➔ see Table 6.1). When assessing the patient, record best motor, best verbal, etc. Record as, for example, E4, V5, M6 = 15.

⚠ Tracheotomy/intubation or oral/facial injuries invalidate verbal assessment.

Coma is defined as GCS of E2, M4, V2, or less.

The British Society of Rehabilitation Medicine defines the scale of head injuries as follows:
- mild—GCS score of 13–15;
- moderate—GCS score of 9–12;
- severe—GCS score of <9.

Pupillary response

Assess pupil size and reaction to light. If pupils are equal and reacting to light and accommodation, record this as 'PERLA'.

Proper assessment of pupils requires a bright light. Ocular injury will affect pupillary responses, as will the use of miotic eye drops. Bear in mind that drugs, such as atropine and dopamine, also have an effect on pupillary reactions. Unequal pupils with a sluggish reaction may be due to compression of the oculomotor nerve (cranial nerve (CN) III) as a result of raised ICP. Pinpoint pupils may be caused by opiate overdose.

Eye movements

The presence of purposeful eye movements in a patient who is in every other respect unresponsive may indicate a psychogenic cause (e.g. catatonia or locked-in syndrome).

General observation and assessment

Observe for all of the following:
- Facial droop (CN XII), which may indicate a stroke.
- Look in the patient's ears. Any bleeding or leakage of CSF may indicate a fracture of the base of the skull.
- Periorbital bruising ('raccoon eyes') and bruising around the mastoid process (Battle's sign) may also be indications of a basilar skull fracture.
- Any palpable depression of the skull may indicate a depressed skull fracture.
- Observe skin colour and sensation. Clammy skin may indicate hypoglycaemia. Hot, dry skin may indicate fever.
- Observe for needle marks, which may indicate recent drug use.
- Observe for any sign of trauma or bruising to the face or skull. Look for any lacerations, and consider the need for tetanus prophylaxis.
- Incontinence is a common presentation in stroke or seizure.

- Check for the smell of alcohol, but never assume that a reduced GCS score is due to alcohol.
- Check for the smell of acetone, as this may indicate ketosis.

Palpation

Assess the patient's reflexes and motor responses.

- Note any abnormal motor activity, such as the Babinski reflex (the great toe moves upward, whilst the other toes curl downward when the sole of the foot is stimulated), indicating damage to the CNS.
- Unequal strength may occur in stroke. Flaccid responses and decerebrate movement (adduction, extension, and hyperpronation of the arms) or decorticate movement (flexion of the arms at the elbows, wrists, and fingers) indicate severe injury and a poor prognosis.

Table 6.1 Glasgow Coma Scale

	Score
Eye opening (E)	
Nil	E1
In response to pain	E2
In response to verbal cue	E3
Spontaneous	E4
Motor response (M)	
Nil	M1
Abnormal extension	M2
Abnormal flexion	M3
Weak flexion	M4
Localizing	M5
Obeys commands	M6
Verbal response (V)	
Nil	V1
Incomprehensible	V2
Inappropriate	V3
Confused	V4
Orientated fully	V5

Adapted from Teasdale, G. and Jennett, D.B. (1974). Assessment of coma and impaired consciousness. A practical scale. *Lancet* vol 304, issue 7872, 81–4 with permission.

Initial nursing interventions

Airway and breathing

- Establish and protect the airway.
- Airway adjuncts or intubation may be necessary.
- If the GCS score is <8, the patient will require intubation.
- Intubated patients will require capnography (➔ see Capnography, p. 670).
- Gently suction to remove any secretions, and remove dentures.
- If the patient's gag reflex is reduced or absent, they will require intubation.

▶▶ Call for the anaesthetist.

- If there is any suggestion of trauma, immobilize the C-spine. Remember that up to 10% of patients with a head injury also have an associated neck injury.
- Once the airway has been secured, administer high-flow O_2.

▶ Remember that inadequate resuscitation may lead to the development of a 2° brain injury.

Circulation

- Establish venous access using a wide-bore cannula, and collect blood samples for FBC, group and save, U&E, coagulation studies, toxicology screening, and, if appropriate, prescribed medication screening.
- CBG levels should be determined on arrival in the ED, and corrected accordingly.
- Attach the patient to a monitor, and commence meticulous recordings of vital signs.
- Record a 12-lead ECG.
- If the patient is hypotensive, give IV fluids as prescribed.
  - ▶ Be careful, as fluid overload can exacerbate cerebral oedema. However, this has to be balanced against the need to maintain adequate cerebral perfusion pressure.
  - A urinary catheter may be necessary to ensure accurate monitoring of fluid balance.
- A gastric tube may be indicated to empty the stomach, but the nasal route is contraindicated if there is any suggestion of facial or base of skull fractures.

⚠ Do not underestimate the potential for massive haemorrhage (some of which may not be immediately obvious) from a scalp laceration.

Neurological monitoring

Record the GCS score, and ensure that the neurological status is frequently reassessed. Meticulous monitoring and frequent reassessment are vital for detecting any further deterioration in conscious level (➲ see Table 6.1 on the Glasgow Coma Scale, p. 177).

▶ Remember that changes in the GCS score may be more significant than the overall score. If the GCS score is <8, the patient requires intubation.

Investigations

- Blood tests.
  - Immediate checking of blood glucose levels when the patient arrives in the ED is imperative.
  - Other blood tests, such as FBC, U&E, cross-matching, and clotting screen, will be required if the patient is on anticoagulant therapy or is perceived as vulnerable to bleeding (e.g. due to excessive alcohol consumption).
  - Blood cultures should be considered if the patient is pyrexial.
- In line with NICE guidelines, traditional X-rays are now increasingly being replaced by CT scanning (for guidelines relating to head injuries in children, ➲ see Chapter 4).
- CT scanning is used to identify brain injury, especially conditions, such as haematomas, that may be responsive to surgical intervention and treatment.
- In a patient with a ↓ conscious level, localizing neurological signs, or papilloedema, a CT scan should precede lumbar puncture. Lumbar puncture may be performed where there is suspicion of infection of the CSF (e.g. in meningitis) and to conclusively rule out subarachnoid haemorrhage following a negative CT, but this procedure should take place on the ward.

Skull fractures

The brain is well protected by the skull, CSF, and meninges, and it takes a significant trauma to cause a skull fracture and cerebral contusion. Skull fractures are usually classified as linear, depressed, or base of skull.

- A linear skull fracture is a simple fracture that may be seen in the occipital, temporal–parietal, or midline areas of the skull. These fractures are caused by a significant trauma to the skull and may cause an underlying haematoma.
- A depressed skull fracture is more complicated and may be associated with a scalp laceration. The depressed segment may be evident on examination, and neurosurgical intervention may be required to elevate the segment to prevent further damage to neural tissue.
- A fracture of the basilar bone of the skull occurs in the floor of the skull. Fractures in this bone can cause tears in the sac compartments that hold the brain, resulting in leakage of CSF and thus exposing the cranial vault to the outside environment and potential infection. Prophylactic antibiotics may be considered.

Signs of a basilar skull fracture may include:
- eye bruising ('raccoon eyes');
- bruising around the mastoid process (Battle's sign);
- blood in the ear canals or behind the tympanic membrane (TM).

Patients may complain of:
- visual disturbance;
- facial muscle weakness;
- loss of hearing;
- balance problems;
- altered facial sensation;
- loss of sense of smell;
- nasal drip caused by leaking CSF.

Complications of head injury

Intracranial haematoma

- Deteriorating level of consciousness after a head injury may be due to an intracranial haematoma.
- Accurate observation and monitoring are essential for identifying such developments early on, as surgical intervention may be lifesaving.
- ↑ agitation or confusion, increasingly severe headache, or persistent vomiting require reassessment by a senior clinician.
- ⚠ Patients on anticoagulants or those with bleeding disorders are at ↑ risk of developing an intracranial haematoma after a head injury.

Extradural haematoma

Extradural haematoma results from rupture of one of the meningeal arteries that run between the dura and the skull. The commonest cause is a linear fracture of the temporal–parietal bone, with associated injury to the middle meningeal artery.

Injury to, or laceration of, this artery may result in a rapidly expanding haematoma that, if not evacuated, may be fatal. These patients may be difficult to assess, as the initial injury will often be relatively minor. More than 50% of cases occur in people under 20y of age. The patient may report a period of unconsciousness, followed by full coherence, and there may be a subsequent ↓ in GCS score.

Signs and symptoms will be due to rising ICP. The nurse's role in caring for these patients is accurate neurological assessment and consistent monitoring.

Subdural haematoma

A subdural haematoma is a blood clot that forms beneath the dura mater. This type of venous bleed is usually caused by trauma such as a fall, an assault, or the acceleration–deceleration patterns associated with a road traffic accident.

There are two main types of subdural haematoma:

- acute—develops within 24h of the initial trauma and is associated with severe brain insult;
- chronic—develops over a period of several days after the initial trauma and often occurs in the elderly or in alcoholics. The patient may present with a fluctuating level of consciousness, and there may be a vague (or sometimes no) history of trauma.

A poor prognosis is likely if the subdural haematoma is bilateral, if it accumulates rapidly, or if there is a delay of >4h in achieving definitive neurosurgical management.

Diffuse axonal injury

This is a severe brain injury, often caused by rapid deceleration, and it is the commonest cause of coma and subsequent disability. Patients with diffuse axonal injury are often in a deep coma immediately after injury, despite an initially normal ICP and normal CT scan.

Minor head injury

⚠ Never assume that a patient is drunk or attribute a ↓ GCS score to alcohol alone. Always consider other possible causes.

Most patients who present with a minor head injury can be safely discharged from the ED. However, assessment of these patients is far from straightforward, and caution should be exercised if the patient is elderly or epileptic, or there is a history of substance or alcohol misuse.[1] Although these patients may not have a severe head injury, it is important to obtain a clear history, especially any history of unconsciousness, and to assess the GCS score.

- Patients with significant neurological symptoms (e.g. vomiting, dizziness, visual disturbance, severe headache) or a history of unconsciousness may need admission for observation. Ensure frequent reassessment and monitoring in the ED, and report any deteriorating symptoms.
- If the patient is being discharged, ensure that a responsible adult will be staying with the patient overnight, and that they are given comprehensive instructions about head injury and advice about analgesia.

Cerebral concussion

The number of people who sustain a mild head injury and experience subsequent post-concussion symptoms is very high. In the UK, each year, 250–300 hospital admissions per 100 000 members of the population involve head injuries, of which only a small minority (around 8%) are severe.

Concussion is an injury to the brain that usually occurs following a blow or jolt to the head. In most cases, consciousness is not lost. Common causes include head injury due to a road traffic accident, a fall, a sports injury, or an assault.

People who fall often (e.g. because of difficulties with walking or balance) and those involved in contact sports are most at risk.

Post-concussion symptoms include:
- headaches (which may be severe and persistent);
- dizziness;
- nausea;
- vision disturbance;
- poor balance;
- confusion;
- amnesia (retrograde or post-traumatic);
- poor concentration;
- tiredness;
- irritability;
- anxiety;
- low mood.

Post-concussion syndrome may occur with symptoms persisting for weeks or months after the initial injury. These patients need reassurance that this condition will eventually resolve spontaneously, although it can last for up to 6 months.

Reference

1 National Institute for Health and Care Excellence (2014). *Head injury: assessment and early management*. CG176. National Institute for Health and Care Excellence, London. Available at: http://www.nice.org.uk/guidance/CG176.

Stroke

Stroke is the fourth commonest cause of death in the UK after cancer, heart disease, and respiratory disease. It is also the single commonest cause of severe disability. Around 70% of strokes occur in people over 65y of age, but stroke can occur at any age. Around 80% of strokes are due to occlusion of an artery that carries blood to the brain. The development of specialist stroke units across the UK, as well as greater public awareness of stroke, has improved outcomes for stroke patients.

Stroke is a medical emergency, and there should be no time delays in assessing these patients to exclude other possible causes, such as hypoglycaemia or head injury, that need other specific treatments.

Stroke may be caused by:
- a cerebral thrombosis, as a result of atherosclerosis or hypertension;
- cerebral embolism, as a result of atrial fibrillation (AF), MI, or valve disease.

Around 20% of strokes are caused by haemorrhage into the brain. This may be due to:
- an intracerebral haemorrhage, when a blood vessel ruptures within the brain;
- a subarachnoid haemorrhage, when a blood vessel on the surface of the brain bleeds into the subarachnoid space;
- carotid artery dissection.

Risk factors for stroke
- Hypertension.
- Age >70y.
- Trauma.
- Hyper- or hypocoagulable state.
- Smoking.
- AF or MI.
- Diabetes.
- Oral contraceptives.
- Ethnicity.

Signs and symptoms of stroke
- Varying levels of consciousness.
- Motor weakness (opposite side to cerebrovascular accident (CVA)).
- Incontinence.
- Speech deficits.
- Facial drooping and/or loss of tongue control.
- CN involvement (same side as CVA).

The Face Arm Speech Test (FAST)
The FAST was developed in Newcastle, UK, in 1998 and consists of three key elements—facial weakness, arm weakness, and speech disturbances. FAST was designed for assessment of a seated subject, and so does not assess leg weakness. It is considered a reliable tool for paramedics identifying stroke in the community, optimizing the potential for thrombolysis.

Immediate management of non-haemorrhagic stroke

Patients with suspected stroke should be assessed for thrombolysis treatment. If clinically indicated, there must be no delay in administering this treatment and admitting the patient directly to a specialist acute stroke unit.

Brain imaging should ideally be performed immediately, and definitely within 1h of admission, if any of the following are present:

- indications for thrombolysis or early anticoagulation treatment;
- the patient is on anticoagulant treatment;
- the patient has a known bleeding tendency;
- a depressed level of consciousness (GCS score of <13);
- unexplained progressive or fluctuating symptoms (e.g. papilloedema, neck stiffness, or fever);
- severe headache at onset of stroke symptoms.

Inclusion criteria

- Any patient, regardless of age or stroke severity, where treatment can be started within 3h of known symptom onset and where an intracerebral haemorrhage or other contraindications have been excluded, should be considered for treatment using alteplase.
- Between 3 and 4.5h after known stroke symptom onset, patients under 80y of age who have had an intracerebral haemorrhage or other contraindication excluded should be considered for treatment with alteplase.
- Between 3 and 6h after known stroke symptom onset, patients should be considered for treatment with alteplase on an individual basis, recognizing that the benefits of treatment are likely to be smaller than in those treated earlier, but that the risks of a worse outcome, including death, will, on average, not be ↑. However, great care should be taken when deciding whether to thrombolyse a patient who has significant pre-stroke co-morbidity.

Thrombolysis in 'brain attack'

Alteplase should only be administered within a well-organized stroke service, with staff trained in the delivery of thrombolysis and the monitoring and management of post-thrombolysis complications.

It is essential that there are pathways in place which also include the management of any post-thrombolysis complications.

Immediate nursing interventions

- Assess and resuscitate the patient, as needed. Summon senior help, and perform a full neurological assessment.
- Position the patient to avoid aspiration, and establish IV access.
- Collect blood samples, and ensure that these are sent to the laboratory.
- Record CBG levels, and correct them if blood glucose concentration is <4mmol/L.
- Record an ECG, and request a chest X-ray (CXR). Keep the patient NBM, until their swallowing has been assessed.
- An NG tube may be indicated, but a urinary catheter should not be routinely sited.

- Assist medical staff in conducting a full examination of the patient, and provide reassurance to the patient throughout any procedure.
- Ensure personal hygiene and pressure area care, and keep the patient's mouth clean and moist.
- Provide emotional support for the patient and their relatives, who will be very anxious and upset. If the patient has lost their speech or is having difficulty communicating, advise the relatives that he or she may still understand what is being said.
- If the patient is restless or agitated, ensure that the cot sides are kept in place on the trolley to prevent further injury. Make every effort to establish the cause of restlessness, and remedy it where possible.

Immediate management of intracerebral haemorrhage

In about 10% of all patients who present with acute stroke, primary intracerebral haemorrhage (PIH) is the cause. These patients should be closely monitored for deterioration in consciousness by specialists in a neurosurgical or stroke care unit.

Transient ischaemic attack

Patients with a transient ischaemic attack (TIA)—that is, whose acute symptoms and signs resolve within 24h—should be seen by a specialist in neurovascular disease (e.g. in a specialist neurovascular clinic or an acute stroke unit).

Further reading

Intercollegiate Stroke Working Party (2012). *National clinical guideline for stroke*, fourth edition. Royal College of Physicians, London. Available at: ℞ https://www.rcplondon.ac.uk/guidelines-policy/stroke-guidelines.

Subarachnoid haemorrhage

Subarachnoid haemorrhage is the sudden rupture of a blood vessel over the surface of the brain. It occurs under the arachnoid membrane and is another form of stroke. Spontaneous bleeds follow the rupture of a (berry) aneurysm in the circle of Willis. A subarachnoid haemorrhage can also occur when blood leaks from an abnormal tangle of blood vessels called an arteriovenous malformation (AVM). Subarachnoid haemorrhage occurs more often in people with hypertension and smokers. It is commoner in women and older people. Head trauma is also a common cause.

Signs and symptoms

The headache usually starts very suddenly (like a 'blow to the head') and, within seconds, becomes the most intense headache the patient has ever felt. After minutes to hours, the headache spreads to the back of the head, neck, and back, as blood tracks down the spinal subarachnoid space.

Up to 70% of patients present with a severe 'worst ever' headache, often at the back of the head, which then eases off, followed by nausea and vomiting. Neck stiffness is a feature but is not always evident. A rising BP and bradycardia are indicative of raised ICP. In the most severe cases (30–40%), the patient may lose consciousness, and some (10%) may have a seizure.

Nursing assessment and interventions

- Immediate resuscitation may be indicated if the patient is unconscious.
- ►► If the patient is conscious and gives a history of the 'worst ever' headache, summon senior help.
- Perform a complete neurological assessment and nursing interventions (➲ see Neurological assessment, p. 175; Initial nursing interventions, p. 178). Record all observations meticulously.
- If the patient is unconscious, or has a GCS score of <8 and is agitated and restless, intubate to secure the airway.
- Ensure that blood samples are obtained and sent urgently.
- Request a CXR.
- Ensure that the patient is given appropriate analgesia, and monitor the effect.
- Prepare to accompany the patient to the CT department. If the CT scan is normal, lumbar puncture should be considered. This procedure should be performed on the ward, rather than in the ED.
- Reassure and comfort the patient's relatives and carers, who will be very anxious. Keep them informed, and, where appropriate, allow them to stay with the patient.

Meningitis

- Meningitis is an infection of the membranes that cover the brain (the pia mater and arachnoid mater), collectively known as the meninges.
- Meningitis also involves the CSF and ventricles. The cause of the infection can be bacterial, viral, or occasionally fungal.
- Viral meningitis is usually considered to be benign and is a fairly common complication of viral infection. There is no specific treatment, but initial assessment and management are the same as for suspected bacterial meningitis.
- Fungal meningitis occurs in patients who are immunosuppressed (e.g. due to acquired immune deficiency syndrome (AIDS), lymphoma, or steroid therapy).
- The three main causes of bacterial meningitis have historically been:
  - Hib;
  - *Meningococcus*;
  - *Pneumococcus*.
- In recent years, the introduction of Hib vaccination has led to the virtual eradication of Hib meningitis, so *Meningococcus* and *Pneumococcus* are now the main causes of bacterial meningitis.

Symptoms

- Malaise.
- Fever.
- Neck and back stiffness.
- Oversensitivity to light (photophobia).
- Severe headache.
- Drowsiness.
- Nausea and vomiting.

Signs

Meningitis may start like a flu-like illness and may be difficult to diagnose. It should be considered in any febrile patient with the above symptoms, any neurological signs, and any reduced conscious level and/or irritability. In addition, there will be varying degrees of pyrexia as high as 41°C. A very specific meningeal sign is a positive Kernig's sign (straightening the knee, whilst the hip is flexed, causes ↑ discomfort in the presence of meningeal irritation). Meningococcal meningitis has a rapid onset and can result in septicaemia and death within a few hours. Diarrhoea and/or a rash may be evident, and sometimes a seizure may occur.

If there is a rash, it is worth trying the 'glass test'. This involves pressing a glass tumbler against the rash to see whether the red/purple lesions disappear under pressure. The rash of meningococcal septicaemia does not disappear on application of pressure.

Nursing assessment and interventions

- Assess airway, breathing, and circulation, and administer O_2.
- Summon help.
- Establish IV access as a priority, and, if the patient is shocked and deteriorating and/or there is a suspicion of meningococcal infection, administer IV antibiotics as prescribed.

- Give IV fluids as prescribed.
- Ensure that the patient is given analgesia, and an anti-emetic if they are vomiting.
- Collect blood samples for FBC, U&E, blood cultures, and glucose screen. A sample should also be taken for PCR, as well as a clotting sample that can be used for meningococcal serology. Ensure that these samples are sent to the laboratory without delay.
- In addition to assessing and monitoring the patient with regard to GCS score, BP, pulse, SpO_2, and temperature, evaluate the effect of analgesia given.
- Prepare for, and assist, medical staff with lumbar puncture. Make sure that samples of CSF are sent to the laboratory without delay. A CT scan should be performed before a lumbar puncture, if there are focal neurological signs or evidence of papilloedema.
- Ensure pressure area care and personal hygiene.
- As far as possible, the same nurse should care for the patient and accompany them to the X-ray or CT department or, if indicated, on transfer.
- Remember that patients with meningitis are frequently young, and their parents and carers will be very worried. Make sure that they are kept fully informed and involved where appropriate.
- ▶ When caring for the patient, nursing and medical staff should be diligent in their efforts to prevent further spread of infection.

Prophylaxis for meningococcal infection

Prophylactic antibiotics may be needed by the patient's family and those who have had close contact with the patient. Hospital and paramedic staff may also need prophylactic treatment, depending on the degree of contact they have had with the patient, and in accordance with local policy.

▶ Meningococcal infection is a notifiable disease, and the local public health department must be informed.

Further reading

National Institute for Health and Care Excellence (2012). *Meningitis (bacterial) and meningococcal septicaemia in under 16s: recognition, diagnosis and management*. CG102. National Institute for Health and Care Excellence, London. Available at: ℠ http://www.nice.org.uk/guidance/CG102.

Encephalitis

Encephalitis is inflammation of the brain, which is frequently caused by a virus. It is a rare disease that occurs most commonly in children, the elderly, and people who are immunosuppressed.

In mild cases of encephalitis, signs and symptoms may mimic flu or even go unnoticed. In more severe cases, a person is more likely to experience high fever and have symptoms that relate to the CNS, including:

- severe headache;
- nausea and vomiting;
- neck stiffness;
- drowsiness;
- personality changes;
- seizures;
- problems with speech or hearing;
- hallucinations;
- amnesia;
- confusion;
- coma.

Because encephalitis can follow or accompany common viral illnesses, there are sometimes characteristic signs and symptoms of these illnesses beforehand. Often, however, encephalitis occurs spontaneously.

Causes

- Encephalitis can be caused by many types of organisms. One of the most dangerous of these is the herpes simplex virus (HSV). Fortunately, HSV encephalitis is very rare.
- Encephalitis can be a complication of Lyme disease which is transmitted by ticks, or of rabies which is spread by rabid animals.
- Nursing assessment and management of encephalitis will be the same as for meningitis, but treatment may differ, depending on the causative organism.

Seizures

A seizure occurs as a result of a sudden surplus of electrical activity in the brain producing an abnormal neuronal discharge within cerebral tissue. The type of seizure that a person has depends on the area of the brain where this activity occurs. Grand mal seizures that produce repetitive tonic–clonic movements are those most frequently seen in the emergency setting. Epileptic seizures are classed as partial or generalized. Partial seizures involve part of the brain, whereas generalized seizures involve the whole brain. It is possible for partial seizures to become generalized if the epileptic activity spreads to the whole brain.

- After a seizure, a post-ictal state ensues, characterized by muscle relaxation and deep respiration. This may last from a few minutes to several hours.
- In 'status epilepticus', there are multiple seizures without respite or recovery between seizures. This is an emergency condition, and it can result in respiratory difficulties or irreversible cerebral damage if it is not treated immediately. Nurses must remember that seizures are a manifestation of an underlying condition.

Disorders that give rise to seizures include:
- epilepsy;
- stroke;
- metabolic disorders;
- pregnancy-induced hypertension;
- alcohol withdrawal;
- overdose of barbiturates, cocaine, or benzodiazepines;
- previous neurological trauma.

Symptoms
- Aura—taste, smell, or sounds preceding the seizure.
- Fever and/or tremors.

Signs
- Active seizure—tonic–clonic seizure.
- Deep respiration.
- Possible cyanosis.
- Raised temperature.
- Incontinence.

Nursing assessment and interventions
The immediate aim of treatment is to stop the seizure and to protect the patient during the seizure.
- Position the patient in the recovery position.
- Check airway, breathing, and circulation, and give high-flow O_2.
- Use suction, if necessary.
- Keep the cot sides up on the trolley.
- Obtain IV access; check CBG levels, and administer anticonvulsant medication as prescribed (IV, or per rectum (PR) if there is no IV access) or according to local policy.

- Record vital signs as soon as the seizure ceases, and maintain frequent observations, whilst the patient is post-ictal.
- Continually reassure the patient, who may feel very confused and frightened after a fit.
- Other investigations that may be indicated if this is the patient's first fit include FBC, U&E, blood glucose levels, ECG, and CXR.

Nurses must remember that any disorder of the CNS is very frightening for the patient, so, when caring for the patient, they must be calm and reassuring.

Post-ictal psychosis

Post-ictal psychosis is a rare, but serious, complication following seizures, characterized by auditory and visual hallucinations, delusions, paranoia, affective change, and aggression. Following the conclusion of the seizure, the patient feels the typical confusion and lethargy of the post-ictal state, and then gradually recovers to a normal state.

A lucid period, lasting for 12h to 6 days, after the termination of seizure activity precedes the onset of psychiatric symptoms, which often remit spontaneously within days or weeks. This psychosis is treatable with standard antipsychotic drugs and ceases when the patient is no longer experiencing seizures.

Useful websites

National Institute for Health and Care Excellence (NICE). Available at: ℘ http://www.nice.org.uk.
National Stroke Association. Available at: ℘ http://www.stroke.org.

Respiratory emergencies

Overview

A significant proportion of patients who attend the ED will have a respiratory problem. Breathlessness as a PC is extremely common and can indicate a physiological problem in any system, not just the respiratory system. For example, an ↑ in RR is a compensatory mechanism in DKA. Classically, deep sighing respirations are seen in an attempt to ↑ the elimination of CO_2. Conversely, a reduced RR is often seen in CNS depression or opiate drug overdose.

△ A change in RR indicates either a physiological or psychological problem. The respiratory system is usually the first system to respond to altered homeostasis, and changes in the rate and depth of respiration occur within seconds of a problem that may be remote from the respiratory system.

The measurement of RR in clinical practice continues to be omitted or, if recorded at all, serial measurements are often absent. The ↑ use of EWS systems in recent years has seen an improvement in the recording of RRs.

▶ *Always* record RRs for ED patients other than those with the most minor injuries.

The respiratory system

The respiratory system (➲ see Fig. 7.1) can be divided into the upper airway, which consists of the nose, pharynx, and larynx, and the lower airway, consisting of the trachea, bronchus, bronchioles, and alveoli.

Other structures crucial to normal ventilation are the ribs, intercostal muscles, and diaphragm. If any of these are injured, respiratory function can be adversely affected.

Respiration is a collective term that refers to several functions, namely ventilation, gas exchange, and cellular respiration.

Ventilation

Ventilation is the term used to describe the mechanical element of breathing. Ventilation consists of two phases—inspiration and expiration.

Inspiration

This begins with the stimulation of the diaphragm by the phrenic nerve. The diaphragm contracts and flattens, which ↑ the longitudinal dimension of the thorax. The external intercostal muscles pull the chest wall out, which ↑ the diameter of the thoracic cavity. As the lung capacity ↑, the intrathoracic pressure becomes lower than atmospheric pressure, and air is drawn into the lungs until the pressures are equal.

Expiration

This occurs passively. The diaphragm relaxes and moves upwards; the intercostal muscles compress the chest, and the lungs recoil passively. The intrathoracic pressure becomes greater than atmospheric pressure, and air is forced out of the lungs.

Gas exchange

This occurs at the interface between the alveoli and pulmonary capillaries. O_2 in the alveoli is exchanged for CO_2, and O_2-rich blood is then transported to the tissues for cellular metabolism.

ABG sampling measures the O_2 and CO_2 concentrations in arterial blood, and assesses the effectiveness of lung function (➜ see Arterial blood gas sampling, pp. 656–7).

Cellular respiration

This is the consumption of O_2 and production of CO_2 by the mitochondria of cells.

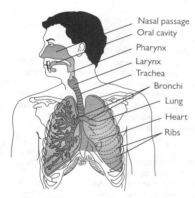

Nasal passage
Oral cavity
Pharynx
Larynx
Trachea
Bronchi
Lung
Heart
Ribs

Fig. 7.1 The respiratory system.

Nursing assessment: overview and history

▶▶ Some patients with respiratory problems require immediate resuscitative interventions. Always undertake an ABC assessment. This will identify those patients with actual or impending airway obstruction and those with absent or ineffective respirations (➜ see Box 7.1).

History

Any of the following features that are present should be recorded in the nursing documentation:
• when the difficulty in breathing started;
• breathlessness on exertion;
• nocturnal dyspnoea;
• orthopnoea;
• cough;
• sputum—colour, amount, and presence of blood;
• breathlessness or inability to take a deep breath—patients with a chest injury often state that they are breathless, but questioning may reveal that they are unable to take a deep breath due to pain;
• chest pain—site and quality. Differentiate between pleuritic and cardiac-type pain, if possible; this can often be difficult, but, if in doubt, consider that the pain could be cardiac, and manage it appropriately;
• any trauma—elicit a clear mechanism if the patient has been injured;
• fever, rigors;
• smoking;
• exercise tolerance—how many stairs can be climbed, or how far the patient can walk on the flat without breathlessness;
• treatment at home or before arriving at the hospital—patients with asthma or COPD may have ↑ their own medication before attending the ED. If there was no improvement after ↑ their own inhaled therapy, this is significant.

For patients with existing respiratory disease, it is important to document:
• medication;
• recent admissions;
• any ICU admissions, intubation, or ventilation;
• non-invasive ventilation (NIV);
• annual flu vaccination;
• previous pneumothoraces.

Box 7.1 Respiratory distress or difficulty

Patients with any number of respiratory problems may present acutely short of breath and exhibit some, or all, of the following signs and symptoms that require immediate intervention:
- marked tachypnoea (RR >30 breaths/min);
- altered conscious level, agitation, confusion, moribund;
- marked accessory muscle use;
- inability to speak due to breathlessness;
- cyanosis;
- exhaustion.

Physical assessment

Inspection

- Observe for pursed lip breathing.
- ▶▶ Drooling indicates an upper airway problem that requires immediate attention.
- ▶▶ Cyanosis (central or peripheral) requires immediate intervention.
- Check the patient's ability to talk in complete sentences. Inability to complete a sentence indicates a severe problem.
- Record the RR, respiratory depth and pattern.
- Note the patient's posture. Patients with partial or impending upper airway obstruction will adopt a posture that maximizes ventilation. Usually they lean forward.
- Observe chest rise and fall, noting any asymmetry or paradoxical movement. Following trauma, paradoxical chest rise and fall may indicate a flail segment.
- Inspect the chest wall for any signs of surface trauma such as abrasions, bruises, wounds, FBs, and scars.
- Observe for accessory muscle usage, which indicates ↑ work of breathing.
- Observe and document the patient's conscious level and degree of agitation, confusion, and restlessness.

Palpation

- ▶▶ Feel the position of the trachea to check that it is in the midline. A deviated trachea is a very late clinical sign and indicates a tension pneumothorax, which is a life-threatening emergency and requires immediate treatment.
- Palpate the clavicles, sternum, and ribs in patients with a chest injury. This may reveal crepitus, surgical emphysema, or tenderness.
- ▶ Patients with a lower chest injury may also have sustained a significant upper abdominal or retroperitoneal injury.

Auscultation and percussion

Listening to breath sounds and percussing the chest is increasingly being undertaken by registered nurses in the ED. Auscultation, in particular, is a relatively simple and useful skill to acquire, and can be mastered with practice and supervision.

- Listen for breath sounds. Are they equal and clear bilaterally? Are there any added sounds such as wheeze or crepitations? Fig. 7.2 shows the landmarks for anterior and posterior chest auscultations.
- ▶▶ A silent chest in an asthmatic patient is life-threatening and requires immediate action. Summon senior help.
- Is there any stridor or an audible wheeze?
- Is the percussion note normal? Dullness indicates fluid or consolidation, whereas hyper-resonance indicates air in the pleural cavity.

Vital signs

Record the following vital signs:
- RR;
- pulse;
- BP;
- O_2 saturations;
- temperature;
- peak flow (in patients with asthma);
- GCS score.

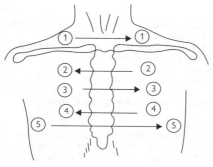

Fig. 7.2 Landmarks for chest auscultation.

Investigations and nursing interventions

Investigations
- ABGs in patients with SpO_2 of <93% on air.
- Sputum for culture and sensitivity (C&S).
- FBC if there is a clinical indication (e.g. infection, anaemia).
- U&E if there are signs of dehydration (may be seen in asthma through insensible losses).
- Blood cultures, if indicated.
- Pain score.
- CXR.
- ECG, if indicated.

Nursing interventions
- Positioning. Patients should be nursed in an upright position. Those with severe respiratory distress often want to sit with their legs over the side or edge of the ED trolley. It can be comfortable for patients to be supported in this position by a bedside trolley.
- Venous access. Some patients will require IV steroids and/or bronchodilators. Not all patients will require IV access.
- O_2 therapy. All patients who are unable to maintain normal O_2 saturations on air will require O_2 therapy. ▶▶ ➡ See Oxygen therapy below.
- Inhaled therapies.
- Psychological support. It can be extremely distressing to be breathless. A calm, reassuring manner will help to reduce the patient's anxiety.
- Analgesia. Pleuritic chest pain can respond well to NSAIDs. Patients with severe pain may require opiate analgesia.

Oxygen therapy

⚠ All patients with respiratory problems must be protected from the dangerous effects of hypoxia and hypercarbia.

▶▶ Only premature infants and COPD patients with a hypoxic drive require controlled O_2 therapy. All other patients should receive enough supplemental O_2 to maintain a normal saturation.

There continues to be some controversy over delivering O_2 to patients with COPD. Normally, respiratory drive is stimulated by an ↑ in CO_2 levels. For example, in a healthy individual, a rise in CO_2 will stimulate an ↑ RR to remove the excess CO_2. In a small group of patients with COPD, CO_2 levels are chronically elevated, and this drive is lost. These patients depend on hypoxia to drive respiration (hypoxic respiratory drive). For this group of patients (remember that not all patients with COPD have a hypoxic respiratory drive), ↑ levels of O_2, which may be given in an emergency, switch off their hypoxic drive to breathe, and they will develop worsening respiratory depression, hypercapnic acidosis, and reduced conscious level, and will require ventilation.

- Give supplemental O_2 by mask to all patients with SpO_2 of <95%.
- In patients with known COPD, give a controlled amount of O_2 by mask, starting at 24–28% and gradually ↑ to achieve a target saturation range of 88–92%. O_2 concentrations should be reduced if the patient becomes drowsy or saturations reach ≥93%. *Obtain an ABG as soon as possible*, as O_2 therapy should be titrated to ABGs, not saturations.
- For patients not known to have COPD, give O_2 to achieve a target saturation of 94–98%.
- If the patient is found to have type II respiratory failure, which is defined as $PaCO_2$ of >6kPa, the cause should be sought and treated.

Asthma: introduction

Asthma is a reversible disease of the airways which still causes in excess of 1200 preventable deaths per year. The evidence suggests that patients with a combination of severe asthma and adverse behavioural or psychosocial factors are more likely to die.

Asthma literally means 'panting' and is characterized by acute exacerbations interspersed by symptom-free periods. The airways become inflamed, narrow, and hyper-responsive. Wheeze tends to be regarded as the principal symptom of asthma. Other symptoms are cough, breathlessness, chest tightness, and accessory muscle usage. These symptoms are variable, intermittent, and often worse at night. When patients are symptom-free, all objective signs of asthma are absent.

Intrinsic asthma has no known allergic cause and tends to occur later in life. Extrinsic asthma has allergic triggers such as pollen, animal hair, certain foods, or certain drugs. Emotion and exercise can also trigger an exacerbation.

The BTS and SIGN *British guideline on the management of asthma* describes in detail the assessment of severity and the treatment required for acute asthma exacerbations in the ED (● see Table 7.1).

Table 7.1 BTS and SIGN levels of severity of acute asthma exacerbations

Moderate asthma	↑ symptoms	
	PEF >50–75% best or predicted	
	No features of acute severe asthma	
Acute severe asthma	Any one of:	
	PEF 33–50% best or predicted	
	RR ≥25/min	
	HR ≥110/min	
	Inability to complete sentences in one breath	
Life-threatening asthma	Any one of the following in a patient with severe asthma:	
	Clinical signs	**Measurements**
	Altered conscious level	PEF <33% best or predicted
	Exhaustion	SpO_2 <92%
	Arrhythmia	PaO_2 < 8kPa
	Hypotension	'normal' $PaCO_2$ (4.6–6.0kPa)
	Cyanosis	
	Silent chest	
	Poor respiratory effort	
Near-fatal asthma	Raised $PaCO_2$ and/or requiring mechanical ventilation with raised inflation pressures	

Assessment of the asthmatic patient

Although the general assessment approach for the breathless patient has already been described (➔ see Nursing assessment: overview and history, p. 198; Physical assessment, pp. 200–1; Investigations and nursing interventions, pp. 202–3), it is worth reinforcing the importance of the following observations. These help to establish the severity of asthma on arrival in the ED and also enable the success of treatment interventions to be evaluated:

- RR;
- pulse;
- SpO_2;
- ABG if SpO_2 is ≤92%;
- temperature;
- BP;
- CXR if a pneumothorax or consolidation is suspected, or if there is life-threatening asthma or failure to respond to treatment;
- peak expiratory flow rate (PEFR);
- pain score;
- AVPU and GCS score.

▶ PEFR is the only objective measurement of lung function available in the ED. It *must* be measured on arrival, and the percentage of best or predicted value calculated and recorded. Fig. 7.3 can be used to compare the PEFR recorded in the ED with the expected best value for gender and height.

Following assessment of the patient with asthma, it is crucial to determine the severity of the asthma (➔ see Table 7.1), as this guides treatment and the need for admission for inpatient treatment.

▶▶ If any features of severe or life-threatening asthma are present, summon help *immediately*. Give high-flow O_2, and commence inhaled bronchodilator therapy, as per the BTS guideline.[1]

Reference

1 British Thoracic Society. *Asthma guideline*. Available at: ℘ http://www.brit-thoracic.org.uk/guidelines-and-quality-standards/asthma-guideline/.

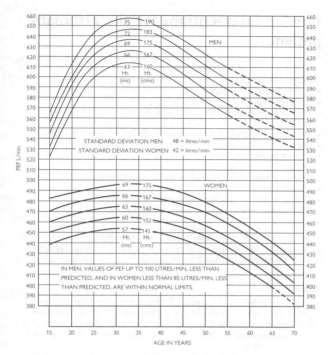

Fig. 7.3 Peak expiratory flow in normal adults.
(Reproduced from Wyatt, J. et al., Oxford Handbook of Emergency Medicine, 4th edn, 2012, p.105, with permission from Oxford University Press.)

Nursing interventions for the asthmatic patient

Once the severity of the asthma exacerbation has been diagnosed, some, or all, of the interventions listed below may be required (➔ see Fig. 7.4). Management priorities will depend on the severity of the asthma.

- Nurse the patient upright.
- Continuous SpO_2 and HR monitoring.
- RR should be recorded every 30min at the very minimum, until it is stable.
- Supplemental high-flow O_2 to maintain saturations above 94–98%.
- Nebulized bronchodilators (may be required 'back-to-back').
- Oral or IV steroids.
- IV Mg^{2+}.
- IV bronchodilators (if advised by senior medical staff).
- ABG analysis.
- CXR if pneumonia or pneumothorax is suspected.
- PEFR should be recorded 30min post-nebulization.
- Analgesia.

Asthma severity may improve rapidly with treatment or worsen significantly despite treatment. Therefore, it is important to reassess severity following any intervention that is given, and to treat any change in condition accordingly.

Admission

- *Patients who show any features of life-threatening or near-fatal asthma must not be discharged from the ED.* Any patient with a persistent symptom of a severe attack despite treatment should not be discharged. Admission *must* be considered for those with psychosocial risk factors (e.g. the socially isolated).
- High dependency unit (HDU) or ICU admission is indicated in type II respiratory failure or if near-fatal or life-threatening features fail to respond to treatment.

Discharge

The BTS guidelines provide details of those patients who may be suitable for discharge (➔ see Fig. 7.4).

Smoking cessation

The opportunity to give smoking cessation advice/brief intervention should not be dismissed because of current pressures to transfer or discharge patients from the ED. Nurses are increasingly taking on the role of the treating and assessing clinician, and may enter into discussions with the patient about various lifestyle choices during the consultation. Equally, there may be opportunities, whilst they are caring for a patient, when the topic of smoking arises. There is evidence that patients are more receptive to

MANAGEMENT OF ACUTE ASTHMA IN ADULTS

ASSESSMENT OF SEVERE ASTHMA

B Healthcare professionals must be aware that patients with severe asthma and one or more adverse psychosocial factors are at risk of death.

INITIAL ASSESSMENT

MODERATE ASTHMA

- increasing symptoms
- PEF >50–75% best or predicted
- no features of acute severe asthma

ACUTE SEVERE ASTHMA

Any one of:
- PEF 33–50% best or predicted
- respiratory rate ≥25/min
- heart rate ≥110/min
- inability to complete sentences in one breath

LIFE-THREATENING ASTHMA

In a patient with severe asthma any one of:
- PEF <33% best or predicted
- SpO_2 <92%
- PaO_2 <8 kPa
- normal $PaCO_2$ (4.6–6.0 kPa)
- silent chest
- cyanosis
- poor respiratory effort
- arrhythmia
- exhaustion
- altered conscious level
- hypotension

NEAR-FATAL ASTHMA

Raised $PaCO_2$ and/or requiring mechanical ventilation with raised inflation pressures

INITIAL ASSESSMENT OF SYMPTOMS, SIGNS AND MEASUREMENTS

Clinical features	Severe breathlessness (including too breathless to complete sentences in one breath), tachypnoea, tachycardia, silent chest, cyanosis or collapse. *None of these singly or together is specific and their absence does not exclude a severe attack*
PEF or FEV$_1$	PEF or FEV_1 are useful and valid measures of airway calibre. PEF expressed as a % of the patient's previous best value is most useful clinically. In the absence of this, PEF as a % of predicted is a rough guide
Pulse oximetry	Oxygen saturation (SpO_2) measured by pulse oximetry determines the adequacy of oxygen therapy and the need for arterial blood gas measurement (ABG). The aim of oxygen therapy is to maintain SpO_2 94–98%
Blood gases (ABG)	Patients with SpO_2 <92% or other features of life-threatening asthma require ABG measurement
Chest X-ray	Chest X-ray is not routinely recommended in patients in the absence of: - suspected pneumomediastinum or pneumothorax - suspected consolidation - life-threatening asthma - failure to respond to treatment satisfactorily - requirement for ventilation

Fig. 7.4 Management of acute severe asthma in adults.   *(Contd.)*

(Reproduced from *Thorax*, British Thoracic Society Scottish Intercollegiate Guidelines Network, 69, pp.13–14, 2014, with permission from BMJ Publishing Group Ltd.)

MANAGEMENT OF ACUTE ASTHMA IN ADULTS

CRITERIA FOR ADMISSION

B Admit patients with any feature of a life-threatening or near-fatal asthma attack.

B Admit patients with any feature of a severe asthma attack persisting after initial treatment.

C Patients whose peak flow is greater than 75% best or predicted one hour after initial treatment may be discharged from ED, unless there are other reasons why admission may be appropriate.

TREATMENT OF ACUTE ASTHMA

OXYGEN

C • Give supplementary oxygen to all hypoxaemic patients with acute severe asthma to maintain an SpO_2 level of 94–98%. Lack of pulse oximetry should not prevent the use of oxygen.

A • In hospital, ambulance and primary care, nebulizers for giving nebulized β_2 agonist bronchodilators should preferably be driven by oxygen.

STEROID THERAPY

A Give steroids in adequate doses in all cases of acute asthma attack.

✓ Continue prednisolone 40–50 mg daily for at least five days or until recovery.

OTHER THERAPIES

A Nebulized magnesium sulfate is not recommended for treatment in adults with acute asthma.

B Consider giving a single dose of IV magnesium sulfate to patients with acute severe asthma (PEF <50% best or predicted) who have not had a good initial response to inhaled bronchodilator therapy.

✓ Magnesium sulfate (1.2–2 g IV infusion over 20 minutes) should only be used following consultation with senior medical staff.

B Routine prescription of antibiotics is not indicated for patients with acute asthma.

β_2 AGONIST BRONCHODILATORS

A Use high-dose inhaled β_2 agonists as first line agents in patients with acute asthma and administer as early as possible. Reserve intravenous $\beta 2$ agonists for those patients in whom inhaled therapy cannot be used reliably.

In patients with acute asthma with life-threatening features the nebulized route (oxygen-driven) is recommended.

A In severe asthma that is poorly responsive to an initial bolus dose of β_2 agonist, consider continuous nebulization with an appropriate nebulizer.

IPRATROPIUM BROMIDE

B Add nebulised ipratropium bromide (0.5 mg 4–6 hourly) to β_2 agonist treatment for patients with acute severe or life-threatening asthma or those with a poor initial response to β_2 agonist therapy.

REFERRAL TO INTENSIVE CARE

Refer any patient:
• requiring ventilatory support
• with acute severe or life-threatening asthma, who is failing to respond to therapy, as evidenced by:
  - deteriorating PEF
  - persisting or worsening hypoxia
  - hypercapnia
  - ABG analysis showing ↓ pH or ↑ H^+
  - exhaustion, feeble respiration
  - drowsiness, confusion, altered conscious state
  - respiratory arrest.

FOLLOW UP

✓ • It is essential that the patient's primary care practice is informed within 24 hours of discharge from the emergency department or hospital following an asthma attack.
• Keep patients who have had a near-fatal asthma attack under specialist supervision indefinitely.
• A respiratory specialist should follow up patients admitted with a severe asthma attack for at least one year after the admission.

Fig. 7.4 (*Contd.*)

lifestyle changes during periods when their behaviours have contributed to a health problem—the so-called 'teachable moment'. All patients who smoke should be advised to stop and offered referral to, or information about, the local smoking cessation support programme.

Further reading

British Thoracic Society. *Asthma guideline*. Available at: ℜ http://www.brit-thoracic.org.uk/guidelines-and-quality-standards/asthma-guideline/.

Pneumonia

Infection of the substance of the lungs is most commonly caused by bacteria. The terms 'pneumonia' and 'chest infection' are often used interchangeably. It is important to use the term 'pneumonia' with caution when discussing the illness with patients and their relatives, as this term causes more alarm than 'chest infection'. Community-acquired pneumonia (CAP) is the name given to a chest infection that was contracted, whilst the patient was at home, as opposed to hospital-acquired pneumonia, which refers to a chest infection contracted within 48h of hospital admission. The commonest causative agent of CAP is *Streptococcus pneumoniae*, which accounts for 1/3 of infections. Hospital-acquired pneumonia is usually contracted by patients who are already vulnerable to infection (e.g. immunocompromised, critically ill, intubated, or ventilated). Hospital-acquired pneumonias usually have a different bacterial origin and tend to be more resistant to standard antibiotic therapy. Patients may present to the ED with signs of a chest infection after a recent admission, and this is worth noting. Mortality from all pneumonias continues to be significant in the elderly population and those with HIV.

Signs and symptoms
• Breathlessness.
• Cough.
• Purulent sputum.
• Fever, shivers, aches, and pains.
• Pleurisy.
• Haemoptysis.
• Hypoxia.
• Signs of consolidation either on CXR or on auscultation and percussion of the chest.

⚠ The elderly can often present 'atypically' with a chest infection or UTI, and may attend the ED with acute confusion or reports of being 'off their legs'.

The patient's signs and symptoms will vary, depending on the infecting pathogen. As *S. pneumoniae* is the commonest cause of bacterial pneumonia, it is worth mentioning its typical onset. There is often a precipitating viral infection, followed by a temperature of >38°C, dry cough, and pleuritic chest pain. The elderly do not usually develop a pyrexia. Several days later, there is rust-coloured sputum, breathlessness, and reduced chest wall movement on the affected side.

In the ED, initial management of the patient with pneumonia is based on an assessment of its severity. A decision is made as to whether the patient can be discharged on oral antibiotics or needs to be admitted for oral or IV treatment. Once the infecting pathogen has been isolated, treatment can be adjusted.

Assessment of the patient with pneumonia

As well as the standard respiratory assessment (→ see Nursing assessment: overview and history, p. 198; Physical assessment, pp. 200–1; Investigations and nursing interventions, pp. 202–3), note should be made of the following:

- any immunocompromise;
- recent hospital admission;
- signs of dehydration;
- signs of hypoxia;
- the patient's social circumstances;
- acute confusion.

Investigations

- Sputum for C&S.
- CXR.
- ABG if SpO_2 is <93% on air.
- FBC, U&E, CRP, and LFTs.

Patients with moderate to very severe CAP may need the following additional tests:

- blood cultures;
- pneumococcal urinary antigen test;
- *Legionella* urinary antigen test.

Further reading

For further reading about additional tests, see British Thoracic Society (2009). *Guidelines for the management of community acquired pneumonia in adults.* Available at: ℞ https://www.brit-thoracic. org.uk/document-library/clinical-information/pneumonia/adult-pneumonia/a-quick-reference-guide-bts-guidelines-for-the-management-of-community-acquired-pneumonia-in-adults/.

Nursing interventions for the patient with pneumonia

Scoring the severity of pneumonia

In patients with pneumonia, clinical judgement should be used together with the validated CURB-65 score to assess severity, risk of death, and risk of ICU admission. Scoring in this way can also guide subsequent treatment and the decision about the need for hospital admission.[2]

One point is given for each of the following:

- Confusion;
- Urea >7mmol/L;
- Respiratory rate ≥30 breaths/min;
- Blood pressure low (systolic <90mmHg or diastolic ≤60mmHg);
- Age ≥65y.

Patients with relatively mild symptoms (CURB-65 score of 0 or 1) with good social support and no other significant health problems can usually be discharged home. Patients with more severe symptoms (CURB-65 score of 2) are at ↑ risk and should be admitted. Patients with a CURB-65 score of ≥3 are at greatest risk. A score of 3 is associated with a 17% risk of death.

Discharge

- Oral antibiotics.
- Analgesia for pleuritic chest pain—vital for deep breathing exercises and expectoration.
- GP follow-up in 48h to assess whether there has been improvement or deterioration.
- Advice to the patient to rest, to take regular oral fluids, and not to smoke.

Admission

Patients who require hospital admission will need the following interventions.

- Nurse in an upright position.
- Give supplemental O_2 to maintain saturations at >93% (careful administration is required in patients with COPD) (➔ see Investigations and nursing interventions, pp. 202–3).
- Administer IV fluids if the patient is dehydrated.
- Give IV antibiotics.
- Give analgesia.
- Give an antipyretic.

Antibiotics

The hospital formulary or local antibiotic guidelines should be followed to ensure that the appropriate empirical treatment is commenced.

Sepsis

The elderly are particularly vulnerable to developing sepsis from pneumonia, and general assessment of the breathless patient should identify any signs of sepsis (➜ see Shock, pp. 278–9).

Reference

2 British Thoracic Society. Available at: ℘ http://www.brit-thoracic.org.uk.

Tuberculosis

Mycobacterium tuberculosis infects 1.5 billion people worldwide, and, in the UK, around 9000 new cases are reported each year, mostly in major cities, especially London. TB is a notifiable disease, and contact tracing is usually done through chest clinics. There are ↑ numbers of strains of multi-drug-resistant (MDR) TB.

1° TB is the initial infection. It usually infects the lungs. TB is spread by inhaling droplets containing the bacteria coughed or sneezed by an infected person. TB can infect any organ but is usually only infectious when it infects the lungs. Because TB can infect many sites, the symptoms can be varied and diagnosis difficult. However, pulmonary TB infection is, by far, the commonest type and should be considered in patients who have the following risk factors:

- living in ethnic minority community;
- immunocompromised;
- poor health and nutrition, homelessness, drug or alcohol use;
- overcrowded living accommodation;
- close household contact with an infected person;
- a history of travel to countries where TB is common.

It should also be considered in those who present with the following signs and symptoms:

- cough;
- fever;
- night sweats;
- haemoptysis;
- weight loss.

TB should be considered as a possible diagnosis in any patient with fever, weight loss, and other unexplained symptoms.

Investigations

- Specific investigations include CXR, which shows classical changes.
- Culturing TB bacteria from sputum or other samples confirms the diagnosis.

Nursing interventions for the patient with suspected TB

Not all patients will need to be admitted. Only those who are ill or highly infectious, or where the diagnosis is uncertain will require admission. Consider isolation measures, whilst the patient is in the ED.

Treatment

The most important factor in treatment is continuous antibiotic therapy for 6 months. The homeless or transient population may need special consideration in relation to maintenance of therapy and follow-up.

Chronic obstructive pulmonary disease

COPD is an umbrella term that is used to describe various diseases (e.g. chronic bronchitis, emphysema, chronic asthma). It is a slowly progressive and irreversible disease, although some patients may show a degree of reversibility with bronchodilator treatment. It usually occurs in people over 50y of age, and smoking is a major factor in the development of the disease.

Assessment of the breathless patient with COPD

Useful information about the severity of the disease can be gained from the patient's history. In mild disease, a 'smoker's cough' is the only abnormal sign. In moderate disease, there is breathlessness and/or wheeze on moderate exertion, cough, and generalized reduction in breath sounds. In severe disease, there is breathlessness at rest, cyanosis, prominent wheeze and/ or cough, and lung overinflation. Also consider and record the following:

- current treatment—inhalers, nebulizers, antibiotics, steroids, O_2, and theophyllines;
- exercise tolerance;
- previous admissions, especially intensive care or treatment with NIV;
- the reason for ED attendance—it is important to identify whether the exacerbation has been accompanied by an ↑ in the amount or type of sputum produced. A recent fall or chest injury may be the cause of the symptoms.

In the ED, assess for the following:

- cough;
- cyanosis;
- sputum—colour and amount;
- wheeze;
- tachypnoea;
- accessory muscle usage;
- lip pursing on expiration;
- chest expansion (which is often poor);
- fever;
- dehydration;
- confusion or reduction in conscious level;
- pain.

Consider whether the patient is septic, and treat any signs of sepsis, severe sepsis, or septic shock immediately.

Investigations

- Continuous monitoring—HR, RR, and SpO_2.
- CXR.
- ECG.
- ABG analysis *as soon as possible*.
- FBC, U&E, and theophylline level (if the patient is taking theophylline).
- Sputum for C&S if purulent.
- Blood cultures if the patient is pyrexial.

Nursing interventions

- Reassurance.
- Nurse the patient in an upright position.
- O_2 therapy to keep saturations in the range of 88–92% (➲ see Investigations and nursing interventions, pp. 202–3).
- Nebulizers (may need to be continuous).
- Steroids.
- IV theophylline (for patients who do not respond to nebulizers).
- Assessment for NIV.
- Mouth care.
- IV fluids if the patient is dehydrated.
- Analgesia.
- AVPU and GCS scores.

Non-invasive ventilation

This is increasingly used in ED resuscitation rooms for the treatment of patients with COPD or heart failure. Evidence suggests that using NIV in patients with COPD reduces mortality and the need for invasive ventilation. NIV should be considered in patients who meet the following criteria[3] (➲ see Ventilation: non-invasive, pp. 766–7):

- respiratory acidosis (pH <7.35, $PaCO_2$ >6kPa) that persists despite maximal medical therapy;
- not moribund, GCS score >8;
- able to protect the airway;
- cooperative and conscious;
- few co-morbidities;
- haemodynamically stable;
- no excess respiratory secretions;
- potential for recovery to a quality of life acceptable to the patient.

Ideally, patients should have an anaesthetic assessment prior to the commencement of NIV, in order to determine their suitability and outline what the ceiling treatment should be. A 'do not attempt resuscitation' (DNAR) order may be completed at this time if the patient is not suitable for invasive ventilation (➲ see Intensive care below).

Intensive care

Patients with exacerbations of COPD should not be automatically excluded from invasive ventilation if all other treatments are failing. The assessing anaesthetist will consider the following:

- quality of life, ideally involving the family in the discussion;
- O_2 requirements when stable;
- co-morbidities;
- forced expiratory volume in 1s (FEV_1);
- body mass index (BMI).

Hospital-at-home schemes

↑ numbers of schemes are available to manage patients with exacerbations of COPD in their own home, thereby either avoiding admission altogether or reducing the length of hospital stay. Patients may know of a 'COPD community nurse' who will be able to give useful clinical information about the patient and their treatments. If there is a local community scheme, it would be worth identifying how the ED can become involved in identifying suitable patients.

Ambulatory care pathways may also be available for patients with mild exacerbations.

Reference

3 National Institute for Health and Care Excellence (2010). *Chronic obstructive pulmonary disease in over 16s: diagnosis and management.* CG101. National Institute for Health and Care Excellence, London. Available at: ℬ http://www.nice.org.uk/guidance/cg101.

Pulmonary embolism

PE occurs when a thrombus, which has usually travelled from a distant site (the deep veins), lodges in the pulmonary vasculature. Less commonly, fat (from long bone fracture), air, or amniotic fluid can cause an embolism. There is an incidence of 60–70 per 100 000 members of the population annually. Around 50% of these cases are in hospitalized patients or those in some form of long-term care. Mortality arising from untreated PE is around 30%. PE is the commonest cause of death following elective surgery, and the commonest cause of maternal death.

> ❶ PE is notoriously difficult to diagnose—only about 10% of patients with a suspected PE actually have one. Hypoxia is common, but young healthy patients can have normal saturations and PaO_2. PE should be considered in cases of sudden collapse or cardiac arrest.

Signs and symptoms
- Tachypnoea (>20 breaths/min)—often the only symptom.
- Tachycardia.
- Pleuritic chest pain.
- Haemoptysis.
- Hypotension.

The signs and symptoms of PE are non-specific and are often found in patients without PE.

Massive PE
This causes sudden circulatory collapse with hypotension. It is rare—only about 5% of PEs present in this way. It should be suspected whenever there is hypotension and distended neck veins not caused by MI, tension pneumothorax, or arrhythmia.

Small or medium PE
This presents more classically with breathlessness, pleuritic chest pain, and haemoptysis.

Multiple recurrent PE
This presents as ↑ breathlessness over a period of weeks or months, with associated lethargy, exertional syncope, and occasional angina.

Nursing assessment for patients with possible PE
A careful history may reveal a known significant risk factor such as abdominal or orthopaedic surgery, late pregnancy, Caesarean section, pre-eclampsia, malignancy, lower leg fracture, or varicose veins. Sedentary travel, which is often a reason for patients presenting with concerns about DVT, is only a minor risk factor. Some patients have no obvious risk factors. Assess for the following:
- tachypnoea;
- tachycardia;
- chest pain—site, quality, and severity;

- pyrexia—low-grade fever may be a response to the inflammatory changes in infarcted lung tissue;
- hypotension—can be suggestive of massive PE;
- haemoptysis;
- AVPU and GCS score.

Investigations

- ECG—sinus tachycardia or AF may be present. Signs of right ventricular (RV) strain or rSR in lead V1.
- CXR to rule out other causes.
- SpO_2.
- ABG analysis
- FBC and U&E.
- D-dimer (but see following paragraph).
- Computed tomographic pulmonary angiography (CTPA).

D-dimer testing

D-dimer is a protein found in the blood after the breakdown of a blood clot. It can be detectable in the blood for many reasons. The inappropriate requests for D-dimer that are sometimes made by ED nurses in an attempt to reduce a patient's wait for blood results can lead to incorrect interpretation of the results and may falsely exclude PE.

D-dimer testing should only be done in patients with a low pretest probability score (➔ see Table 7.2).

Table 7.2 Two-level PE Wells score

Clinical feature	Points
Clinical signs and symptoms of DVT (minimum of leg swelling and pain with palpation of the deep veins)	3
An alternative diagnosis is less likely than PE	3
HR >100bpm	1.5
Immobilization for >3 days, or surgery in the previous 4wk	1.5
Previous DVT or PE	1.5
Haemoptysis	1
Malignancy (on treatment, treated in the last 6 months, or palliative)	1
Clinical probability simplified scores	
PE likely	>4 points
PE unlikely	≤4 points

Adapted from Wells PS et al. (2000), NICE CG144 (2012).

Patients with a higher probability *should not* have a D-dimer requested but are commenced on low-molecular-weight heparin (LMWH), whilst imaging is arranged.

❶ D-dimer is useful *only* for excluding PE and should *only* be used in conjunction with clinical pretest probability scoring. If D-dimer is not detectable or is below a threshold preset by your laboratory, PE can usually be excluded.

Nursing interventions for the stable patient with a high probability of PE

- Continuous monitoring.
- O_2.
- Analgesia.
- LMWH.
- Imaging.
- Low-risk patients are increasingly managed on an outpatient basis, using locally developed ambulatory pathways, so long as they have no clinical or social risk factors.

Interventions for patients with massive PE

Massive PE is highly likely if there is collapse and/or hypotension that is otherwise unexplained, together with hypoxia and engorged neck veins.

- Thrombolysis—IV alteplase (see *BNF* for further information).
- In cardiac arrest, a bolus dose of 50mg of alteplase can be considered, and CPR should be continued for at least 30min.
- If the patient is stable (alert, RR 10–30 breaths/min, systolic BP >100mmHg, and O_2 saturation <92% on air), treat with LMWH.
- Urgent echocardiography or CTPA. If PE is confirmed, give IV alteplase (see *BNF* for further information).

Heart failure

Patients with mild, moderate, or severe heart failure may present to the ED with breathlessness. The incidence of heart failure ↑ with age, and, despite advances in treatment, mortality remains high. Around 50% of patients die within 5y. Acute heart failure can result from MI, arrhythmia, anaemia, infection, medication changes, or patients reducing their diuretic therapy.

Features within the history that may point to heart failure as the cause of dyspnoea include:

- fatigue;
- breathlessness on exertion;
- nocturnal breathlessness;
- orthopnoea (breathlessness when lying flat).

Patients with acute heart failure often present to the ED in early morning and are severely breathless with pulmonary oedema. For more details on the assessment and interventions for heart failure, ➔ see Assessment of the cardiovascular system, p. 234.

Seasonal influenza

Influenza, or 'flu', is a viral respiratory illness that normally occurs in winter, with a peak incidence between December and March. Most people recover after 2wk, but, for some, the complications of flu require hospital admission and can be life-threatening. Those at highest risk from flu are the elderly, children under 5y old, asthmatic patients, pregnant women, and individuals with generally poor health. Most deaths occur in those aged 65y or over. People in at-risk groups should have an annual flu vaccination, as should all health-care workers.

Infectious influenza particles can be transmitted for up to 24h from hands or contaminated surfaces, and for up to 2h on tissues or clothing.

As flu is transmitted by droplets, patients suspected of having flu should be isolated and ideally placed in a single room. Strict hand hygiene and PPE are required when caring for anyone with suspected influenza.

Signs and symptoms

- Fever.
- Headache.
- Myalgia.
- Malaise.
- URTI—non-productive cough, sore throat, and nasal discharge.

Complications

Pneumonia is the commonest complication and usually occurs in high-risk groups.

Viral pneumonia has the most severe symptoms but is usually a rare complication.

2° bacterial pneumonia is a common complication in those over 65y of age and is a significant cause of morbidity and mortality. The classic presentation is a relapse with high fever, cough, and purulent sputum after an initial improvement in flu-like symptoms. For the assessment and management of patients with pneumonia, ➜ see Pneumonia, pp. 212–13.

Simple and spontaneous pneumothorax

A pneumothorax is the collection of air in the pleural space that surrounds the lungs (➔ see Fig. 7.5). A tear in the lung tissue causes inspired air to pass though it into the pleural space. It can occur following trauma or as a consequence of lung disease (e.g. COPD, asthma, cystic fibrosis, bullous lung disease), or it can occur spontaneously (usually in tall, thin young men).

Spontaneous pneumothorax

The phenomenon of spontaneous pneumothorax (SP) in tall, thin young men is interesting. The ♂:♀ ratio of SP is 6:1. It is thought that tall, thin men are more prone to the rupture of bullae (blisters on the pleura that arise from a rupture in the alveolar wall) in the apex, because they are subject to more distending pressure as the thorax is longer.

There is also a significant relationship between smoking and the development of SP. This should be emphasized to patients in an attempt to discourage them from smoking. The lifetime risk of SP in ♂ smokers is 12%, compared with 0.1% in non-smokers. The risk of recurrence in the first 4y can be as high as 54%, and smoking is a significant risk factor for this.

Signs and symptoms

- Breathlessness.
- Unilateral pleuritic chest pain.
- Cough.
- Reduced or absent breath sounds on the affected side.
- Hyper-resonance on percussion of the affected side.
- ↓ chest wall movement on the affected side.

Nursing assessment

- PMH.
- Previous SP—the patient may already have had an SP and know their symptoms well.
- Lung disease—patients with underlying lung disease are more likely to need admission for observation, even with a small pneumothorax or one that has been successfully re-inflated with needle aspiration.
- Pulse.
- RR.
- BP.
- SpO_2.
- Temperature.
- Pain score.
- AVPU and GCS scores.

Investigation

- CXR —relatively asymptomatic patients can often be sent directly to X-ray after a brief assessment. Those with abnormal observations will need further assessment or intervention before X-ray.

Nursing interventions

- Reassurance—chest pain and breathlessness can be very frightening. If the patient has had a previous SP, they may be anxious about needle aspiration or chest drain insertion.
- Nurse the patient upright.
- O$_2$—to maintain saturations at >93%.
- Analgesia.

Management

(➜ See Fig. 7.5.)

- Patients who are not breathless, have a small SP (➜ see Box 7.2), and have no underlying lung disease can be discharged home, with clear written and verbal advice to return to the ED if breathlessness occurs. Early follow-up should be arranged.
- Patients with underlying lung disease require observation and high-flow O$_2$ (this improves the rate of re-inflation by 4-fold), if not contraindicated in COPD. These patients are likely to require more active intervention with needle aspiration or a chest drain, even if they have a small SP.
- Symptomatic patients with small SPs will require needle aspiration. If this is unsuccessful, a chest drain is usually indicated (➜ see Chest drains, pp. 684–6).
- For patients with large SPs and no underlying lung disease, needle aspiration is still the treatment of choice. However, patients with underlying lung disease (particularly those >50y of age) usually need a chest drain.

For information about other chest trauma, ➜ see Chapter 15.

Box 7.2 Classification of SP by size

- *Small SP* has a visible rim of <2cm between the lung edge and chest wall.
- *Large SP* has a visible rim of ≥2cm between the lung edge and chest wall.

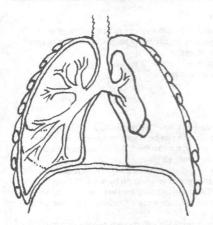

Fig. 7.5 Pneumothorax.

Further reading

MacDuff A, Arnold A, Harvey J; on behalf of the BTS Pleural Disease Guideline Group (2010). Management of spontaneous pneumothorax: British Thoracic Society pleural disease guideline 2010. *Thorax* 65 (Suppl 2), ii18–31.

Cardiovascular emergencies

The heart

A basic understanding of cardiac anatomy and physiology is an essential prerequisite for nurses assessing patients with cardiac-type symptoms. The adult heart is about the size of a fist and sits in the anterior thorax on the left side of the chest in front of the lungs. It is a muscular pump with four chambers:

- right atrium (RA);
- right ventricle (RV);
- left atrium (LA);
- left ventricle (LV).

The atria are the smaller upper chambers of the heart, and the two ventricles are the larger lower chambers of the heart.

The heart is rotated about 30° to the left lateral side, making the RV the most anterior structure of the heart. The LV is about twice as thick as the RV, because it needs greater force to push blood into the aorta and around the body, whilst the RV only needs to push blood through the lungs.

The heart has four valves.

- The tricuspid valve lies between the RA and RV.
- The pulmonary valve lies between the RV and pulmonary artery.
- The mitral valve lies between the LA and LV.
- The aortic valve lies between the LV and aorta.

Healthy valves ensure that blood only flows in one direction.

Beating of the heart

Heartbeats follow a sequential pattern. Contraction of the atria (atrial systole) is followed by contraction of the ventricles (ventricular systole). All chambers then relax during diastole. Simultaneous pressure characteristics occur in the aorta, LA, and LV through one cardiac cycle. The cardiac conduction system arises at the SA (sinoatrial) node and depolarizes through the atrioventricular node, the bundle of His, and the Purkinje system. Depolarization of the myocardium through this route generates a pulsed beat, shown on an ECG as a sinus rhythm (➜ see Fig. 8.3).

The cardiovascular system

The function of the cardiovascular system is to transport O_2 and nutrients to the cells and remove CO_2 and metabolic waste products from the body. The right side of the heart pumps deoxygenated blood to the lungs where gas exchange takes place and then returns the oxygenated blood to the LA through the pulmonary veins (PVs). The left side of the heart pumps blood to the rest of the body through the aorta, arteries, arterioles, and systemic capillaries, and then returns blood to the RA through the venules and great veins.

The heart has its own blood supply via the coronary arteries. The left and right coronary arteries, which originate in the aortic valve annulus, branch into a network of arteries that supply both the right and left side of the heart. It is worth noting that the coronary arteries fill during diastole. Disease processes that affect the cardiovascular system can interfere with the body's ability to maintain tissue oxygenation and cardiac output.

The cardiovascular patient

Cardiovascular emergencies are a common presentation in the ED, and the number of deaths from heart disease remains high. Most patients with chest pain arrive by ambulance, but a significant number arrive by public and private transport. Any patient presenting with chest pain that appears to have a cardiac origin should have an ECG recorded without delay to ensure that a cardiac cause is either identified in a timely way or ruled out.

Typically, patients with chest pain of cardiac origin present with anterior wall pressure/discomfort, which can radiate to the left or right arm and shoulder/neck and be associated with nausea and vomiting. Patients can also complain of epigastric pain and pain between the shoulder blades. (▶ Patients can present with pain radiating to either their left or right arm.) ED nurses need to be mindful that patients who are having a cardiac event may present with atypical symptoms such as nausea and vomiting, shortness of breath, or generally feeling unwell. Equally, patients presenting with a cardiac event may complain of pain in the left side of the neck, jaw, shoulder, or arm, but no chest pain. These are not uncommon presentations of cardiovascular problems, particularly in diabetic patients, and failure to recognize a cardiac cause may result in possible treatment delay. It should be noted that some ethnic groups have a higher propensity to cardiac disease.

Cardiac problems are very frightening for the patient and family, as mortality in this area is still high. Nurses need to demonstrate not only competence and speed, but also empathy and understanding, when caring for this group. Walk-in centres and minor injury units must have the capability to respond to common cardiovascular emergencies, whilst waiting for additional emergency assistance. Due to the ↑ in cardiac centres, many patients may be conveyed directly by ambulance to one of these centres.

Assessment of the cardiovascular system

Use a systematic approach—follow ABCDE.

- A. Ensure a patent airway. If at risk, summon help immediately.
- B. Record the respiratory rate, rhythm, and depth. Note the use of accessory muscles and abnormal noises. Record SpO_2, and administer O_2 therapy as indicated—*aim at achieving SaO_2 >94% or 88–92% if the patient has COPD.*
- C. Record the BP; attach to a cardiac monitor, and manually record the pulse. Note the pulse pressure—avoid the recording rate directly from the cardiac monitor. Obtain a 12-lead ECG promptly.
- D. Assess the conscious status—consider AVPU or GCS. Note any limb weakness or altered sensation.
- E. Ensure the patient is undressed to enable a full assessment (remember to keep the patient warm). Record the temperature. Do not forget to record the blood sugar, and correct any abnormality.

Obtain an 'AMPLE' at the same time as assessing the patient:

- *A*llergies;
- *M*edication—prescribed/over-the-counter/herbal/supplements;
- *P*ast (relevant) medical history;
- *L*ast meal;
- *E*vents leading up to admission; duration of pain.

Assess pain 'PQRST'.

- *P*rovokes. What causes the pain/makes it better or worse?
- *Q*uality. What does it feel like, e.g. sharp/dull?
- *R*adiates. Does it radiate/is it only in one place/did it start in one place and then move location?
- *S*everity. How severe on a scale of 0 (no pain) to 10 (worst pain ever)? Remember to assess how the pain was at its worst, compared to now. (➔ see Pain assessment and management, p. 732)
- *T*ime. Onset and how long did it last/when was it at its worst?

Nursing intervention

- Attach cardiac monitoring, and obtain a 12-lead ECG promptly.
- Establish IV access, and collect blood for FBC, U&E, clotting, appropriately timed TnI or TnT (early may be negative).
- Ensure pain relief.
- For acute coronary syndrome (ACS), consider aspirin and clopidogrel (unless contraindicated).
- Request CXR, if indicated.
- Reassure, and offer support and comfort to the patient and family, minimizing anxiety as much as possible.

ECG

ECG interpretation by pattern recognition is acceptable, but all ECGs must be reviewed by a clinician empowered to commence treatment within 10min of the patient arriving in the ED. Remember that the ECG cannot be interpreted in isolation—the key is always in the history. Ensure ECG leads are correctly placed and electrodes are attached to the bare chest—sweaty and hairy patients can cause difficulties. Dry, then clean the skin with an alcohol wipe. If required, shave chest hair.

Precordial or chest leads

Attach the chest leads, which are labelled V1–V6. The correct positions for the chest leads are as follows (→ see Fig. 8.1):
- V1: fourth intercostal space (ICS), right sternal border;
- V2: fourth ICS, left sternal border;
- V3: midway between V2 and V4;
- V4: fifth ICS, left mid-clavicular line;
- V5: left anterior axillary line at the same horizontal* level as V4;
- V6: left mid-axillary line at the same horizontal* level as V4 and V5.

* At right angles to the mid-clavicular line.

To avoid the common error of counting the space between the clavicle and first rib, locate the angle of Louis (sternal angle). To find the angle of Louis, find the sternal notch (top of the sternum), run your finger down to find a ridge). To find the fourth ICS, with a finger on this ridge, slide the finger down and to the side to locate the second ICS, then count down to the third and fourth space.

When recording an ECG on a ♀ patient, the priority is to apply the electrodes in the correct anatomical areas. If significant breast tissue is resulting in a poor-quality trace, position the electrodes under the breast, and record which ICS this is on the ECG. Although it is acknowledged that attenuation of the signal does not change when electrodes are placed over the breast, there is insufficient published evidence to support this.

For further information, see → ECG recording, pp. 698–700.

Limb leads Fig. 8.2 shows the placement of the limb leads, which are either colour-coded or labelled:
- red lead—right arm (RA);
- yellow lead—left arm (LA);
- green lead—left leg (LL);
- black lead—right leg (RL).

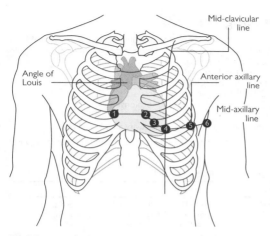

Fig. 8.1 ECG chest lead placement.

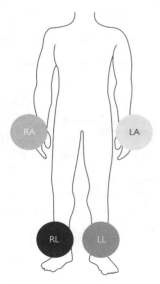

Fig. 8.2 ECG limb lead placement.

Interpreting the ECG

A systematic approach will enable the practitioner to identify normal ECG parameters and, over time, recognize abnormalities and their clinical significance (➲ see Table 8.1 and Fig. 8.3).[1]

- Is there any electrical activity?
- What is the ventricular (QRS) rate?
- Is the QRS rhythm regular or irregular?
- Is the QRS complex width normal or prolonged?
- Is atrial activity present?
- Is atrial activity related to ventricular activity and, if so, how?

▶ Remember: *all* ST segment deviation is abnormal until proven otherwise!

Table 8.1 Common ECG changes

ECG change	Possible cause
ST segment elevation	Possible STEMI I, II, III, aVL, aVF (1mm or one small square) and V1–V6 (2mm or two small squares) (NB. Two contiguous leads required)
T wave inversion	ACS (NB. Two contiguous leads required)
ST segment depression	ACS (NB. Two contiguous leads required)
Tachycardia (HR >100bpm)	Numerous. Significance depends on haemodynamics and clinical history
Bradycardia (HR <60bpm)	Numerous. Significance depends on haemodynamics and clinical history
Narrow complex tachycardia (HR >100bpm)	Numerous. Significance depends on haemodynamics and clinical history
Broad complex tachycardia	Possible VT
AF (HR >120bpm, irregularly irregular)	Numerous. Significance depends on haemodynamics and clinical history. Consider infection, shock, dehydration, etc.
Irregular	Numerous. Significance depends on haemodynamics and clinical history
LBBB	Nearly always pathological in origin. Possible AMI
RBBB	May be normal. Significance depends on haemodynamics and clinical history (e.g. PE)

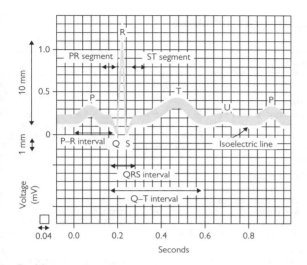

Fig. 8.3 Pulsed beat displayed on ECG.

(Reproduced with permission from Wyatt, J., et al. (2012). *Oxford Handbook of Emergency Medicine*, 4th edn, p. 65. Oxford University Press, Oxford.)

Reference

1 Nolan J (ed) (2010). *Advanced life support*, sixth edition. The Resuscitation Council, London.

Rhythm disturbances

These are commonly treated in the ED. Not all are life-threatening, but they may require intervention or admission. Arrhythmias are classified as originating from the atria or the ventricles, and, whilst usually a symptom of more chronic cardiovascular disease, they may also present acutely in a young person with no previous history of cardiac problems.

Tachycardia

By definition, tachycardia = HR >100bpm. It can be subdivided into broad or narrow complex, with the commonest tachycardias being sinus or AF and the most life-threatening being VT. Patients presenting with arrhythmias should be assessed in an area where resuscitation equipment is readily available.

Atrial fibrillation

AF is a rapid and disorganized atrial activity associated with an inconsistent ventricular response. It is increasingly common due to the ageing population. By definition, it is a narrow-complex tachycardia, but it is often incorrectly referred to as supraventricular tachycardia (SVT). The incidence of AF ↑ with age, but that of SVT ↓ with age.

Acute causes
Acute AF may be triggered by underlying disease pathologies, including:
• heart disease (failure, ACS);
• structural abnormalities (including mitral valve disease);
• substance abuse (alcohol, drugs);
• dehydration;
• medication-induced (e.g. 2° to digoxin toxicity);
• hypoxia;
• infection;
• PE;
• endocrine abnormalities (e.g. thyrotoxicosis);
• post-cardiac surgery.

Chronic AF has numerous causes, ranging from alcohol to thyroid malfunction, although it is often idiopathic/age-related.

ECG diagnosis The ECG is irregularly irregular without organized atrial activity. Fibrillation waves are best seen in V1 (also V2 and II).

Treatment is designed to either slow the ventricular rate or to cardiovert the rhythm. The decision is based on the clinical condition (➔ see Fig. 8.4) and the duration of AF (<48h or >48h). Patients may spontaneously revert, particularly if underlying conditions, such as dehydration, infection, or hypoxia, are treated.
   Assess thromboembolic risk, and consider anticoagulation.

Nursing intervention
Utilize the ABCDE approach.
• Vital signs: temperature; BP; pulse; RR; SpO₂—*aim at achieving SaO₂ >94% or 88–92% if the patient has COPD.*

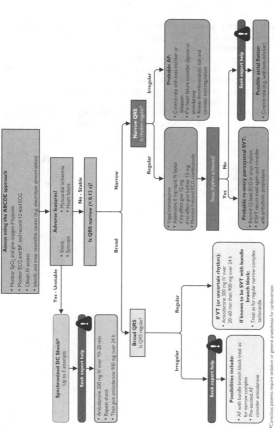

Fig. 8.4 Adult tachycardia algorithm (with pulse).
(Reproduced with the kind permission of the Resuscitation Council (UK). 2015 Guidelines.)

- Attach the patient to a cardiac monitor with a defibrillator nearby, and ensure serial ECGs.
- Assess pain, and give analgesia and an anti-emetic as prescribed.
- Request CXR.
- Establish IV access, and collect blood for FBC, U&E (Mg^{2+} priority), CK, appropriately timed TnI or TnT (early may be negative), coagulation screen, and thyroid function.
- Patients on digoxin: check digoxin levels.
- Consider the need for IV fluids (in absence of cardiac failure) to hydrate and correct electrolyte imbalance.
- Ensure the administration of other drugs as prescribed.

▶ Remember the patient may feel unwell and anxious—the need for empathy and reassurance to reduce anxiety is paramount.

Ventricular and narrow-complex tachycardias

Ventricular tachycardia

VT is a clinical emergency requiring immediate medical review. Its causes are variable, but an acute cardiac cause must be considered in all patients. Treatment will be dictated by haemodynamic compromise (➲ see Fig. 8.4) and may require immediate cardioversion.

Diagnosing VT on an ECG

The following are common features of VT:
- Wide QRS >3 small squares.
- Rate >100bpm.
- Capture beats (a normal QRS within the VT) or fusion beat, which is a single bizarre beat not resembling the previous broad complex (the underlying rhythm and the VT are 'fused together').
- V lead concordance: all pointing the same direction (↑ or ↓).

Nursing intervention

These patients are very unstable, as sudden deterioration is a risk with VT. The monitoring of BP/pulse is mandatory. If patient is compromised, immediate cardioversion is required.
- A defibrillator must be immediately available, and the patient should not be left unattended.
- All patients with VT should be admitted to a monitored area (typically coronary care unit (CCU) or cardiology ward) for ongoing management and close observation.
- During transfer, the ED nurse must ensure immediate access to a defibrillator.

Common drugs used

Amiodarone is a commonly used anti-arrhythmic.
- Ideally, amiodarone should be administered via a large vein, as opposed to a peripheral line, as thrombophlebitis can occur.
- Amiodarone may induce hypotension/bradycardia/heart block. This risk is ↑ if administered fast or administered with other anti-arrhythmic agents.

⚠ Complex arrhythmias may occur following an overdose. Specific management is required. There is no role for generic anti-arrhythmic therapy.

Narrow-complex tachycardia

The term supraventricular tachycardia (SVT) has been superseded by 'narrow-complex tachycardia'. Assessment and basic treatment are as for AF/VT—specific treatment is in accordance with local policy and the tachycardia treatment protocol (➲ see Fig. 8.4).

Treatment options

Vagal stimulation
- Should only be undertaken following specific training and with monitoring/IV access.

- Ask the patient if a specific manoeuvre has worked in the past.
- The most effective treatment is the Valsalva manoeuvre (raising intrathoracic pressure). This can be performed by instructing the patient to attempt to blow out the plunger of a 20mL syringe. The rhythm will not change until *after* the stimulus has stopped.
- Carotid sinus massage is the least effective manoeuvre and is potentially dangerous (↑ risk of embolic stroke) in the elderly. Record the rhythm strip for at least 1min post-manoeuvre.

Adenosine

- Blocks the AV node, inducing temporary AV block.
- Adenosine has a very short half-life and must be rapidly administered and followed by a saline bolus.
- A rhythm strip of any rhythm change must be recorded.
- Adenosine can make patients feel unwell and may induce bronchospasm.
- Adenosine is contraindicated in second- or third-degree AV block and sinus node disease. Effects of adenosine are antagonized by methylxanthines such as caffeine and theophylline. Larger doses may be required, if these are present.

▶ Be careful to warn patients that they may feel unwell after adenosine, but that this will pass quickly.

Cardioversion

Defibrillation and cardioversion share common processes, especially regarding operator safety and paddle/pad position. The principal differences in cardioversion are lower direct current (DC) energy selection, mandatory use of the synchronized function on the defibrillator, and patient sedation. For more information, ➋ see Cardioversion, pp. 674–5.

Bradycardia

Bradycardia is defined as a ventricular rate of <60bpm. Treatment is directed by adverse clinical signs (➔ see Fig. 8.5). Remember that bradycardia may be normal in people who are physically fit.

Causes

- SA or AV node ischaemia, e.g. cardiac disease.
- Raised ICP.
- Pre-terminal hypovolaemia.
- Hypoxia.
- Vagal stimulus, e.g. vasovagal/faint.
- Drugs, e.g. β-blockers.

Atrioventricular block

First-degree AV block is demonstrated by a prolonged PR interval (>5 small squares/>0.2s). It does not require treatment but may indicate pathological disease. It can also be 2° to medication (e.g. β-blockers and some calcium channel antagonists).

Second-degree AV block is subdivided into Möbitz type 1 (Wenckebach) and Möbitz type 2. Both indicate AV node disease.

- Type 1 is demonstrated by increasingly lengthening PR interval until a QRS complex is dropped. It can be remembered by saying 'going, going, gone, and walking (Wenckebach) back'.
- Type 2 is demonstrated by the loss of a QRS complex non-conducted P wave. This can be predicted (e.g. 2:1 block (two atrial contractions to one ventricular contraction), etc.) or can be unpredictable. It indicates an ↑ risk of third-degree AV block or asystole.

Third-degree AV block is demonstrated by dissociation between the atria (P waves) and the ventricles (QRS complexes). Ventricular rate is generated at the AV node or below. The width of the QRS complexes will be dependent on the site of the ventricular stimulus. Within the bundle of His, they will be narrow; below the bundle of His, they will be broad. Generally, the broader the complex, the more unstable.

Treatment

Follow the Resuscitation Council treatment guidelines (➔ see Fig. 8.5), and treat the underlying cause.

- Atropine remains the most commonly used drug. It is particularly effective for narrow bradycardias but is unlikely to work in third-degree AV block.
- Acute MI (AMI) can present with third-degree AV block, either due to AV ischaemia (inferior AMI) or destruction of the bundle branch (anterior AMI). Prompt reperfusion is required to reperfuse ischaemic tissue and should not be delayed in an attempt to introduce a pacing wire.
- External pacing is an emergency technique that can stabilize haemodynamically unstable patients. Patients will need to be informed that the procedure is uncomfortable, even with sedation (➔ see Cardiac pacing, pp. 672–3).

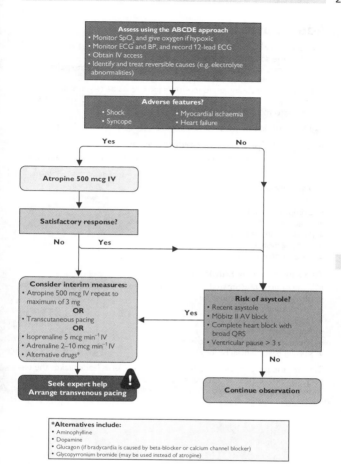

Fig. 8.5 Adult bradycardia algorithm (includes rates inappropriately slow for haemodynamic state).

(Reproduced with the kind permission of the Resuscitation Council (UK). 2015 Guidelines.)

Adult basic life support

ED nurses may be called to perform resuscitation procedures within the ED or within the community—the principles are the same.

- Cardiac arrest may happen anywhere in the ED. Resuscitate patient where they arrest; do *not* move to the resuscitation room.
- The ED may be summoned to emergencies outside (e.g. hospital car park). The priority is to instigate effective resuscitation. Do *not* delay moving to the ED.

(→ See Basic life support—adult, p. 662, and Fig. 21.7 on p. 663.)

Receipt of a prehospital cardiac arrest

Confirm who is going to 'run' the arrest, e.g. the cardiac arrest team or run 'in-house' (according to local policy).

Nominated roles

- Team leader.
- Compressions/CPR
- IV access.
- Airway management.
- Defibrillation and/or drugs.
- Care of next-of-kin.

Ambulance crew handover

- Time of arrest/estimated downtime (this can be unreliable).
- Establish if any bystander CPR.
- Drugs administered.
- Defibrillator shocks given.
- Any return of circulation.
- Special circumstances (e.g. overdose).
- Known past medical history

Transfer the patient to the ED trolley, whilst the team leader takes the history. Confirm cardiac arrest. Interruption to compressions should be minimized. Attach a monitor/confirm ETT placement or assist with intubation.

Advanced life support

➔ See Defibrillation, pp. 690–1, p. 692. Fig. 8.6 gives the adult ALS algorithm.

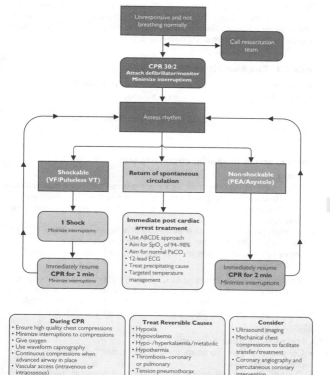

Fig. 8.6 Adult advanced life support algorithm.

(Reproduced with the kind permission of the Resuscitation Council (UK). 2015 Guidelines.)

Cardiac arrest

Causes of cardiac arrest

The commonest cause of adult cardiac arrest is thromboemboli (AMI/PE), but the 'four Hs and four Ts' (→ see Box 8.1) should be considered in all cardiac arrests. These cause cardiac arrest, and not just non-VT/VF, as it is possible to have a tension pneumothorax presenting in VF.

> #### Box 8.1 The four Hs and four Ts
>
> - Hypoxia
> - Hypovolaemia
> - Hyper-/hypokalaemia/metabolic disorders
> - Hypothermia
>
> - Tension pneumothorax
> - Tamponade
> - Toxins
> - Thrombosis (coronary or pulmonary)

Cardiac arrest in special circumstances

Pregnancy

Cardiac arrest during pregnancy is rare but requires significant modification to BLS. Physiological changes during pregnancy result in high risk of aspiration, ↑ difficulties in airway management, and difficulty in performing chest compressions.

- All visibly pregnant patients need to be resuscitated, whilst tilted 15° to the left to displace the uterus and ease caval compression.
- Higher hand positions may be required to adjust for the displacement of the internal organs.

ALS remains the same, including ABCDE/early defibrillation with consideration of early intubation. Emergency Caesarean section, ideally within 5min (>23wk to maximize mother/fetal survival), should also be considered. At <20wk, the uterus is unlikely to compromise maternal cardiac output.

Poisoning/overdose

- May be accidental or deliberate.
- Consider the agent. Some are toxic to the rescuer (e.g. cyanides, organophosphates).
- The ABCDE approach should be followed to prevent cardiopulmonary arrest.
- Effective compressions and ventilations (early intubation) are the principal treatments during resuscitation 2° to poisoning.
- Success following a prolonged cardiac arrest is reported, regardless of the presenting rhythm, utilizing the 'four Hs and four Ts' approach.
- Identification of the poison may enable the use of an appropriate antidote (e.g. naloxone for opioids).

Trauma

Cardiac arrest 2° to blunt trauma has a poor outcome.
- Use the normal ABCDE approach with aggressive and prompt treatment of injuries. These may encompass intubation, bilateral needle decompression and bilateral chest drain placement, fluid bolus (± O-negative blood), with compressions supported by adrenaline.
- Thoracotomy should be considered where there is a history of penetrating trauma (➔ see Resuscitative thoracotomy, p. 529).

Electrocution Relatively infrequent, but potentially devastating multisystem injury.
- The normal ABCDE approach should be utilized, with early defibrillation as required.
- Removal of clothing will reduce further burns and allow full inspection for tissue damage/burns/compartment syndrome and 2° injuries from falls, etc.
- Consider IV fluids if extensive tissue damage.

Asthma

Cardiac arrest as a result of a severe asthma attack is often a terminal event. It is linked to bronchospasm, mucus plugging, tension pneumothorax, and arrhythmias. Dehydration is also common.
- The ABCDE/early defibrillation approach should be followed, using the four Hs and four Ts to guide management.
- Ventilation/compressions may be ineffective due to ↑ airway pressures.
- Early intubation assists with oxygenation.
- In tension pneumothorax, needle decompression, if required, should be followed with a definitive chest drain.

Anaphylaxis
➔ See Shock, pp. 278–9.

Electrolyte imbalance
➔ See Table 8.2.

Drowning

Standard ABCDE approach. Common cause of accidental death, typically due to hypoxia. ↑ survival if linked to hypothermia.
- Prolonged CPR should be considered.
- If possible, ascertain history (e.g. intoxication, head injury, chest pain whilst swimming, fall from a height) that led them to be in the water (➔ see Drowning, pp. 576–7).
- Consider acute respiratory distress syndrome (ARDS) for up to 72h.

Hypothermia

Defined as a core temperature <35°C.
- Standard ABCDE approach, but pulse checks should be at 1min intervals, and defibrillation is less effective with body temp <30°C.
- Give initial shock, then review strategy.
- Survival after prolonged CPR is possible.

Table 8.2 Electrolyte imbalance in cardiac arrest

Possible causes	Likely presentation	Potential ECG changes	Treatment considerations
Hyperkalaemia			
Renal failure	Weakness	Prolonged PR interval	IV furosemide
Drugs (ACE, ARB, potassium-sparing diuretics)	Flaccid paralysis	Flat/absent P waves	Calcium resonium
	Paraesthesiae	Peaked T waves	IV glucose/insulin
Rhabdomyolysis	Bradycardia	T wave greater than R wave	Nebulized salbutamol
Metabolic acidosis	Ventricular tachycardia	ST segment depression	Calcium chloride (protects the heart but does not lower K$^+$)
Endocrine disorders (Addison's disease)	Cardiac arrest	Prolonged QRS	Haemodialysis
Diet		Bradycardia	
		Ventricular tachycardia	
		Cardiac arrest	
Hypokalaemia			
GI loss	Fatigue	U waves evident	IV potassium
Drugs (diuretics, laxatives)	Weakness	T wave flattening	IV magnesium (replenishment of magnesium facilitates uptake of potassium)
Renal dysfunction (tubular disorders, diabetes)	Leg cramps	ST segment elevation	
	Constipation	Arrhythmias	
Dialysis	Rhabdomyolysis	Cardiorespiratory arrest	
Endocrine disorders (Cushing's disease)	Ascending paralysis		
Metabolic alkalosis	Respiratory difficulties		
Magnesium depletion			
↓ dietary intake			
Treatment of hyperkalaemia			

Hypercalcaemia			
Hyperparathyroidism	Confusion	Short QT interval	IV fluids
Malignancy	Weakness	Prolonged QRS	IV furosemide
Sarcoidosis	Abdominal pain	Flat T waves	IV hydrocortisone
Drugs	Hypotension	AV block	IV pamidronate
Hypocalcaemia			
Chronic renal failure	Paraesthesiae	Prolonged QT interval	IV calcium chloride
Acute pancreatitis	Tetany	T wave inversion	IV magnesium sulphate
Calcium channel blocker overdose	Seizures	Heart block	
Toxic shock syndrome	AV block	Cardiac arrest	
Rhabdomyolysis	Cardiac arrest		
Hypermagnesaemia			
Renal failure	Confusion	Prolonged PR interval	IV calcium chloride
Iatrogenic	Weakness	Prolonged QT interval	IV furosemide
	Respiratory depression	Peaked T waves	Ventilatory support
	AV block	AV block	Haemodialysis
	Cardiac arrest	Cardiac arrest	
Hypomagnesaemia			
GI loss	Tremor	Prolonged PR interval	IV magnesium sulphate
Polyuria	Ataxia	Prolonged QT interval	
Starvation	Nystagmus	ST segment depression	
Alcoholism	Seizures	T wave inversion	
Malabsorption	Arrhythmias (torsade de pointes)	Flat P waves	
Drugs (diuretics)	Cardiac arrest	Prolonged QRS	
		Torsade de pointes	

- Rewarming required, ideally by cardiopulmonary bypass. If unavailable, warmed fluids, air, O_2, and bladder/gastric irrigation or warmed peritoneal/pleural lavage can be used. Administer all fluids at 40°C.
  - During rewarming, vasodilatation occurs, requiring large volumes of IV fluids (➔ see Drowning, pp. 576–7).
  - Active rewarming should be reviewed once body temp 32–34°C, as active hypothermia may be beneficial in the comatose patient.

Massive pulmonary embolism
Is common cause of cardiac arrest (typically PEA)—diagnosis is difficult. Treat with bolus thrombolysis and heparin (a prolonged period of CPR will be required; thrombolytic drugs may take up to 90min to be effective) (➔ see Pulmonary embolism, pp. 222–4).

Drugs for cardiac arrest and post-resuscitation nursing care

Drugs for cardiac arrest
➲ See Table 8.3.

Post-resuscitation nursing care
- Maintain airway.
- O_2 support should initially be in high concentration to achieve rapid restoration; as breathing improves *aim at achieving SaO_2 >94% or 88–92% if the patient has COPD*.
- Maintain neurological monitoring (if GCS <8, patient needs intubation).
- Observe for any seizures as this may indicate cerebral hypoxia and possible raised ICP (an indication for intubation).
- Monitor rhythm/BP/pulse/RR/O_2 saturations, capnography, blood glucose, and temperature (haemodynamic instability may indicate need for inotropic support).
- Repeat ECG (changes to ECG must be immediately reported). Initial ECG may be undiagnostic. CPR is not a contraindication for thrombolysis.
- CXR.
- Check U&E (to include Mg^{2+}), FBC, and clotting.
- ABG.
- Maintain accurate fluid balance and observe urine output.
- Cool the patient according to local guidelines. Research into post-arrest cooling is ongoing.
- Confirm admission area/bed.
- Debrief the resuscitation team.
- Keep family informed and involved.

Cooling
- Follow local guidelines.
- External cooling blankets; cold fluid bolus (4°C); ice packs to the groin/axilla/forehead are initially effective.

Table 8.3 Drugs that may be used in cardiac arrest

Drug	Dose and rationale	Comments
Adrenaline	1mg every 3–5min. ↑ systemic vascular resistance during CPR, resulting in relative ↑ of cerebral and coronary perfusion	↑ cardiac O_2 demand; can be arrhythmogenic; avoid in cardiac arrest 2° to solvent abuse
Atropine	Titrate 0.5–3mg for symptomatic bradycardia	Blocks effect of vagus nerve on SA and AV nodes. Side effects dose-related
Amiodarone	If VF/VT persists, 300mg by bolus injection (flushed with 20mL of 0.9% sodium chloride or 5% glucose) is given after third shock. Further dose of 150mg may be given for recurrent or refractory VF/VT, followed by 900mg infusion over 4h 300mg over 20–60min (use local protocols); then 900mg infusion over 24h. Use for haemodynamically unstable SVT/VT/tachycardias (broad and narrow). Cell membrane stabilizer	Can be arrhythmogenic. Can cause hypotension/ bradycardia. ↑ warfarin and digoxin plasma levels. Avoid using >1 anti-arrhythmic
Sodium bicarbonate	1mL/kg of 8.4%: typically 50mL. Use for tricyclic overdose; hyperkalaemia; correction of severe acidosis	ABG monitoring. Exacerbates intracellular acidosis. Requires ↑ ventilation. Has limited role—limit to special circumstances
Calcium chloride	10mL of 10%. Use for hypomagnesaemia, hyperkalaemia, hypocalcaemia, and calcium channel blocker overdose. Has role in mechanisms linked to myocardial contraction	Has limited role—limit to special circumstances
Thrombolysis	As for AMI. Used if PE or AMI is suspected. Both have a thromboembolic component	CPR for minimum of 60–90min post-treatment

Chest pain: common causes

This is a common presenting condition; the diagnosis may be cardiac, non-cardiac, or benign. Chest pain is a very frightening experience for the patient, and any patient presenting with this condition should be classed as urgent. Box 8.2 describes cardiovascular emergencies that may present with chest pain, and Box 8.3 gives other possible causes of chest pain.

The type and nature of chest pain support the diagnosis plus associated risk factors. Clinicians need to be alert to the atypical presentations, as failure to consider a cardiac cause can delay treatment. Patients at greatest risk of being missed are the elderly, females, diabetics, patients with poor command of English, and individuals who are alcohol-dependent.

Box 8.2 Cardiovascular emergencies presenting with chest pain

Myocardial infarction
- Pain gradual onset, although may suddenly become worse.
- Band-like pain, tight/crushing/pressure.
- Indigestion/epigastric ache.
- Commonly associated with nausea and vomiting.
- May radiate to arm/neck/back/shoulder.
- May be associated with SOB.
- Beware of atypical presentation plus isolated epigastric/back pain—inferior AMI.

Acute coronary syndrome Presentation as for AMI.

Dissecting thoracic aneurysm
- Immediate onset of pain.
- Severe and/or tearing.
- Predominantly located in, or radiating to, the back and/or shoulder blades.
- Disparity between left and right—BP >20mmHg.

Pulmonary embolism
- Pleuritic in nature.
- Tachycardic and hypotensive.
- Dyspnoea, tachypnoea, and hypoxia.
- Fever, cough, and haemoptysis.
- ECG showing signs of RV strain or rSR in lead V1.

Common pitfalls

- Pain relief with glyceryl trinitrate (GTN) does not exclude AMI.
- Normal ECG at initial assessment.
- Pain relief with antacids.
- Thinking that the patient is 'too young'.

Patients can describe cardiac pain as sharp (indicating intensity—not nature of pain), play down their symptoms, and present without chest pain but with confusion, collapse/stroke, back pain, isolated jaw/neck/arm/epigastric pain, and belching. Many patients perceive it as discomfort, rather than pain. Some patients may deny chest pain but cite shortness of breath (SOB) as their reason for coming to the ED. SOB/confusion/collapse all indicate the need for an immediate ECG.

Box 8.3 Other causes of chest pain

Pericarditis
- Sharp in nature.
- Aggravated by lying down, turning, coughing, and deep inspiration.
- Associated with a fever, cough, and sputum.
- Diminished by sitting up and leaning forward.
- ECG shows saddle-shaped ST segments, often globally.

Pleurisy
- Sharp in nature; worse on inspiration and coughing.
- Can be precisely localized by the patient.
- Anterior wall localization may be accompanied by tenderness of a costochondral junction.

Pneumothorax
- May be acute/chronic.
- COPD.
- Tearing; ↑ by breathing.
- Dyspnoea, tachycardia, agitated.
- ↓ breath sounds, chest wall movement. Sudden onset of pleuritic pain.

Musculoskeletal
- History of trauma.
- Localized tenderness and worse on movement (pain of AMI can also ↑ with application of pressure!).

Oesophagitis/spasm
- Central chest pain/burning.
- Possibly associated with belching (beware of atypical cardiac patient!).

Costochondritis
- Localized pain worse over costochondral junction and with 'springing' of the chest—beware cardiac pain reproducible with chest palpation.

Shingles
- Intense pain—rash often not initially present.
- Dermatome distribution.

Chest pain: assessment and nursing interventions

Patient assessment

Patients presenting with chest pain should be assessed in an area where resuscitation equipment is easily accessible.

- Rapid assessment ABCDE/AMPLE/PQRST.
- Attach the patient to a cardiac monitor.
- Record BP and HR every 15min in the first hour; then reduce to hourly if stable.
- First ECG <10min after arrival and reviewed by a clinician empowered to treat.
- Repeat every 15min in the first hour—each ECG is reviewed in its correct sequence. If ACS suspected, repeat an ECG every 15min and if patient develops additional pain.
- Summon help if ST segment deviation is detected.
- Record temperature.

Nursing intervention

- GTN (according to local patient group direction (PGD)) or as prescribed.
- Aspirin 300mg (unless known allergy) via PGD or as prescribed.
- Establish IV access, and collect blood for U&E (including Mg^{2+}), FBC, cardiac enzymes, appropriately timed TnI/TnT (early may be negative), blood glucose, clotting, lipids (for risk stratification). If tachycardic, request thyroid function.
- Request CXR.
- Assist the assessing clinician in examination and assessment of the patient.
- Reassure the patient, and keep the relatives informed.

Angina

Angina can be defined as pain or chest discomfort due to inadequate coronary blood supply to the myocardium. It is usually brought on by exertion, and the patient presents with central chest pain, sometimes radiating to the jaw, neck, or back. Its onset may be rapid or gradual. Patients presenting to the ED may be experiencing their first episode of angina and be very fearful. Consider MI in pain lasting >15min. Immediate ECG/cardiac monitoring is indicated.

Acute coronary syndrome

The term ACS covers a spectrum of conditions, including unstable angina, non-ST-elevation MI (NSTEMI), and ST-elevation MI (STEMI). Predictable angina is *not* an ACS.

The commonest cause of an ACS is the rupture of a lipid-rich atheromatous plaque within a coronary artery, causing local coronary artery spasm and activation of platelets and fibrin to heal the local damage, resulting in the formation of a thrombus.

This healing process results in total or partial occlusion of the coronary artery, leading to myocardial cell death. The end diagnosis depends on the degree of damage confirmed with serial ECG and cardiac markers.

Unstable angina: diagnosis

Any condition that affects myocardial O_2 demand can worsen existing stable angina, leading to unstable angina (⊃ see Box 8.4).

Unstable angina and MI may be hard to differentiate initially, so the assessment and early management are similar. Unstable angina is a medical emergency with a high 30-day mortality.

Symptoms

- Pain at rest.
- Pain lasting >15min.
- Pain greater than patient's normal angina.
- Pain ↑ in frequency/severity/duration.
- Associated SOB, nausea and vomiting, or other new symptoms.
- Arrhythmia or left ventricular failure (LVF).

Diagnosis

The initial diagnosis is based on clinical history, confirmed by ECG changes and appropriately timed TnI/TnT (early may be negative). A normal ECG does not exclude an ACS, and traditional cardiac enzymes (CK or CKMB-mass) may be normal.

ECG changes in acute coronary syndrome/unstable angina
(⊃ See Figs. 8.7 and 8.8.)
- ST segment changes >0.5mm = 1/2 small square.
- T wave depression/inversion or flattened T wave.
- Significant T wave inversion can be indicative of an NSTEMI.

Box 8.4 Conditions that can cause stable angina to worsen to form unstable angina

- Anaemia. Hb affects O_2 delivery. Obtain FBC.
- Tachycardia, e.g. AF. ↑ myocardial O_2 demand.
- Hypoxia. ↓ O_2 delivery.
- Hypotension. Significant hypotension ↓ coronary artery perfusion.
- Pyrexia. ↑ myocardial O_2 demand—typically by ↑ vasodilatation and thus HR.
- Valve disease. Aortic stenosis ↑ myocardial O_2 demand/workload. All valve disease ↑ the risk of AF.
- Multiple pathologies. A combination of systemic illness (e.g. pneumonia), pyrexia, ↓ oxygenation, and ↑ HR can combine to produce unstable angina.

Normal lead II

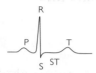

Ischaemic changes in lead II

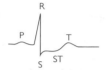

Fig. 8.7 ECG changes in ACS unstable angina.

(Reproduced with permission from Wyatt, J., et al. (2012). *Oxford Handbook of Emergency Medicine*, 4th edn, figs. 3.3 and 3.4, p.69. Oxford University Press, Oxford.)

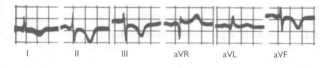

I II III aVR aVL aVF

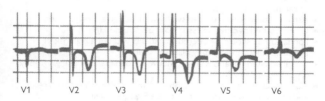

V1 V2 V3 V4 V5 V6

Fig. 8.8 ECG of NSTEMI (subendocardial infarct).

(Reproduced with permission from Wyatt, J., et al. (2012). *Oxford Handbook of Emergency Medicine*, 4th edn, fig. 3.8, p.75. Oxford University Press, Oxford.)

Unstable angina: management and nursing interventions

Immediate management
- Rapid assessment ABCDE/AMPLE/PQRST.
- Attach the patient to a cardiac monitor.
- Record BP and HR every 15min in the first hour; then reduce to hourly if stable.
- After repeating every 15min in the first hour, if the patient develops additional pain, this is an indication of potential instability.
- Review ECGs in their correct sequence.
- Summon help if ST segment deviation is detected.

Nursing intervention
- Supplementary, as indicated.
- GTN (according to local PGD) or as prescribed.
- Aspirin 300mg (unless known allergy) by PGD or as prescribed.
- Establish IV access, and collect blood for U&E (including Mg^{2+}), FBC, cardiac enzymes, appropriately timed TnI/TnT (early may be negative), blood glucose, clotting, lipids (for risk stratification). If tachycardic, request thyroid function.
- Request CXR.
- Assist the doctor in examination and assessment of the patient.
- Reassure the patient, and keep the relatives informed.

Administration of prescribed medications
- Opiate analgesia (draw up 10mg morphine or 5mg diamorphine; dilute in 10mL and 5mL, respectively, and saline flush). Upwards of 15–20mg of morphine may be required. Anti-emetic, if required (avoid cyclizine as can be arrhythmogenic).
- Aspirin 300mg (chewed, then swallowed). Still give if on warfarin.
- GTN 400 micrograms, unless systolic BP <90mmHg.
- Fondaparinux should be offered to patients without a high risk of bleeding, unless angiography planned <24h.
- Unfractionated heparin is an alternative to fondaparinux if angiography is planned within 24h.
- Commence IV nitrates as prescribed; ↑ the rate to achieve pain relief, and record BP every 15min if systolic BP ≥100mmHg.
- Administer clopidogrel 300mg and oral β-blocker (unless contraindicated).
- Patient with ACS should be admitted to CCU or similar environment for ongoing monitoring/pain management and to ensure prompt response to clinical deterioration—arrhythmia or conversion to AMI.

Acute myocardial infarction: types and presentation

The different types of AMI are shown in Table 8.4.

NSTEMI The initial diagnosis, management, and admission are the same as for unstable angina. Formal diagnosis is made at 24h following ECG review and assessment of cardiac enzymes (e.g. TnT/TnI, CK, CK-MB). This type of infarct is becoming commoner, and care is required to ensure early identification and admission to CCU.

STEMI remains the single largest cause of death associated with coronary heart disease (CHD) within the developed world. It is the end of a spectrum of disease following the same process as other ACS but involves total occlusion of a coronary artery. Initial management remains the same for STEMI as for ACS, but the use of reperfusion therapy is a priority. Symptoms are the same as for other ACS, but beware of atypical presentation.

Atypical/pain-free acute myocardial infarction presentation

Symptoms of AMI do not have to include pain. Registries show that up to 30% of patients with STEMI present with atypical symptoms (ESC, 2012).[2] Careful consideration should be given to patients who do not fit the classical AMI picture. Early ECG will help in making the correct diagnosis. There is an ↑ in mortality and morbidity associated with late diagnosis of atypical AMI. Patients can describe cardiac pain as sharp (indicating intensity, not nature, of pain), play down their symptoms, and present without chest pain but with confusion, collapse/stroke, back pain, isolated jaw/neck/arm/epigastric pain, and belching. Many patients perceive it as discomfort, rather than pain. Some patients may deny chest pain but cite SOB as their reason for coming to the ED.

Reference

2 Task Force on the management of ST-segment elevation acute myocardial infarction of the European Society of Cardiology (ESC), Steg PG, James SK, Atar D, Badano LP, et al. (2012). ESC Guidelines for the management of acute myocardial infarction in patients presenting with ST-segment elevation. *Eur Heart J* **33**, 2569–619.

Table 8.4 Types of AMI

ECG changes	Coronary artery	Comments
Inferior AMI		
ST elevation (≥1mm/1 small square): II, III, and aVF	Right coronary	Bradycardia, heart block, and AF. High risk for RV infarction and rupture of papillary muscle
Anterior lateral AMI		
ST elevation: I, aVL (≥1mm/ 1 small square); V1–V6 (≥2mm/2 small squares)	Left main stem or anterior descending	High risk for LV dysfunction
Anterior AMI		
ST elevation: V1–V6 (≥2mm/ 2 small squares)	Anterior descending or sub-branch	High risk for LV dysfunction
Lateral AMI		
ST elevation: I, aVL (≥1mm/ 1 small square); V5–V6 (≥2mm/2 small squares)	Circumflex	ST elevation can be limited to I and V6
Posterior AMI (➔ see Fig. 8.9)		
ST depression: V1–V3 with associated ↑ R wave height. ST elevation V7–V9 (≥1mm/ 1 small square)	Right coronary ± posterior descending	Record posterior ECG leads in all patients with ST depression V1–V3, regardless of presence of ↑ R wave height
RV		
Isolated ST elevation in V1	Right coronary	Record V3–5 (right-sided ECG) in all inferior AMI and hypotensive AMI patients

ST elevation in V1–V6 can be diagnostic of an AMI at 1mm/1 small square, particularly in V4–V6, but the evidence base for treatment supports 2mm/2 small squares.

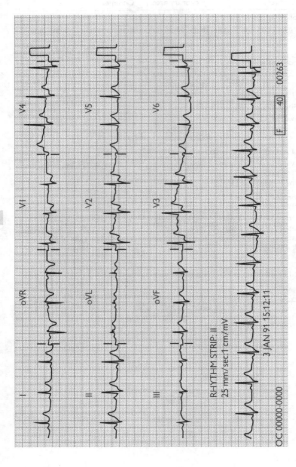

Fig. 8.9 Posterior AMI.

Acute myocardial infarction: diagnosis and management

Diagnosis

Diagnosis is based on the triad of:

- ECG changes (ST segment/LBBB) in two contiguous leads ± reciprocal changes (see Figs. 8.9, 8.10, and 8.11).
- Clinical presentation.
- Changes to cardiac markers.

Immediate interventions

Patients with an MI can be extremely anxious, are likely to be in pain, and may have a sense of impending doom. They will need a calm and competent response from the nurse caring for them.

▶ Local policies and procedures should be followed in all instances.

- Opiate analgesia (draw up 10mg morphine or 5mg diamorphine; dilute in 10mL or 5mL, respectively, and saline flush). Upwards of 15–20mg of morphine may be required. Anti-emetic if required (avoid cyclizine, as it can be arrhythmogenic).
- Aspirin 300mg (chewed, then swallowed). Still give if on warfarin.
- GTN 400–800 micrograms sublingually, unless systolic BP <90mmHg.
- Subcutaneous (SC) low-molecular-weight heparin (LWMH) (enoxaparin 1mg/kg bd) or heparin infusion (800–1000 units/h, activated partial thromboplastin time (aPTT) × 2 control). *Note*: Heparin use will depend on choice of lytic agent (generally not used with streptokinase).
- Commence IV nitrates; ↑ rate to achieve pain relief, and record BP every 15min if systolic BP ≥100mmHg.
- Administer clopidogrel 300mg (unless contraindicated).
- Start oral β-blocker (unless contraindicated).

Treatment

Primary percutaneous coronary intervention or primary angioplasty

Primary angioplasty is increasingly the main or first treatment for patients suffering an MI, as it is the most effective way of re-establishing coronary artery flow, thus limiting damage to the heart muscle. It re-establishes coronary flow in more cases than thrombolysis, but it needs to be delivered quickly or it may lose some of the advantages. There is also evidence of the longer-term benefits of primary angioplasty over thrombolysis, but primary angioplasty facilities are still restricted to some areas due to resources. Where there is local/regional agreement, patients suffering from an MI will be conveyed to the nearest PCI facility, as opposed to the nearest ED. However, it should always be considered for patients in cardiogenic shock or for those for whom thrombolytics are contraindicated.

Preparation for primary coronary intervention

Pre-treatment with clopidogrel 300–600mg and use of glycoprotein IIb/IIIa inhibitors may be requested prior to transfer. In addition, IV β-blockers have additional proven benefit for reducing mortality.

During transfer, ongoing cardiac monitoring and access to a defibrillator and resuscitation equipment are essential. Analgesia may be required (IV nitrates and possibly opiates). ∴ A suitable escort must go with the patient to ensure continuity of care and to offer constant reassurance to the patient. The family and significant others must also be kept informed of the progress, as this can be a stressful event for them as well.

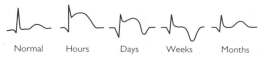

Fig. 8.10 ECG changes following MI.

(Reproduced with permission from Wyatt, J., et al. (2012). *Oxford Handbook of Emergency Medicine*, 4th edn, fig. 3.5, p. 73. Oxford University Press, Oxford.)

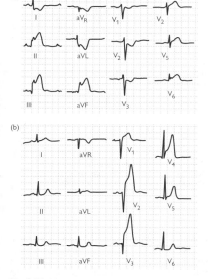

Fig. 8.11 (a) Acute inferolateral infarction with 'reciprocal' ST changes in I, aVL, and V2–V3. (b) Acute anteroseptal infarction with minimal 'reciprocal' ST changes in III and aVF.

(Reproduced with permission from Wyatt, J., et al. (2012). *Oxford Handbook of Emergency Medicine*, 4th edn, figs 3.6 and 3.7, p. 73. Oxford University Press, Oxford.)

Thrombolysis for acute myocardial infarction

Thrombolysis is indicated where:
- symptoms of AMI <12h;
- ECG criteria are met;
- no PCI availability;
- there are no contraindications (for contraindications, ➲ see Box 8.5).

▶ Contraindications warrant immediate senior review for risk assessment and possible PCI.

Box 8.5 Contraindications to fibrinolytic therapy

Absolute contraindications
- Haemorrhagic stroke or stroke of unknown origin at any time.
- Ischaemic stroke in preceding 6 months.
- CNS trauma or neoplasms.
- Recent major trauma/surgery/head injury (within preceding 3wk).
- GI bleeding within the last month.
- Known bleeding disorder.
- Aortic dissection.
- Non-compressible punctures (e.g. liver biopsy, lumbar puncture).

Relative contraindications
- TIA in preceding 6 months.
- Oral anticoagulant therapy.
- Pregnancy or within 1wk post-partum.
- Refractory hypotension (systolic BP >100mmHg and/or diastolic BP >110mmHg).
- Advanced liver disease.
- Infective endocarditis.
- Active peptic ulcer.
- Refractory resuscitation.

Taskforce on the Management of ST-segment elevation, acute myocardial infarction of the European Society of Cardiology (2008). Management of acute myocardial infarction in patients presenting with persistent ST-segment elevation, *European Heart Journal* **29**, 9–45.

Thrombolytic agents

There are two groups of thrombolytic agents: fibrin-specific, e.g. tenecteplase, and non-fibrin-specific, e.g. streptokinase (➲ see Table 8.5). Hospital policy should be reviewed, as practice differs, with some hospitals using only one type of agent for all patients (e.g. tenecteplase) and others using a combination of streptokinase and fibrin-specific agents, depending on the location of the AMI.

Heparin for fibrin-specific agents (check local policy)
- 4000–5000 units IV bolus.
- LMWH, e.g. enoxaparin 1mg/kg bd (NB: Max 100mg bd for tenecteplase in first 24h) or 800–1000 units/h IV, adjusted to aPTT × 2 control.

Nursing care/alerts for patients having streptokinase

Hypotension with streptokinase is common but is rarely 2° to anaphylaxis. Maintain meticulous monitoring of BP and pulse every 2–5min, initially for first 15min and then as the condition dictates. If the patient develops hypotension, do the following.

- Stop the infusion.
- Lie the patient flat (if tolerated).
- Administer a fluid challenge of 250–500mL of 0.9% saline, if required.
- Restart infusion at 50% of the original rate, and ↑ once BP recovers.
- If hypotensive again, call for medical assistance and review lytic agent.
- Treat true anaphylaxis with prompt IM adrenaline. Avoid steroids, if possible, due to ↑ risk of myocardial rupture post-AMI.

Indications of reperfusion

- The most sensitive/specific indication is 50% resolution of ST segment elevation at 90min post-thrombolysis.
- Pain-free (remember opiates given, etc.).
- Arrhythmias (commonly idioventricular) also indicate reperfusion.
- Failure to demonstrate reperfusion is a medical emergency requiring immediate intervention.

Table 8.5 Thrombolytic agents

Drug	Administration	Comments
Streptokinase	Dissolve 1.5 million IU in 100mL of 0.9% saline, and administer over 1h via infusion pump	High incidence of hypotension (20–25%) and anaphylaxis. Slightly lower incidence of haemorrhagic stroke, but less effective agent. Does not require immediate heparin. Can be given only once in patient's lifetime. Avoid if patient hypotensive. Consider a fibrin-specific agent for all anterior AMI
Tenecteplase	Weight-adjusted (increments of 10kg) single-bolus agent. Given over 10s	Requires heparin bolus pre-dose with infusion/SC doses post-administration
Reteplase	Non-weight-adjusted twin-bolus drug, with doses given 30min apart. Given over 2min	Requires heparin bolus pre-dose with infusion/SC doses post-administration
Alteplase (rTPA)	Weight-adjusted infusion administered over 90min. Dose- and rate-dependent on onset of symptoms	Requires heparin bolus pre-/post-administration. Complex regime—has a specific role in PE

Pericarditis

Pericarditis is caused by inflammation of the pericardium, resulting in pain that may be associated with mild pyrexia and an audible 'pericardial rub'.

Causes
- AMI (Dressler's syndrome or large AMI involving atria).
- Bacterial or viral infection.
- TB (± HIV).
- Cancer (typically within chest cavity, e.g. lung).
- Rheumatic fever.
- Uraemia.
- Collagen disease (e.g. systemic lupus erythematosus (SLE)).
- Trauma (e.g. fracture of sternum, cardiac surgery, or local radiotherapy).
- Drugs.

Signs and symptoms
- Patients complain of sharp retrosternal pain that is worse on inspiration, movement, swallowing, or lying down.
- Sitting forward/expanding the thoracic cavity may relieve pain.
- Pain may radiate or be localized.
- Tachycardia.
- A pericardial rub (like walking through snow) may be heard. Its absence does not exclude diagnosis.
- Mild pyrexia.

Investigations
- ECG, FBC, ESR, U&E, CRP, CXR, and, if in AF/flutter, thyroid function.
- Clinical history.

ECG (➲ see Fig. 8.12) classically shows concave ST elevation, which is widespread but in the early stages can be localized. T wave changes are possible (to include flattening/inversion), and PR segment depression has been noted. Careful history and ECG examination are required to avoid misdiagnosis, e.g. AMI.

Treatment
Is primarily pain relief with non-steroidal anti-inflammatory drug (NSAID) (aspirin 600mg or ibuprofen) and assessment for pathological disease. Consider echocardiogram.

Dressler's syndrome is caused by an autoimmune response to damaged cardiac tissue and consists of pericarditis, fever, and pericardial effusion. It can occur 3–14 days post-AMI/cardiac surgery and requires admission—ideally to CCU/cardiology ward.

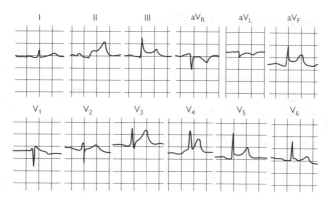

Fig. 8.12 ECG of pericarditis.

(Reproduced with permission from Wyatt, J., et al. (2012). *Oxford Handbook of Emergency Medicine*, 4th edn, fig. 3.10, p. 79. Oxford University Press, Oxford.)

Myocarditis

Is a medical emergency and can present similarly to AMI/pericarditis with ECG ST segment changes. Again the history is the key; myocarditis can be caused by bacterial or viral infection. Diagnosis can be difficult, depending on the severity, but raised cardiac markers (CK/TnT/TnI) mandate admission to CCU/cardiology ward.

Left ventricular failure

This is a common emergency with patients presenting with chest pain, SOB or acute respiratory distress, anxiety/agitation, and, in some cases, with a ↓ GCS.

Nursing assessment/intervention

As for cardiovascular assessment, with specific management guided by the patient's BP.

- Sit upright if GCS/BP allows.
- Give supplementary O₂ as required; *aim at achieving SaO₂ >94% or 88– 92% if the patient has COPD.*
- Record 12-lead ECG, BP, pulse, RR, SpO₂.
- Gain IV access and bloods for U&E, FBC.
- Administer IV nitrates if systolic BP ≥100mmHg.
- Administer IV furosemide.
- Opiates reduce LV pre- and after-load (ventricular stress) and ↓ anxiety.

Hypertensive left ventricular failure

Patients presenting in LVF frequently have hypertension. These patients respond to aggressive management, which may include the following:

- Nitrates: initially sublingual (SL) GTN or 2–9mg buccal nitrates.
- IV nitrates are the main treatment. Record BP every 5min, and titrate GTN according to systolic BP (aim for >100mmHg).
- Administer IV furosemide.
- The hypoxic or tiring patient will benefit from CPAP (consider intubation).
- Nebulized β₂-agonist (bronchospasm is common, but nebulizing β₂- agonist may ↑ HR).
- Treat underlying cause, e.g. AMI or fast AF.

All patients with LVF will require admission and physician review. Patients should be admitted to CCU.

Cardiogenic shock

▶▶ This is a significant medical emergency requiring immediate support from senior medical staff. Cardiogenic shock has a high mortality.

Causes are numerous, with the most common being AMI with marked loss of LV function, development of a ventricular septal defect, or rupture of a papillary muscle. The commonest chronic cause is decompensated heart failure 2° to a systemic illness.

Nursing assessment

These are very unwell patients who will appear clinically shocked.

Signs and symptoms
- Pale, cold, clammy, and cyanosed.
- Severely hypotensive due to reduced cardiac output.
- Tachycardia to compensate initially followed by bradycardia and arrhythmias.
- Dyspnoea.

Nursing intervention

- Administer high-flow O_2—*aim at achieving SaO_2 >94% or 88–92% if the patient has COPD.*
- Vital signs: temperature, BP, pulse, RR, SpO_2.
- Attach the patient to a cardiac monitor with a defibrillator nearby.
- Record ECG. This may show ventricular ectopic beats.
- Assess pain, and give analgesia and an anti-emetic as prescribed.
- Request CXR.
- Establish IV access, and collect blood for FBC, U&E (Mg^{2+} priority), CK, appropriately timed TnI/TnT (early may be negative), and coagulation screen.
- CVP access is desirable.
- Maintain strict fluid balance (urethral catheterization may be necessary).
- IV fluids may be needed but should be titrated to CVP and LV function.
- Ensure the administration of medication as prescribed, i.e. antibiotics, inotropic drugs.
- Offer reassurance and support to the patient and family.

Specific treatment

Depending on the response to resuscitation, admission to the ICU/CCU should be expedited for ongoing management.
- Treatment may include angioplasty or thrombolysis for AMI (angioplasty is preferred, if available).
- Inotropes, nitrates, and vasodilatory drugs may be used to aid and support the cardiovascular system.
- An intra-aortic balloon pump may be required to support the function of the LV.

Shock

By definition, shock is a combination of failure to perfuse and failure to oxygenate vital organs. Shock is a clinical emergency requiring prompt identification. Treatment must be aimed at the cause of shock, and not generic 'blind' fluid resuscitation.

Types of shock

- Compensated shock. The body strives to meet oxygenation and perfusion, and uses compensation mechanisms to achieve this: ↑ RR, vasoconstriction, and tachycardia. At this point, BP is maintained, with 'pulse pressure narrowing' as diastolic BP rises to meet systolic BP.
- Decompensated shock is the failure of the body to support perfusion. It is characterized by hypotension.
- Hypovolaemia may be due to loss of circulating fluid, and not just from trauma, e.g. burns, dehydration.
- Pump failure. Typically cardiogenic 2° to AMI, although drug-induced (e.g. β-blockers) and other causes should be considered.
- Distributive shock. 2° movement of fluid due to vasodilatation primarily due to anaphylaxis or sepsis. It resembles hypovolaemia, but fluid loss is not visible. An early indicator of distributive shock is a widened pulse pressure, as the diastolic BP ↓.
- Neurogenic shock is another form of distributive shock and is caused by stimulation of the autonomic nervous system, resulting in vasodilatation. This is often called spinal shock, although the same process occurs during 'fainting'.
- Obstructive shock is due to 'obstruction of blood flow', e.g. 2° to tension pneumothorax, PE, or cardiac tamponade.

Diagnosis

- The typical picture of tachycardia and hypotension is a late sign and indicates decompensated shock.
- Greater use of RR, capillary refill, pulse pressure, anxiety/confusion, drowsiness, and clinical suspicion is required.
- A key nursing observation is dizziness and/or drop in BP when the patient sits up.
- ABG monitoring of lactate (± base excess) can indicate the degree of inadequate tissue perfusion.
- An ↑ early warning score can indicate shock.

Generic treatment

This is aimed at improving perfusion. Oxygenation and the treatment of the underlying cause of shock are the clinical priorities.

- Administer high-flow O_2—*aim at achieving SaO$_2$ >94% or 88–92% if the patient has COPD.*
- Fluid challenge and/or fluid resuscitation.
- Specific treatment, depending on the cause of shock.
- Blood.

Fluid resuscitation
- Typically a 20mL/kg bolus of crystalloid (0.9% saline) is used to improve perfusion.
- Haemodynamic status post-fluid resuscitation should be assessed.
- Fluid resuscitation has to be carefully managed—senior help is required.
- Over-resuscitation with crystalloid will dilute the circulatory volume and clotting factors.
- Extreme caution is necessary in cardiogenic shock or shock related to dissection of abdominal aortic aneurysm (AAA) or penetrating trauma.

Recent evidence from battlefield resuscitation has identified the need for major trauma transfusion guidelines (➜ see Guides to assessment, pp. 490–6).
- Patients who are at risk of clotting problems through haemorrhage and fluid resuscitation should receive adequate FFP and supplementary platelets, not just packed cells.
- Senior transfusion advice should be sought in fluid resuscitation in major trauma.

Septic shock

Septic shock is defined as sepsis-induced hypotension persisting despite adequate fluid resuscitation. Sepsis is a systemic response to infection, leading to acute organ dysfunction 2° to documented or suspected infection. Similar to polytrauma, AMI, or stroke, the speed and appropriateness of therapy administered in the initial hours after severe sepsis develops are likely to influence outcome. Treatment of septic shock is the same as for all types of shock, but blood cultures and early administration of broad-spectrum antibacterial agents and IV fluids are vital.

▶▶ Do not delay antibacterial therapy if there is difficulty in obtaining blood cultures, as even small delays in administration of antibiotics ↑ mortality.

Systemic inflammatory response syndrome

Systemic inflammatory response syndrome (SIRS) suggests an inflammatory response; it can be used as a screening tool for sepsis. Sepsis is present when infection accompanies at least two of the criteria in Table 8.6 (separate criteria apply for paediatrics). Infection with SIRS has a higher mortality risk than infection without SIRS.

Table 8.6 Adult SIRS criteria: positive if two or more signs present

Sign	Parameters
Temperature	>38°C (100.4°F) or <36°C (96.8°F)
HR	>90
RR	>20 or $PaCO_2$ <32mmHg
WBC	<4000 cells/mm³ or >12 000 cells/mm³ or >10% immature neutrophils (band neutrophils)

Nursing assessment

These are very unwell patients with infection, documented or suspected, and some (not all) of the following.

Signs and symptoms
- Fever (>38.3°C).
- Hypothermia (core temperature <36°C).
- HR >90/min.
- Systolic BP <90mmHg, mean arterial pressure (MAP) <70mmHg, or systolic BP ↓ >40mmHg in adults.
- ↓ capillary refill or mottling.
- Tachypnoeic/dyspnoeic with associated arterial hypoxaemia.
- Altered mental status.
- Ileus (absent bowel sounds).
- Significant oedema or positive fluid balance (>20mL/kg over 24h).
- Acute oliguria (urine output <0.5mL/kg/h for at least 2h, despite adequate fluid resuscitation).
- Hyperglycaemia (>7.7mmol/L) in the absence of diabetes.
- Raised CRP.
- Raised WBCs.
- Raised creatinine.
- Coagulation abnormalities.
- Hyperlactataemia.

Nursing intervention

- Administer high-flow O_2—*aim at achieving SaO_2 >94% or 88–92% if the patient has COPD.*
- Vital signs: temperature, BP, pulse, RR, SpO_2.
- Attach the patient to a cardiac monitor with a defibrillator nearby.
- Record ECG.
- Assess pain, and give analgesia and an anti-emetic as prescribed.
- Request CXR.
- Establish IV access, and collect blood for cultures, FBC, U&E, and coagulation screen.
- CVP access is desirable.
- Maintain strict fluid balance (urethral catheterization may be necessary).
- IV fluids will be needed but should be titrated to CVP and LV function.
- Ensure the administration of medication as prescribed, i.e. antibiotics, inotropic drugs.
- Offer reassurance and support to the patient and family.

Further reading

Dellinger RP, Levy MM, Rhodes A, *et al.*; Surviving Sepsis Campaign Guidelines Committee including the Pediatric Subgroup (2013). Surviving sepsis campaign: international guidelines for management of severe sepsis and septic shock: 2012. *Crit Care Med* **41**, 580–637.

Sudden cardiac death

Sudden cardiac death (SCD) is a direct result of a life-threatening cardiac arrhythmia, normally VF. The result is an abrupt loss of pulse and consciousness caused by an unexpected failure in the heart's ability to function effectively. The only immediate definitive treatment is defibrillation as soon as possible, and, as such, the condition carries a very high mortality rate; CPR should be undertaken, whilst waiting for the definitive treatment (defibrillation) to occur. The chances of survival ↓ ~10% with every minute of delay.

Although pre-existing heart disease is a common cause of cardiac arrest, SCD is unpredictable; 80% of young SCD will occur with no prior symptoms.

When symptoms do occur, they include:
- chest pain (exercise-related is a red flag);
- syncope;
- palpitations;
- breathlessness (disproportionate to the amount of exercise);
- dizziness.

Identified risk factors

- Known coronary artery disease (CAD).
- Poor ejection fraction (EF) <35%.
- Family history of SCD.
- Hypertrophic cardiomyopathy.
- Inherited congenital or structural abnormalities.
- Inherited channelopathies (Brugada syndrome, long QT syndromes, etc.).
- Unexplained syncopal episodes.
- Failed SCD.

The nurse in the ED should be alert to the possibility of identifying this group of patients, where possible, to allow escalation for senior/cardiology review. This would allow thorough investigation to take place and, where necessary, to enable protection to be offered via implantable cardioverting defibrillator (ICD) device, if appropriate.

Further reading

Papadakis M, Sharma S, Cox S, Sheppard MN, Panoulas VF, and Behr ER (2009). The magnitude of sudden cardiac death in the young: a death certificate-based review in England and Wales. *Europace* **11**, 1353–8.

Anaphylaxis

Anaphylaxis is caused by an adverse reaction to a foreign protein; its onset can be rapid or more gradual (min/h) (➔ see Fig. 8.13).

The reluctance to administer adrenaline can be fatal.

Specific reactions

Respiratory
Upper airway involvement is common. Systemic respiratory reactions, such as lip tingling and tongue swelling, are significant. Bronchospasm is common, as the lung is sensitive to histamine. This can be particularly the case in those who suffer from asthma.

Skin
A widespread raised red rash, itching, and angio-oedema. Widely dispersed skin symptoms indicate a systemic reaction.

Gastrointestinal tract
Abdominal pain/cramps ± diarrhoea and vomiting are common and are due to reduced perfusion to the bowel and/or attempts to expel ingested foreign material. The risk of misdiagnosing food poisoning needs to be avoided.

Circulation
Anaphylaxis results in distributive shock, but BP may be maintained due to compensatory strategies. This often results in delayed administration of adrenaline.

Adrenaline

Administration of adrenaline is lifesaving. It should be given immediately if the patient has any life-threatening airway (stridor), breathing (bronchospasm), or circulation (shock) features. Adrenaline is administered by IM injection. IV injection is discouraged. Patients with adrenaline auto-injectors (e.g. Epi-Pen®) will tend to self-administer before arrival. Additional adrenaline may be required.

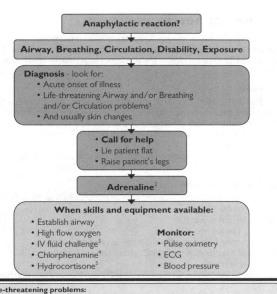

Anaphylactic reaction?

Airway, Breathing, Circulation, Disability, Exposure

Diagnosis - look for:
• Acute onset of illness
• Life-threatening Airway and/or Breathing and/or Circulation problems[1]
• And usually skin changes

• **Call for help**
• Lie patient flat
• Raise patient's legs

Adrenaline[2]

When skills and equipment available:
• Establish airway
• High flow oxygen
• IV fluid challenge[3]
• Chlorphenamine[4]
• Hydrocortisone[5]

Monitor:
• Pulse oximetry
• ECG
• Blood pressure

1 Life-threatening problems:
Airway: swelling, hoarseness, stridor
Breathing: rapid breathing, wheeze, fatigue, cyanosis, SpO_2 < 92%, confusion
Circulation: pale, clammy, low blood pressure, faintness, drowsy/coma

2 Adrenaline *(give IM unless experienced with IV adrenaline)*
IM doses of 1:1000 adrenaline (repeat after 5 min if no better)
• Adult   500 micrograms IM (0.5mL)
• Child more than 12 years: 500 micrograms IM (0.5 mL)
• Child 6–12 years: 300 micrograms IM (0.3mL)
• Child less than 6 years: 150 micrograms IM (0.15mL)

Adrenaline IV to be given **only by experienced specialists**
Titrate: Adults 50 micrograms; Children 1 microgram/kg

3 IV fluid challenge:
Adult - 500–1000 mL
Child - crystalloid 20 mL/kg

Stop IV colloid
if this might be the cause
of anaphylaxis

	4 Chlorphenamine (IM or slow IV)	**5 Hydrocortisone** (IM or slow IV)
Adult or child more than 12 years	10 mg	200 mg
Child 6–12 years	5 mg	100 mg
Child 6 months to 6 years	2.5 mg	50 mg
Child less than 6 months	250 micrograms/kg	25 mg

Fig. 8.13 Anaphylaxis algorithm.
(Reproduced with the kind permission of the Resuscitation Council (UK). 2015 Guidelines.)

Abdominal aortic aneurysm

AAA is a major cause of death, particularly in middle-aged/elderly ♂. Diagnosis is at times difficult, particularly following sudden collapse. Triage nurses need to retain a high index of suspicion in middle-aged/elderly ♂ with back or loin pain. Misdiagnosis of renal colic delays definitive treatment.

Diagnosis

- Abdominal/epigastric or back pain are classic signs, and the presence of a palpable abdominal mass confirms the diagnosis if it is detectable.
- Rupture may present with epigastric pain radiating to the back.
- Abdominal ultrasound is helpful, but abdominal CT provides the definitive diagnosis.
- The risks/benefits of haemodynamically unstable patients going to CT should be assessed thoroughly on a case-by-case basis.

Nursing intervention

- Administer high-flow O$_2$—*aim at achieving SaO$_2$ >94% or 88–92% if the patient has COPD.*
- Assess BP, pulse, and RR.
- Attach a cardiac monitor.
- Obtain senior help immediately: surgeons and anaesthetists.
- Secure IV lines; obtain U&E, FBC, group and save, glucose, LFT, coagulation screen.
- Request blood (follow local protocols) (➔ see Massive haemorrhage, p. 493).
- Maintain a systolic BP of 80–90mmHg, using IV fluids (can be controversial due to risk of rupture).
- Assess pain, and give analgesia.
- Request CXR and abdominal X-ray, and obtain a 12-lead ECG.

▶▶ The priority is to move to theatre. Time in the resuscitation room should not delay transfer. Local policy may dictate that the patient is transferred to a regional hospital or that a vascular surgeon travels to the patient.

Cardiac arrest following AAA is either due to massive hypovolaemia following rupture and is rapidly fatal without surgical intervention or is due to parasympathetic activity following the tearing of the inner aortic wall—this responds promptly to atropine ± low-level fluids.

Thoracic aortic dissection

This is tearing of the thoracic aorta and is classified as type A involving the ascending aorta and/or aortic arch, or type B involving the descending aorta. It is most commonly associated with hypertension and connective tissue disorders. The highest incidence occurs in individuals 50–70y old, with a ♂:♀ ratio of 2:1. In 96% of presentations, pain is typically sudden, severe, and tearing in nature—radiating to the patient's back. Severe hypotension on presentation is evidence of a poor prognostic outcome. Patients with types A and B can present with either hyper- or hypotension.

Investigation (to confirm diagnosis)

- CXR (this can be normal) may show pleural effusion, widened mediastinum, and/or calcified aorta.
- ECG. No specific changes associated with dissection, but 30% of the time will show evidence of LV hypertrophy. A further 30% will be normal. ECG may show ischaemic changes if the coronary arteries are involved.
- Echocardiogram may enable type A to be identified.
- CTPA/MRI are necessary for a definitive diagnosis.

Nursing intervention

- Administer high-flow O_2—aim at achieving SaO_2 >94% or 88–92% if the patient has COPD.
- Attach the patient to a cardiac monitor.
- Maintain frequent monitoring of all vital signs, especially BP (beware pseudohypotension due to involvement of the brachiocephalic and left subclavian arteries supplying the right and left arms, respectively).
- BP should be recorded for both the left and right side. All pulses should be checked.
- Ensure the patient is given opiate analgesia and an anti-emetic.
- Secure IV access. Obtain U&E, FBC, and group and save. Cross-match for at least 6 units, and inform the lab by phone of probable diagnosis.
- Assist in the insertion of an arterial line (➲ see Arterial line insertion and invasive blood pressure monitoring, pp. 658–9).
- Offer support to the patient, and keep the family informed.
- Specific treatment involves BP control (e.g. IV β-blockers) and advice from cardiologists/cardiothoracic team.
- Accompany the patient to theatre if surgery is decided on.

Deep venous thrombosis

DVT is an increasingly common presentation in the minors area of the ED due to an ↑ public knowledge of the risks. It is difficult to diagnose, leading to under- and overdiagnoses. The principal clinical concern is development of PE.

Diagnosis

This is initially based on risk factors:
- immobility (do not forget flights or chair/bed rest);
- recent surgery (particularly lower leg/pelvis);
- cancer;
- IV drug use;
- smoking;
- pregnancy/pelvic mass;
- contraceptive pill;
- overweight;
- previous DVT/PE;
- thrombophilia.

Clinical features

- Calf pain and local swelling are the classic signs of a DVT, along with tenderness, warmth, and distension of superficial veins.
- Clinical signs also resemble those of cellulitis (which may coexist with a DVT), muscular injury, or ruptured Baker's cyst.

∴ Clinical examination and history may be insufficient to exclude DVT. Final diagnosis is typically based on a combination of D-dimer with Doppler ultrasound/venogram and risk assessment, e.g. Wells criteria (➲ see Table 8.7). This will depend on local policy.

Treatment

Depending on the risk, treatment may be started before formal diagnosis and with GP follow-up for ongoing management ± oral warfarin therapy.

Further reading

National Institute for Health and Clinical Excellence (2012). *Two level Wells score template for deep vein thrombosis and pulmonary embolism.* CG144. National Institute for Health and Care Excellence, London.

Table 8.7 Two-level DVT Wells score

Clinical feature	Points	Patient score
Active cancer (treatment ongoing, within 6 months, or palliative)	1	
Paralysis, paresis, or recent plaster immobilization of the lower extremities	1	
Recently bedridden for 3 days or more, or major surgery within 12wk requiring general or regional anaesthesia	1	
Localized tenderness along the distribution of the deep venous system	1	
Entire leg swollen	1	
Calf swelling at least 3cm larger than asymptomatic side	1	
Pitting oedema confined to the symptomatic leg	1	
Collateral superficial veins (non-varicose)	1	
Previously documented DVT	1	
An alternative diagnosis is at least as likely as DVT	−2	
Clinical probability simplified score		
DVT likely	2 points or more	
DVT unlikely	1 point or less	

NICE Clinical Guideline 144: Two level Wells score template for deep vein thrombosis and pulmonary embolism – June 2012.

Musculoskeletal injuries

Introduction

Patients with musculoskeletal injuries represent ~25% of the ED workload.

These injuries may be simple fractures or can be life- or limb-threatening. ED nurses should be able to assess musculoskeletal injuries and identify life- or limb-threatening trauma, some of which may not be immediately apparent. ENPs will be expected to assess, diagnose, treat, or refer many straightforward fractures.

This chapter differs from other chapters in that it takes into account that many patients presenting with musculoskeletal injuries and ailments may be managed solely by an ENP.

An understanding of the anatomy is essential for the accurate assessment and management of musculoskeletal injuries.

Anatomy

The skeletal system provides the shape and form for our bodies, in addition to providing support and protection, allowing bodily movement, producing RBCs, and storing minerals. The human skeleton is divided into two distinct parts.

- The axial skeleton consists of bones that form the axis of the body, which supports and protects the organs of the head, neck, and trunk. These bones include the skull, sternum, ribs, and vertebral column.
- The appendicular skeleton consists of the upper limbs, lower limbs, and pelvic girdle. The sacrum and coccyx are considered to be part of the vertebrae.

The internal organs are protected by the skeletal system, and fracture of any bony structure may cause associated damage to the soft tissue and viscera. Blood cells are produced by the marrow located in some bones. Fractures to long bones, in particular, can result in a significant loss of circulating volume.

- *Joints* are the point where articulating bones meet. They are encased in a capsule and lubricated with synovial fluid. Joint movements include abduction, adduction, flexion, extension, and rotation.
- *Muscle* is the contractile tissue that attaches to a tendon or bone to aid movement.
- *Tendon* is the fibrous tissue that connects muscle to bone.
- *Ligament* is the fibrous connective tissue that connects bone to bone.

Fractures

A fracture is a partial or complete breach in the continuity of a bone. Fractures can be open or closed, and displaced or undisplaced. They are also classified in relation to their anatomical location (e.g. proximal, distal, shaft, head, or base).

Any of the following types of fracture may occur.

- *Simple*—single transverse fracture of bone, with only two main fragments.
- *Transverse*—at 90° to the axis of the bone.
- *Oblique*—at 45° to the axis of the bone, with only two main fragments.
- *Spiral*—seen in long bones as a result of twisting injuries and twists around the bone shaft. Consider the possibility of NAI and the need for safeguarding in adults and children.
- *Comminuted*—complex fracture resulting in >2 fragments.
- *Crush*—loss of bone due to compression.
- *Wedge*—compression to one area of bone resulting in a wedge shape (e.g. vertebra).
- *Burst*—comminuted compression fracture with scattering of fragments.
- *Impacted*—bone ends driven into each other.
- *Avulsion*—bony attachment of a ligament or muscle is pulled off.
- *Hairline*—barely visible lucency, with no discernible displacement.
- *Greenstick*—buckling or bending of immature bones, most commonly seen in children.
- *Pathological*—fracture due to underlying disease (e.g. osteoporosis, Paget's disease).
- *Stress*—certain bones are prone to fracture after repetitive minor injury (e.g. metatarsal).
- *Fracture dislocation*—fracture adjacent to, or in combination with, a dislocated joint.

Musculoskeletal assessment

When assessing patients with musculoskeletal injury, always consider spinal injury, and act to prevent further injury. Advanced trauma life support (ATLS) guidelines should take precedence, and life-threatening injuries should be dealt with immediately.

History taking

This should include the following:
- recent trauma;
- underlying orthopaedic condition;
- relevant medical history;
- current medications;
- known allergy.

Ask about the mechanism of injury, the degree of force used, and how long the patient was exposed to the force. Inconsistencies between the history and injury should raise suspicion of abuse, especially if the patient is a child or vulnerable adult.

Ask about, and document, pain or sensory loss—pain distal to the injury may suggest vascular involvement. Likewise, any sensory loss distal to the injury may indicate neurological insult.

The five Ps

When assessing an injured extremity, use the 'five Ps':
- Pain;
- Pallor;
- Pulselessness;
- Paraesthesiae;
- Paralysis.

Inspection

- Observe the skin colour, and note any bruising, abrasions, laceration, puncture wounds, or critical skin.
- Note any deformity, swelling, or oedema around the wounded area, and compare it with the uninjured limb.
- Observe for pain and the patient's ability to move the affected limb.

▶▶ If there is gross deformity (e.g. joint dislocation), summon help immediately. This is an orthopaedic emergency.

Palpation

Carefully palpate the injured area to assess skin temperature and specific areas of pain; feel for pulses, and assess capillary refill. Absence of pulses or sensation, particularly if distal to the injury, suggests neurovascular compromise. Crepitus may be felt with movement of the injured limb.

▶▶ If neurovascular compromise is identified, summon help immediately.

Nursing interventions

Life-threatening features must be dealt with before limb-threatening features. General nursing management of musculoskeletal injuries should focus on the following.

- Pain. Immobilizing the area may give initial relief, but opiate analgesia is usually indicated in bony injuries.
- Vital signs. Record BP, pulse rate, RR, temperature, and O_2 saturation. If there is a history of dizziness or blackout prior to the injury, record ECG and CBG.
- Establishing IV access, and blood tests for FBC, U&E, coagulation studies, and group and save. Commence infusion of fluids, as prescribed, and chart accordingly.
- Immobilization. Various splints may be used, but vascular status needs to be established prior to application, and access to pulse points must be ensured for ongoing monitoring. If there is no apparent neurovascular injury, the injured limb should be immobilized in its presenting position.
- Elevation of the injured limb aids venous return and helps to minimize swelling.
- Remove jewellery and tight clothing. If jewellery needs to be cut off, where possible, obtain written consent from the patient or a relative.

Additional interventions

- Where appropriate, the assessing nurse should request X-rays.
- Any open wounds should be covered with sterile dressings, until they can be thoroughly aseptically cleaned.
- Patients who have open fractures should be given IV antibiotics. Ensure that medications are given, as prescribed.
- The patient's tetanus status should be established, and, where there is doubt, a booster should be given (➋ see Box 9.3).
- Assist with manipulation of the fracture and the application of a plaster cast or traction.
- Ensure pressure area care for vulnerable patients (assess the Waterlow score).
- Reassure and comfort the patient, and keep their relatives informed.
- Administer analgesia, as prescribed, and evaluate its effect.

Fractures of the thoracic and lumbar spine

These are classified according to the pattern of injury.
- Compression fracture—the anterior aspect. The vertebra breaks and loses height. This type of fracture is usually stable and is rarely associated with neurological problems.
- Axial burst fracture—often caused by a fall from a height, with the patient landing on their feet.
- Flexion/distraction fracture—the vertebra is literally pulled apart (e.g. in a head-on car crash, in which the upper body is thrown forward, whilst the pelvis is stabilized by the seat belt).
- Transverse process fracture—this type of fracture results from rotation or extreme sideways bending, and usually does not affect stability.
- Fracture dislocation—this is an unstable injury involving bone and/ or soft tissue, in which one vertebra may become displaced from the adjacent one.

Treatment

This is aimed at protecting nerve function, and restoring alignment and stability of the spine. Compression fractures and some burst fractures are treated conservatively. Some injuries, such as an unstable burst fracture, flexion–distraction injury, or fracture–dislocation, may require surgical intervention. Surgery realigns the spinal column and holds it together, using metal plates and screws (internal fixation) and/or spinal fusion.

Torticollis

Torticollis is an acquired condition, in which the neck appears to be in a twisted or bent position. It is caused by involuntary contractions of the neck muscles, leading to abnormal postures and movements of the head. If there is a history of trauma, refer the patient for a full clinical assessment.

If there is no history of trauma, exclude neurological signs and symptoms.

- Reassure the patient.
- Advise the patient on analgesia.
- Refer them to physiotherapy services.

Traumatic neck sprain (whiplash)

Traumatic neck sprain (commonly referred to as 'whiplash') is a common presentation in the ED. It occurs when the soft tissues in the neck are strained as a result of a sudden jerk. It most commonly occurs after road traffic accidents but can also occur in sporting injuries.

History and examination

If there is a significant mechanism of injury (e.g. fall from a height, axial loading injury) or there are abnormal neurological signs (e.g. numbness, paraesthesiae), or if there is cervical bony tenderness or marked pain in the midline, immobilize the C-spine, and refer the patient immediately. In the absence of any of the above signs or symptoms:

- give analgesia and NSAIDs;
- encourage the patient to resume normal routine as soon as possible;
- refer them to physiotherapy services;
- be meticulous in documenting findings, as these injuries are often the subject of insurance claims. Avoid using the term 'whiplash'.

High-risk features

- Significant mechanism of injury.
- Tenderness over spinous processes.
- Neurological signs and symptoms.
- Severe pain.
- Patient holding their own head.

If these features are present, immobilize the patient, and refer them for immediate medical assessment.

▶ Traumatic neck sprain is a diagnosis that is only made after significant injury has been ruled out. Formal rules for C-spine clearance should be used to assess the need for X-ray (➲ see C-spine assessment, pp. 688–9).

Shoulder and clavicle injuries

Clavicle fractures

Most clavicle fractures can be treated conservatively, often requiring simple analgesia, a broad arm sling, and orthopaedic follow-up. Occasionally, when there is severe displacement of the clavicle or tenting of the skin, orthopaedic intervention may be required.

Shoulder injuries

Dislocation of the shoulder is common in adults. This follows an injury that is compatible with shoulder displacement (e.g. fall on to an outstretched arm). Anterior dislocation is commoner than posterior dislocation. Consider posterior dislocation if the mechanism of injury is attributed to a fit or a direct blow to the shoulder. Diagnosis can often be made clinically, as the patient will have severe pain in their shoulder and will be holding their arm to their chest at the elbow.

On examination, the contours of the shoulder appear different and less defined. Careful examination for the integrity of the axillary nerve must be performed, assessing sensation to touch and pinprick over the 'regimental badge area' (the lateral aspect of the proximal humerus) and assessing the integrity of the radial nerve, looking for wrist drop.

Patients with a dislocated shoulder should be given analgesia and encouraged to relax. An X-ray should be taken to confirm the diagnosis and identify any accompanying fractures.

▶ Be aware that posterior dislocations are fairly difficult to diagnose, so always seek senior support if you are uncertain.

Reduction of shoulder dislocations

- There are three common methods used to reduce shoulder dislocations—Kocher's method, the Hippocratic method, and use of gravitational traction.
- The key to reduction is good analgesia and adequate sedation to ensure relaxation of the patient.
- Post-reduction neurovascular examination must be carried out to ensure that no entrapment of the axillary nerve has occurred during the reduction procedure.
- Post-reduction films should be taken.
- It is important to note that humeral head fractures can be a complication of overenthusiastic reduction procedures, so proceed with caution.

Evidence suggests that immobilization of the limb in a collar and cuff for 3wk is beneficial. The patient should be referred to the fracture clinic for follow-up.

Acromioclavicular joint injury

These are reasonably common injuries associated with a fall or a heavy blow directly to the shoulder. Occasionally, they result from a fall on to an outstretched hand (FOOSH). The patient will complain of pain and tenderness directly over the acromioclavicular joint (ACJ). On examination, there is normally a step deformity over the ACJ, with a marked loss of mobility. ACJ injuries are classified into three groups:

- minimal separation between the clavicle and acromion;

- obvious subluxation of the joint;
- complete dislocation of the ACJ.

Treatment involves effective analgesia and a broad arm sling. The patient should be given advice about shoulder exercises. Often physiotherapy follow-up can be helpful. For the more severe joint disruption injuries, an orthopaedic outpatient appointment should be obtained.

Soft tissue shoulder injuries

Soft tissue shoulder problems are a common presentation in the ED, as they can be very painful, restricting daily activity. Nurses should be cautious when assessing shoulder problems, bearing in mind that the shoulder is a complex joint and vulnerable to injury due to its wide range of movement.

The rotator cuff muscles consist of the following:

- supraspinatus;
- infraspinatus;
- subscapularis;
- teres minor.

These muscles strengthen the shoulder capsule and prevent dislocation. Disease of, or injuries to, the rotator cuff apparatus can be due to degeneration (old age), trauma (impingement of the supraspinatus), or acute calcification.

Minor rotator cuff strains commonly occur in athletes. They usually present with a 'twinge' that is felt in the shoulder area and show limitation in function.

Treatment consists of rest, ice, and analgesia, and then exercise and physiotherapy. If untreated, there is a risk of muscle thickening and scarring that may predispose the patient to rotator cuff tear. Complete and partial tears are more frequently seen in older patients, in whom they are caused by a process of degeneration within the tendon.

Patients complain of pain on specific range of motion (ROM) and of being unable to lie on the affected side.

Acute tendinitis/acute calcification

Deposits of calcium hydroxyapatite appear on the tendon of the supraspinatus muscle. This causes an acute vascular reaction, swelling, and pain.

- History—acute pain worsening over days, and then gradually resolving.
- X-ray may show calcification on the supraspinatus tendon.
- Treatment—NSAIDs, or perhaps none, as pain subsides over a period of several days.

Adhesive capsulitis ('frozen shoulder')

This is the spontaneous onset of pain and sensitization of the shoulder, caused by inflammation of the glenohumeral joint and its surrounding capsule. It sometimes follows an injury. There is pain and severe limitation of all movements. It also occurs after a stroke and is commoner in people with diabetes.

Subacromial bursitis

This is inflammation of the subacromial bursa. There is pain and weakness when the arm is abducted through a 60° arc and pain on deep palpation.

- If it is the tendon that is injured, rather than the bursa, there is likely to be more pain when the arm is abducted against resistance.
- Treatment consists of rest, ice, and analgesia. NSAIDs may be helpful.

Upper limb injuries

Rupture of the long head of the biceps

The tendon may rupture during activity involving the biceps muscle. The patient gives a history of sharp pain and a tearing sensation. Despite obvious deformity ('popeye deformity'), which ↑ with contraction of the biceps, the biceps strength is often maintained. Treatment consists of rest, ice, NSAIDs, and physiotherapy. Complete tears require orthopaedic referral.

Bicipital tendinitis

This often occurs as a result of injury, overuse, or ageing (as the tendon loses elasticity). Bicipital tendinitis is a fairly common complaint of swimmers, rowers, throwers, golfers, and weightlifters. The patient complains of pain and tenderness along the bicipital groove. The pain is worse during movement or activity and at night.

> ❶ Any injured limb should be assessed for the presence of the 'five Ps' that might indicate neurovascular compromise:
> * pain;
> * pallor;
> * pulselessness;
> * paraesthesiae;
> * paralysis.

Humeral shaft fractures

Fractures to the neck and shaft of the humerus are commoner in older ♀, due to osteoporosis. The integrity of the radial nerve should be assessed.
* If any deficit or displacement is found, the patient should be referred to the orthopaedic team immediately.
* If the fracture is minimally displaced and there is no neurological deficit, place in a collar and cuff, and refer to the fracture clinic.
* Severe angulation or displacement of the humeral head should be referred to the orthopaedic team.
* The practitioner who is assessing the patient should be aware that humeral fractures have been associated with elder abuse, and a careful history must be taken to determine how the injury has occurred.

Elbow injuries

Elbow injuries are a common presentation in the ED. Full range of movement usually excludes serious injury. A recent study[1] suggests that, if the patient has normal extension, flexion, and supination, they do not require emergency elbow radiographs.

Supracondylar humeral fracture

This is relatively rare in adults and often results from a FOOSH.

- Assess the neurovascular status of the limb. Give special consideration to the integrity of the radial and median nerves, as well as the brachial artery.
- Normally, the arm is very swollen and deformed around the elbow.
- On initial assessment, give analgesia; place the patient in a comfortable position, and request an X-ray.
- Most patients will require further intervention and MUA.
- Place in above-elbow back slab, and refer to the orthopaedic team.

Dislocated elbow

Elbow dislocation, which is normally associated with significant force, will be obvious on examination, as there will be significant loss of the normal triangular contours between the olecranon and epicondyles.

- Make the patient comfortable; give IV analgesia, and request X-ray.
- Perform neurovascular observations throughout.
- Obtain senior support, as urgent reduction will be needed under controlled conditions.

Olecranon bursitis

There are many causes of olecranon bursitis, but the main ones are direct trauma and infection.

- Most cases settle without any treatment—simple analgesia and rest normally suffice.
- If there are signs of infection, treat with appropriate antibiotics. (Follow local guidance on antibiotic use.)
- Very occasionally, if infection is severe, orthopaedic intervention is needed.

Epicondylitis

Commonly known as 'tennis elbow' or 'golfer's elbow', this results from overuse or strain of the common tendinous insertions of the extrinsic extensor and flexor muscles of the lateral and medial epicondyles of the humerus. Treatment includes analgesia, rest, and supportive measures. If symptoms persist, physiotherapy and referral to a soft tissue clinic for steroid injections may be required.

Reference

1 Lennon RI, Riyat MS, Hilliam R, Anathkrishnan G, and Alderson G (2007). Can a normal range of elbow movement predict a normal elbow x ray? *Emerg Med J* **24**, 86–8.

Radial head fractures

Radial head fractures are usually caused by a FOOSH. The patient may complain of pain on pronation and supination of the forearm. Fractures may not be obvious on X-ray, but evidence of an effusion (fat pad sign) is indicative of a bony injury. Loss of full extension of the forearm should also raise the suspicion of a fracture. Treatment consists of a collar and cuff or broad arm sling, analgesia, and follow-up in the fracture clinic. If there is significant angulation, seek an orthopaedic opinion.

Radial and ulnar shaft fractures

These fractures cause significant deformity or angulation of the forearm. They require immediate assessment and analgesia. Ensure that there is no neurovascular deficit, and place the arm in a broad arm sling or rest on a pillow. Refer the patient for X-rays. Always ensure that X-rays are taken of the whole forearm, thus ensuring that Monteggia and Galeazzi fractures are not missed. It is important to note that neurovascular injury is common in adults. These patients will require referral to an orthopaedic surgeon.

- A Monteggia fracture is a fracture of the ulna with associated dislocation of the radial head within the elbow joint.
- A Galeazzi fracture is a fracture of the radius with an associated injury to the distal radioulnar joint of the wrist.

Wrist injuries

Fractures within the wrist are commonly associated with a FOOSH and are often age-dependent:

- <10y: often present with greenstick/buckle fractures, with transverse fractures through the metaphysis;
- 10–16y: associated with a fracture through the epiphysis, usually Salter–Harris type II fracture (➲ see Fig. 4.11);
- 17–40y: more likely to be a scaphoid fracture;
- ≥40y: more likely to present with a Colles' or Smith's fracture.

Colles' fracture

This is usually associated with obvious clinical signs—the wrist is often deformed and swollen; the patient is unable to pronate or supinate their wrist, and they are in a great deal of discomfort or pain.

- Give analgesia.
- Place the wrist in a broad arm sling.
- Perform neurovascular observations.
- Send the patient to X-ray.
  - This fracture is associated with dorsal angulation, which produces the classical 'dinner fork deformity' on the lateral view. It is normally associated with an avulsion of the ulnar styloid process.

If displaced, or if there is notable impaction, manipulation under LA with sedation and analgesia is often required.

- Manipulation under LA is usually performed using either a haematoma block or a Bier's block.
  - A Bier's block procedure must be performed in a controlled environment. An ECG and consent must be obtained before the procedure.
  - If a Bier's block is the procedure of choice, two doctors must be present.
- Apply a back slab, and take a post-reduction X-ray.
- If the fracture is successfully reduced, the patient may be discharged and followed up in the fracture clinic.

Undisplaced fractures can be treated conservatively with a dorsal back slab and follow-up in the fracture clinic.

Smith's fracture

Smith's fracture of the wrist is associated with a palmar or volar angulation of the distal radius. It often requires surgical intervention and must be discussed with the orthopaedic team.

Barton's fracture

This is a fracture of the joint of the anterior margin of the distal radius, with proximal displacement. Treat in a volar slab, and refer to the orthopaedic team.

Hutchinson's fracture

This is an undisplaced fracture of the ulnar styloid, commonly seen in the anteroposterior (AP) projection. Patients present with a history of a

FOOSH injury and complain of pain over the ulnar styloid. Treat with analgesia, a dorsal back slab, a broad arm sling, and follow-up in the fracture clinic.

Wrist sprain

This should be treated with analgesia, wrist and hand exercises, and, if required, a wrist splint. Instruct the patient to exercise the wrist and not to keep it in the splint all the time.

Tenosynovitis

This is often associated with repetitive activity. Over a period of time, the patient develops swelling over the wrist. The wrist becomes very painful on movement, and crepitus can often be palpated. Treatment includes wrist splintage and analgesia (NSAIDs) for 7–10 days. Occasionally, physiotherapy can be useful. The patient should be taught progressive exercises and given adequate advice about recurrence.

Scaphoid fracture

This is usually caused by a FOOSH. Signs and symptoms include:
- pain over the anatomical snuffbox and on telescoping of the thumb;
- pain directly over the scaphoid tubercle when palpated;
- pain on flexion and ulnar deviation of the wrist.

Scaphoid fractures may not always be apparent initially, and requesting specialist scaphoid views may be helpful.
- Around 70% of scaphoid fractures involve the waist and can be associated with avascular necrosis.
- The remainder occur in the dorsal and proximal poles, and are associated with fewer complications.

If there is clinical suspicion of a fracture, but no definite fracture on the X-ray, it is usual practice to treat as a fracture and immobilize the wrist in a splint or POP. Review the patient at 10–14 days, either in the ED or fracture clinic (depending on local policy). The wrist should then be X-rayed again, by which time the fracture should be more evident due to new callus formation. Analgesia advice should be given, and analgesia prescribed, if required. Some departments use small-limb MRI scanners to detect these fractures.

Lunate and perilunate dislocations

These often follow a FOOSH. Clinically, the patient will present with pain and swelling over the anterior aspect of the wrist. These dislocations are rare and often difficult to detect on X-ray. The AP will appear normal; therefore, a close inspection of the lateral view is imperative. If there is any suspicion of a dislocation, give the patient adequate analgesia, and seek senior advice.

Other carpal bone fractures

These are rare and often associated with direct trauma. Patients with a significant mechanism of injury and associated wrist trauma need careful assessment and imaging. If there is evidence of dislocation, the patient must be referred to the on-call orthopaedic team. Small avulsions and fractures of the hook of the hamate or triquetrum can be treated with a back slab or wrist support and analgesia, and referred to the fracture clinic.

Hand injuries

Hand injuries are a common presentation in the ED and require meticulous assessment, as injuries to nerves and tendons can be quite subtle in presentation. It is essential that the ENP who is examining the hand has a sound understanding of the anatomy.

- Always document the dominant hand, occupation, and social circumstances of the patient, as these have a bearing on treatment decisions.
- Uncomplicated lacerations and fractures will be managed by ED clinicians, with specialist follow-up, if needed.
- Complicated hand injuries where there is neurovascular or tendon damage or injuries with a cosmetic implication should be referred to the hand surgeon, as these injuries can result in significant loss of function.

The hand is made up of multiple compartments and planes. Because of its intricate anatomical structure and wide range of function, it is essential that the examination is thorough and the ENP documents all structures examined.

- Examination should include the radial, ulnar, median, and digital nerves.
- Establish and document the integrity of extensor tendons and deep and superficial flexor tendons.
- Note any vascular deficit.

Damage to any of these structures requires specialist assessment. Initial assessment and treatment of any hand wound should include:

- analgesia;
- removal of any rings;
- temporary splinting and elevation of the injured limb.

Metacarpal fractures

Fractures of the fifth metacarpal are sometimes referred to as a 'boxer's fracture', as they frequently result from punching. If the fracture is very displaced or if there is rotational deformity, it needs to be referred. Treat undisplaced fractures with no rotational deformity with a high sling, neighbour strapping of the affected finger, and fracture clinic follow-up. Some metacarpal fractures may be managed more comfortably in a volar slab.

Distal phalangeal fractures

Manage closed fractures to the distal phalanx with elevation and analgesia. Refer open fractures/burst fractures to the hand surgeon.

Proximal and middle phalangeal fractures

Treat undisplaced fractures with analgesia, neighbour strapping, and elevation. Angulated fractures require manipulation under digital block, followed by neighbour strapping.

Volar plate injuries

A volar plate injury is caused by hyperextension injury to the proximal interphalangeal joint (PIPJ). It may be just a sprain to the ligaments, or it may be more serious, involving an avulsion fracture where the ligament has pulled off a piece of bone. Simple sprains may be treated with rest, ice, compression, and elevation (RICE) and neighbour strapping. Refer more complex injuries to the hand surgeon.

Ulnar collateral ligament injury

This is also known as 'gamekeeper's thumb' or 'skier's thumb.' A partial or complete tear to the ulnar collateral ligament is most often the result of sporting injuries but can be caused by a fall. The patient will complain of pain over the base of the thumb and will have difficulty grasping objects. Partial tears may be immobilized in a cast and followed up in the fracture clinic. Complete tears may require surgical intervention.

Mallet deformity

Mallet finger is a closed injury to the extensor mechanism near its insertion into the distal phalanx. It is often associated with an avulsion fracture at the base of the distal phalanx. Mallet finger is a characteristic flexion deformity of the distal interphalangeal joint (DIPJ). Apply a mallet splint or Zimmer splint, and refer the patient for orthopaedic follow-up. The patient will require instructions on how to maintain full extension of the digit whilst changing the splint.

Avulsion and degloving injuries

These are often the result of high-velocity RTCs and industrial accidents. Degloving injury, which can result in extensive avulsion of the skin and subcutaneous tissues, is a serious injury in which an extensive area of skin is sheared from its underlying blood vessels and nerves. These patients need immediate analgesia and urgent referral to a plastic surgeon. Any delay in referral must be avoided to ensure the best outcome for the patient. The injured limb should be covered in a sterile saline dressing and elevated.

Amputation of the distal phalanx

Refer patients who present with partial or complete amputation of the fingertips to the hand surgeon. Place the amputated portion in a saline-soaked swab surrounded by ice. Some may be suitable for reimplantation. Give the patient effective analgesia, as these injuries are very distressing. Also give IV antibiotics, and establish the patient's tetanus status.

Paronychia

This is an infection of the lateral border of the nail that is usually attributable to simple trauma such as nail biting. Artificial nails are also thought to be a cause of paronychia. A paronychia usually starts as a cellulitis but often progresses to abscess formation, which requires incision and drainage. Infection can sometimes spread under the nail, causing a subungual abscess that requires trephining.

Subungual haematoma

This is the result of direct trauma to the distal phalanx that causes bleeding under the nail. The presence of a subungual haematoma is suggestive of a nail bed injury and an underlying distal phalangeal fracture. It is important to identify such injuries, as inappropriate management can damage nail plate regeneration. Formation of a nail bed scar may prevent plate adherence to the bed and lead to the subsequent development of onycholysis of the newly formed nail plate. Trephining the nail provides instant pain relief and is not contraindicated, even in the presence of a fracture to the distal phalanx. However, it should be done under sterile conditions, and it is important to consider appropriate wound care, tetanus prophylaxis, and antibiotic therapy.

Tendon sheath infections

Tendon sheath infections of the hand are usually the result of direct inoculation of bacteria from penetrating trauma. This is a very painful condition and needs urgent referral to a hand surgeon for irrigation, IV antibiotic therapy, elevation, and further management.

Trigger finger

Trigger finger, also known as stenosing tenosynovitis, is a painful condition that affects the tendons in the hand. It can affect one or more fingers, and symptoms can include pain, stiffness, clicking, and a small lump of tissue (known as a nodule) at the base of the affected finger or thumb. It is commoner in:

- women;
- individuals over 40y of age;
- those with certain medical conditions such as diabetes.

Trigger finger may get better without treatment. However, treatment options include:

- rest and analgesia;
- NSAIDs, which may be used to reduce the swelling;
- splinting, which involves strapping the affected finger to a plastic splint to relieve pain and aid recovery;
- corticosteroid injections, which may be used to reduce the swelling;
- surgery on the affected sheath, which involves releasing the affected sheath to allow the tendon to move freely again.

Back pain

Simple backache is a common presentation in the ED and may be managed by an ENP with appropriate training. This pain is usually attributed to heavy lifting or manual work, and must be differentiated from nerve root pain or back pain that is attributed to a more serious pathology. Simple back pain is usually attributable to muscle or ligamentous 'strain'. The patient may present as follows:

- presentation between the age of 20 and 55y;
- pain in the lumbosacral region;
- no tenderness in the spinous process;
- pain that is 'mechanical' in nature;
- pain that varies with physical activity and over time;
- the patient is generally well;
- no numbness or tingling in the legs;
- no bowel or bladder problems.

Simple back pain accounts for about 90% of all episodes of back pain. Around 90% of patients make a full recovery within 4–6wk.

Management of simple back pain

- If the patient has no 'red flags', reassure them, and provide positive information about the prognosis.
- Encourage early light activity.
- Educate them about the nature of back pain, and address psychosocial features, as this has prognostic importance.
- Advise them to use NSAIDs, muscle relaxants, and simple analgesia (this is as effective as opiates).
- Refer them for early physiotherapy.

Nerve root pain

Nerve root pain is a more complex condition, which requires a medical assessment. The patient may present with the following:

- unilateral leg pain that is worse than low back pain;
- pain generally radiating to the foot or toes;
- numbness and paraesthesiae in the same distribution;
- nerve irritation signs;
- reduced straight leg raising (SLR), which reproduces back pain;
- motor, sensory, or reflex change;
- limited to one nerve root.

Around 50% of patients recover from an acute attack within 6wk.

▶ Red flags: possible serious pathology

These patients must be seen by a doctor or an advanced practitioner.

- Presentation under 20y of age, or onset over 55y of age.
- Violent trauma (e.g. fall from a height, road traffic accident).
- Constant, progressive, non-mechanical pain.
- Thoracic pain.
- PMH of neoplasm.
- Patient is taking systemic steroids.
- Drug abuse.
- HIV.
- Patient is systemically unwell.
- Weight loss.
- Persistent severe restriction of lumbar flexion.
- Widespread neurological signs and symptoms.
- Structural deformity.
- Bowel and bladder disturbance.

Fracture of neck of femur

This is common in the elderly, especially in women, following relatively minor trauma. The risk ↑ because of osteoporosis and osteomalacia, and also because of the higher incidence of falls.

Many hospitals have fast-track policies for these patients.

- As these fractures can frequently be diagnosed clinically, give patients with suspected fractures effective analgesia (e.g. morphine sulfate) prior to X-ray.
- An inpatient bed should also be arranged at this time.
- Blood loss is significant, particularly with intertrochanteric fractures, so establish IV access and commence fluids, as early hydration reduces mortality.
- Take blood samples for FBC, U&E, and cross-matching.
- Monitor vital signs regularly to ensure haemodynamic stability is maintained.
- Record the ECG to exclude MI or other arrhythmia.
- Obtain a Waterlow score, and initiate pressure area care in the ED, as these patients are very vulnerable to pressure ulcers.
- Apply skin traction early if the patient is not going to theatre (➔ see Skin traction: application, p. 754).

Supracondylar fractures

Supracondylar fractures of the femur are assessed in the same way as shaft fractures. The mechanisms of injury are similar, with pain usually localized to the knee. These fractures do not cause the same extent of blood loss as shaft fractures and are repaired by either long leg casting or surgery.

Dislocated hip prosthesis

Hip dislocations most commonly occur in people with total hip replacements or femoral head replacements.

The patient may present in severe pain, with an internally rotated, flexed leg. Early limb relocation is indicated, so long as there is no associated fracture. This may be done in the ED under sedation. Once relocated, the patient should be admitted for traction. If relocation attempts are unsuccessful with sedation in the ED, urgent transfer to theatre for closed or open reduction under general anaesthetic is indicated.

Lower limb injury: triage

History taking and examination at triage need to be brief and should focus on ensuring neurovascular function, relief of pain, and, if appropriate, referral to X-ray. A more thorough examination will be performed by the ENP or the doctor.

Knee injuries

When assessing the injury, the nurse or ENP should consider the following factors.

- Mechanism of injury—a twisting injury may suggest injury to the menisci.
- Valgus or varus strain may cause damage to the medial or lateral collateral ligament, respectively.
- Rapid swelling of the knee after injury is usually an acute haemarthrosis and implies significant injury.
- A more gradual swelling suggests an effusion.
- Medical history taking should include pre-existing injuries to that limb, medical conditions that affect the musculoskeletal system or bone density, and factors that would influence recovery.
- Ask about current medications and any known allergies.
- It is also important to establish a social history, as limb injuries may adversely affect a younger person's ability to work and may limit an older person's ability to care for himself or herself. These factors need to be taken into consideration in any treatment plan.

Examination

For examination of the knee, the patient needs to be partially undressed and lying on a trolley. Examine both legs for comparison.

- Look for swelling, bruising, redness, abrasions, and any breaks in the skin.
- Feel the skin temperature, and compare it with the other joint. Feel for crepitus, and look and feel for an effusion.
- An examination for effusion should be performed with the injured knee in extension. The suprapatellar pouch should be milked to determine whether an effusion is present.
- Assess the tone and bulk of the quadriceps for any sign of wasting. Compare the painful knee with the asymptomatic knee. The musculature should be symmetrical bilaterally.
- Feel for joint line tenderness, which may suggest injury to the menisci.
- Feel for bony tenderness over the patella, tibial plateau, and femoral condyles.
- Assess the collateral and cruciate ligaments.
- Ask the patient to straight leg raise. Ability to do this against resistance generally excludes quadriceps or patellar tendon rupture or transverse patellar fractures.

Medial collateral ligament

The valgus stress test is performed with the patient's leg slightly abducted. Place one hand on the lateral aspect of the knee joint and the other hand at the medial aspect of the distal tibia. Then apply valgus stress at both 0° (full extension) and 30° of flexion to assess for pain or laxity in the medial collateral ligament.

Lateral collateral ligament

To perform the varus stress test, place one hand at the medial aspect of the patient's knee and the other hand at the lateral aspect of the distal fibula. Apply varus stress at both 0° (full extension) and 30° of flexion to test for pain or laxity in the lateral collateral ligament.

Anterior cruciate ligament

This may be injured in a twisting or hyperextension movement. Use the drawer test to assess the cruciate ligaments. For the anterior drawer test, the patient's knee must be flexed to 90°. Fix the patient's foot in slight external rotation (by sitting on the foot), and then place your thumbs at the tibial tubercle and your fingers at the posterior calf. Ensure that the patient's hamstring muscles are relaxed, and then pull anteriorly and assess anterior displacement of the tibia (anterior drawer sign).

Lachman's test

This is another method of assessing the integrity of the anterior cruciate ligament (ACL). The injured knee is flexed to 15°. Stabilize the distal femur with one hand, grasping the proximal tibia in the other hand. Then attempt to sublux the tibia anteriorly. Lack of a clear endpoint indicates a positive Lachman's test.

Posterior cruciate ligament

The posterior cruciate ligament (PCL) is less frequently injured than the ACL. For the posterior drawer test, the injured knee must be flexed to 90°. Standing at the side of the trolley, observe for posterior displacement of the tibia ('posterior sag sign'). Then fix the patient's foot in the neutral position (by sitting on it); position your thumbs at the tibial tubercle, and place your fingers on the posterior calf. Push posteriorly, and assess for posterior displacement of the tibia.

Ottawa knee rules

An X-ray is only required for acute knee injuries with one or more of the following findings:
• age ≥55y;
• tenderness at the head of the fibula;
• isolated tenderness of the patella;
• inability to flex to 90°;
• inability to weight-bear at the time of injury and in the ED.

However, consider X-raying patients aged >18y and <55y who are intoxicated with alcohol or have a history of degenerative bone disease.

Patellar fracture

This occurs as a result of a fall on to the knee. An indirect twisting injury or a direct blow to the joint can also result in a fracture. The patient presents with pain, swelling, crepitus, effusion, and extension block. Inability to straight leg raise may suggest rupture of the quadriceps or patellar tendon. Do not confuse a bipartite patella with a fracture.

Treatment
- Immobilize in a non-weight-bearing cast, and ensure that the patient is given written instructions about the plaster cast.
- Ensure that adequate analgesia is provided.
- Give the patient crutches and advice on how to use them.
- Arrange early follow-up in the fracture clinic.

Patellar dislocation

This results from a direct blow to the medial aspect of the knee. The patient presents with lateral deformity, medial tenderness, and pain on attempted movement. Haemarthrosis may also be evident.

Treatment
- The patella can be relocated by extension of the knee. Analgesia and muscle relaxants should be used to relieve pain prior to the procedure.
- Once the patella has been relocated, a supportive bandage, such as a Robert Jones bandage, or a cricket pad splint should be applied.

Soft tissue knee injuries

Soft tissue injuries to the knee are a common presentation in the ED. Such injuries are now frequently managed by ENPs. Patients may present with an acute or chronic problem, and this should be elicited in the history.

History taking

- Ask about the time and date of injury.
- What is the mechanism of injury?
- Was there a cracking or popping sound at the time of injury?
- Degree and site of pain, and referral of pain.
- Ability to weight-bear.
- Instability or locking since the injury.
- Swelling and speed of onset.
- Any other joint affected (e.g. hip, ankle).
- Is the condition long-standing?
- Ask about exacerbating factors (e.g. using stairs, rising from a sitting position).

Prepatellar bursitis

People who spend a lot of time on their knees often present with swelling in the front of the knee. The constant friction aggravates the bursa (lubricating sac), which is situated in front of the kneecap (patella). The bursa allows the kneecap to move smoothly under the skin. If the bursa becomes inflamed, it fills with fluid and causes swelling of the knee. This condition is called prepatellar bursitis.

Symptoms

- Pain usually with activity.
- Rapid swelling on the front of the kneecap.
- Tender and warm to touch.

If there is any history of trauma, it may be necessary to X-ray the knee to exclude a fracture. Conservative treatment is usually effective, so long as the bursa is only inflamed and not infected.

Treatment

- The patient should rest until the bursitis settles.
- Apply ice at regular intervals, three or four times a day, for 20min at a time. Do not apply ice directly on to the skin.
- Elevate the affected leg as much as possible.
- Advise the patient to take anti-inflammatory medication such as aspirin or ibuprofen.

Some clinicians may decide to aspirate the bursa. Chronic bursitis may require orthopaedic referral.

Compartment syndrome

The muscles of the limbs are organized into compartments and divided by thick fascia. Compartment syndrome occurs when the pressure inside a compartment is ↑ above 30–40mmHg, compressing the nerves and blood vessels within that space. It can occur in upper or lower limbs as the result of high-energy trauma and bony injury. It can also result from tight bandages or casts. Compartment syndrome is commonest in the lower leg and forearm, although it can also occur in the hand, foot, thigh, and upper arm.

The classical sign that should alert nurses to the possibility of compartment syndrome is extreme pain in the compartment that is out of all proportion to the injury and is not relieved with analgesia and elevation. The skin overlying the compartment will be critical, swollen, and shiny. As the pressure continues to rise, there may be diminished sensation, weakness, and paleness of the skin. This condition is diagnosed by inserting a needle attached to a pressure meter into the compartment. When the compartment pressure is >45mmHg or when the pressure is within 30mmHg of the diastolic BP, the diagnosis is made.

Treatment for both acute and chronic compartment syndrome is usually surgery.

Nursing interventions for compartment syndrome

- Ensure adequate opiate analgesia.
- Elevate the limb.
- Remove any constricting dressings or POP.
- Prepare for, and assist, medical staff in measuring compartment pressure.
- Prepare the patient for surgery.
- Maintain frequent monitoring.
- Offer support and reassurance to the patient.

Ankle injuries

Ankle fractures refer to fractures of the distal tibia, distal fibula, talus, and calcaneus. The true ankle joint consists of the tibia (medial wall), the fibula (lateral wall), and the talus, the base upon which the tibia and fibula sit. The joint allows dorsiflexion and plantar flexion movement at the ankle.

The subtalar joint consists of the talus and calcaneus. The subtalar joint allows inversion and eversion.

- Excessive inversion stress is the commonest cause of ankle injuries. This is due to the medial malleolus being shorter than the lateral malleolus, thus allowing the talus to invert more than evert. Also the deltoid ligament gives more support to the medial malleolus than do the less substantial lateral ligaments.
- The ankle is much more stable and resistant to eversion injury than it is to inversion injury. However, when eversion injury does occur, the patient often sustains significant damage to bony and ligamentous supporting structures and joint instability.

The ankle joint may be destabilized either by a fracture to one of the bones or by injury to a ligament. Most ankle injuries occur during sports activities or when walking or running on an uneven surface. Forced rotation or angulation of the joint can result in a fracture and/or associated ligament injury. Fractures of the ankle are serious because of the implications for weight-bearing and mobility. They can be very painful and heal slowly.

Ottawa ankle rules

Fractures account for only 15–20% of all ankle injuries, so X-rays are not indicated in all cases. The Ottawa ankle rules[2] have been demonstrated to be very accurate in identifying patients who may have sustained a fracture, and applying the rules will assist the triage nurse in making decisions about whom to refer for X-ray.

The Ottawa ankle rules are based on the assessment of the ability to bear weight at the time of injury and subsequently in the ED. They also specify areas of bony tenderness that allow the clinician to determine accurately which patients are at negligible risk of fracture.

Management of ankle fractures

Management depends on clinical and radiological findings. It is important to exclude neurovascular compromise and to establish the integrity of the ankle mortise. Note any talar shift on the X-ray.

- Simple undisplaced lateral malleolar fractures can usually be immobilized in a below-knee back slab and followed up in the next fracture clinic. Large avulsion fractures of the lateral malleolus should be managed in the same way.
- Displaced fractures of the lateral or medial malleolus should be referred immediately to orthopaedics, as they need open reduction and internal fixation (ORIF).
- Bimalleolar, trimalleolar, and intra-articular fractures of the distal tibia (pilon fractures) need urgent orthopaedic assessment, as they require ORIF.

Box 9.1 Weber ankle fracture classification

Type A
- Below the level of the ankle joint.
- Tibiofibular syndesmosis intact.
- Deltoid ligament intact.
- Medial malleolus often fractured.
- Usually stable, but occasionally requires an ORIF.

Type B
- Fracture of the fibula at the level of the syndesmosis.
- At the level of the ankle joint, extending superiorly and laterally up the fibula.
- Tibiofibular syndesmosis intact or only partially torn, but no widening of the distal tibiofibular articulation.
- Medial malleolus may be fractured or deltoid ligament may be torn.
- Variable stability.

Type C
- Fracture of the fibula proximal to the syndesmosis.
- Above the level of the ankle joint.
- Tibiofibular syndesmosis disrupted, with widening of the distal tibiofibular articulation.
- Medial malleolus fracture or deltoid ligament injury present.
- Unstable—requires ORIF.

Skinner, H, *Current diagnosis & treatment in orthopedics*, 5/e © 2013. With permission from McGraw-Hill Global Education Holdings, LLC.

The Weber ankle fracture classification (➔ see Box 9.1) is a simple system for the classification of lateral malleolar fractures, relating to the level of the ankle joint, and determining treatment.

Reference
2 Ottawa Hospital Research Institute. *Ottawa ankle rules for ankle injury radiography*. Available at: http://www.ohri.ca/emerg/cdr/docs/cdr_ankle_poster.pdf.

Ankle dislocation and sprain

Ankle dislocation

▶▶ Ankle dislocations are an orthopaedic emergency and are the result of significant trauma. Do not delay in getting specialist help.

Because of the large amount of force required and the inherent stability of the joint, dislocation of the ankle joint alone is uncommon without an associated fracture. In addition, there is disruption of the lateral or medial ligaments on the tibiofibular syndesmosis. Examination of the joint shows obvious swelling and deformity. Tenting of the skin by the malleoli may be present. Palpation of the joint reveals tenderness along the joint line, consistent with ligamentous injury. Early reduction is imperative, as any delay ↑ the risk of neurovascular compromise. In patients with vascular compromise, perform a reduction prior to radiological examination.

When requesting X-rays, request AP, lateral, and mortise/oblique views.

Nursing interventions
- Establish venous access, and collect blood for FBC and U&E.
- Ensure the administration of IV opiate analgesia. Entonox® can also be administered.
- If opiate analgesia is administered, monitor RR and SpO$_2$.
- Assist in reducing the dislocation. Support and reassure the patient, as this can be very painful.
- Apply the plaster, whilst the alignment of the joint is maintained. When dry, a window needs to be cut in the plaster, so that pedal pulses can be checked.
- Record baseline observations and pedal pulses.
- Accompany the patient to X-ray.
- Prepare the patient for admission.

Ankle sprain

A sprain is caused by stretching of a ligament that may be torn or partially torn (❸ see Fig. 9.1). The signs of an ankle sprain are not dissimilar to those of a fracture and can include:
- pain or tenderness;
- swelling;
- bruising;
- inability to walk or bear weight on the joint;
- stiffness.

Ankle sprain is a very common injury. The severity depends on the mechanism of injury and how badly the ligaments are stretched or torn. Ankle sprains are graded as follows.
- Grade I, mild sprain—stretch and/or minor tear of the ligament without laxity (loosening).
- Grade II, moderate sprain—tear of the ligament plus some laxity.
- Grade III, severe sprain—complete tear of the affected ligament (very lax).

Treatment for ankle sprains is as follows.
- Rest the ankle, either completely or partly, depending on the severity of the sprain. Use crutches for as long as it is painful to weight-bear.
- NSAIDs.
- Use ice packs, ice massages, or even a bag of frozen peas to help to relieve the swelling, pain, bruising, and muscle spasms. Keep using ice for up to 3 days after the injury.
  - ▶ Never apply ice directly to the skin—always wrap in a cloth or towel before applying.
- Acute phase. There is little evidence to support the use of compression bandages or products in the acute phase.
- Rehabilitation. It may be of benefit to strap or brace significant sprains during rehabilitation. This should be under the supervision of the physiotherapy/orthopaedic team.
- Elevation. Raising the ankle to, or above, the level of the heart will help to prevent the swelling from getting worse and will also help to reduce bruising. Try to keep the ankle elevated for about 2–3h a day, if possible.

Although most patients make a full recovery from their injury, some may experience long-term problems and recurrent sprains. Where possible, patients with moderate to severe sprains should have physiotherapy follow-up. Patient education and advice about what to expect are very important aspects of care.

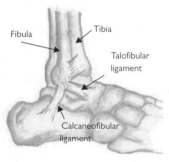

Fig. 9.1 Lateral ankle ligaments.
(Reproduced with permission from Bulstrode, C., et al. (2002). *Oxford Textbook of Orthopaedics and Trauma*, p. 1307. Oxford University Press, Oxford.)

Gastrocnemius muscle tears

Tears to the lateral or medial bellies of the gastrocnemius are very common. They are acutely painful and commonly occur during sports or other activity. There is sudden onset of calf pain, with a feeling of 'tearing.' The calf may be bruised and/or swollen. There is tenderness laterally or medially to the muscle bellies. The integrity of the Achilles tendon should be assessed, and the fibula examined to identify signs of tenderness. X-rays are only necessary if there are signs of bony tenderness over the calcaneus or fibula. Treatment of a rupture is symptomatic—rest and NSAIDs, with or without the use of crutches, and walking with a slightly raised heel may provide dramatic relief. Symptoms usually settle within 2wk.

Achilles tendon injuries

The Achilles tendon is the tendon that connects the calf muscle (gastrocnemius) to the calcaneus.

- Achilles tendinitis is an inflammation of the tendon that causes it to become swollen, painful, and less flexible than usual.
- A ruptured tendon may occur when the tendon has been structurally weakened by untreated tendinitis, or due to unaccustomed activity. Patients often report hearing a pop at the back of the ankle. Symptoms include pain, swelling, and loss of function.
  - As the calf muscle is no longer attached to the calcaneus, the patient finds weight-bearing difficult and may be unable to stand on their toes.

Examination

- The area of the rupture may be swollen, tender, and bruised.
- A gap in the tendon may be palpable.
- Although X-rays do not show the tendon injury, they show the calcaneus. In some cases, the tendon may not tear but may cause a small avulsion fracture of calcaneal bone.
- If the tendon has not ruptured, the patient may have sustained only a pulling injury to the tendon, causing tendinitis.
- The most reliable diagnostic test for a suspected rupture of the Achilles tendon is the Simmonds' test (also called the Thompson test or Simmonds–Thompson test). The patient lies face down, with their feet hanging off the edge of the bed. If the test is positive, there is no movement of the foot (plantar flexion) on squeezing the corresponding calf, indicating likely rupture of the Achilles tendon.

Treatment

The treatment options are surgical or conservative, and the choice of treatment is often dependent on the clinician and local policy. Both treatments may require an initial period of equinus casting. The cast may be changed at 2- to 4wk intervals to slowly stretch the tendon back to its normal length. Casting may be combined with early movement (1–3wk) to improve overall strength and flexibility.

Equinus cast

This is usually a below-knee cast (occasionally extended to above the knee), done with the patient's leg hanging over the end of the bed. It is designed to take the stretch off the tendon. The requirements are exactly the same as for a below-knee cast, and the same method is used except for the slab, which is applied to the anterior aspect of the lower leg from the knee end first. The foot should be plantar flexed.

Plantar fasciitis

This is inflammation of the plantar fascia of the foot. It is an overuse injury which causes heel pain that may radiate forward into the foot. Pain is usually worse first thing in the morning, eases as the day wears on, and becomes more painful again in the evening, especially after walking. Treatment usually consists of rest and NSAIDs. Patients with persistent pain may need referral to orthopaedics for steroid injections.

Fracture of the lateral process of talus

This is more commonly known as 'snowboarder's ankle', and the injury is indeed commoner in snowboarders than in the general population. Most patients present with unremitting pain and swelling and what they believe is a sprained ankle. Diagnosis is usually made when the person is referred to an orthopaedic doctor and a CT scan of the ankle is performed.
- If the fracture fragments are undisplaced, treatment is conservative, in a cast for 6wk and non-weight-bearing on crutches.
- Displaced fractures usually require surgical intervention.

Calcaneal fractures

Fractures of the hindfoot, particularly the os calcis (calcaneus), are not unusual and are the result of an axial load type of injury (e.g. jumping from a height). Calcaneal fractures are serious, because 2° arthritis of the subtalar joint can occur. Examine both calcanei, as these fractures are often bilateral and frequently involve the subtalar joint. They are also often associated with burst fractures of the spine, and, for this reason, it is important to examine the cervical spine, lumbar spine, pelvis, and hips. X-rays show a ↓ in Böhler's angle to <20%.

Metatarsal fractures

These are common sporting injuries caused by direct trauma, excessive rotational forces, or overuse. Avulsion fractures of the base of the fifth metatarsal are caused by inversion injuries where the base of the fifth metatarsal is avulsed by the peroneus brevis tendon. The Ottawa ankle rules also provide guidelines on when to request foot X-rays following an ankle injury (➲ see Ankle injuries, pp. 320–1). The treatment of metatarsal fractures varies, depending on the nature and location of the fracture, and, in some cases, the occupation of the patient (e.g. footballer, ballet dancer). If the fracture fragments are well aligned, the treatment is an elastic support bandage or POP back slab and restricted weight-bearing for 6–8wk. However, avulsion fractures of the base of the fifth metatarsal are sometimes slow to heal and, for this reason, should be followed up in the fracture clinic.

Jones fracture

This is a fracture at the base of the fifth metatarsal at the metaphyseal–diaphyseal junction. It must be differentiated from the commoner avulsion fracture of the fifth metatarsal styloid process. Jones fractures are sometimes treated in a below-knee plaster cast for 4–6wk, but very often surgical intervention is required.

Fractured toes

As treatment of undisplaced fractures of toes is symptomatic, X-rays are only required if there is a deformity that may require reduction or there is an overlying wound that would indicate a compound fracture. Always X-ray a suspected fracture in the great toe.

Where there is no bony injury to toes, reassure the patient, and advise them to wear sensible shoes. Occasionally, relief may be obtained from two-toe neighbour strapping.

- Undisplaced fracture of the toe.
  - Neighbour strapping and analgesia. No follow-up is necessary.
  - Fractures to the great toe (first toe) require supportive splinting. The patient should be non-weight-bearing using crutches and must be given a follow-up appointment in the fracture clinic.
- Dislocated or displaced fracture of toes. Reduce, using Entonox® or a digital nerve block, and neighbour strap. Follow-up at the fracture clinic is required.

Wounds: introduction

The stages of wound healing

Assessment and management of acute wounds are an essential component of emergency nursing. It is important that nurses working in any urgent care setting have a sound understanding of the healing process.

Vascular inflammatory phase: 0–3 days

Within seconds of the injury, blood vessels constrict to control bleeding at the site. Platelets unite to form clots and arrest bleeding. Neutrophils enter the wound to fight infection and attract macrophages. Macrophages break down necrotic debris and activate the fibroblast response.

Destructive migratory phase: 2–5 days

Dead tissue and bacteria are removed during this stage. Where cells die due to injury, the body acts to dissolve and eliminate necrotic matter. Macrophages migrate into the wound and play a vital role in this stage by engulfing bacteria, any FBs, and necrotic tissue. With neutrophils, the macrophages attract fibroblasts and influence the growth of new blood vessels into the wound.

Proliferative phase: 3–24 days

Fibroblasts proliferate in the deeper parts of the wound, synthesizing small amounts of collagen, which facilitates further fibroblast proliferation. Granulation tissue also appears in the deeper layers of the wound. The proliferation phase lasts for 24–72h.

Maturation phase: 24 days to 1y

During this phase, fibroblasts leave the wound; there is a ↓ in vascularity, and collagen is remodelled into a more organized matrix. The wound changes from a red granulation tissue to a pink epithelialization phase. Finally, a white, relatively avascular tissue develops, and the epidermis is restored to normal thickness.

Wound contraction, which starts during the proliferative phase and continues into this final phase of healing, is powerful and may, in certain individuals, cause contracture. In some individuals, the healing process can lead to the formation of excessive amounts of scar tissue, resulting in keloid scarring. Although healed wounds never regain the full strength of uninjured skin, they can regain up to 70–80% of the original strength.

Wound categorization

Wounds may be categorized as acute or chronic.

- Acute wounds seen in the ED include surgical, traumatic, and thermal injuries.
- Chronic wounds include malignant wounds, pressure sores, leg ulcers, and diabetic foot ulcers (➔ see Leg ulcers, p. 425). These wounds are attributable to systemic disease processes that require specialist intervention beyond the emergency setting, and such patients must be referred on to either the appropriate specialty or the primary care provider.

Pre-tibial lacerations

These are lacerations to the anterior aspect of the lower leg. They are a common presentation, particularly in elderly women, and are sometimes associated with long-term corticosteroid treatment. Because of this and also the anatomical position, healing may be impaired and very slow. Increasingly, these patients are being referred to plastic surgery for early skin grafting, but, where this is not immediately available, skilled initial management can have successful outcomes.

- The flap often appears concertinaed backwards, leaving an open wound. The flap needs to be gently smoothed over the wound, after gentle cleaning with saline and removal of any haematoma.
- The skin edges of the flap should be brought together and held in position with Steri-Strips™, covering as much of the wound as possible. These wounds should not be sutured, as this can lead to necrosis of the flap. Steri-Strips™ ensure a better outcome for the patient.
- Once the Steri-Strips™ have been applied, the wound should be covered with a non-adherent well-padded dressing and a support bandage. The bandage should be applied from the toes to below the knee to encourage even circulation.
- The patient should be advised to mobilize as necessary, but also to elevate the limb, where possible, to aid venous return and to prevent the development of a chronic, non-healing leg ulcer.
- Consider the patient's tetanus status and the need for antibiotic prophylaxis.
- Simple analgesia, such as paracetamol, is advisable to control any pain.
- Discharge to the care of the GP and practice nurse is the most appropriate option, where continuity of care is more likely than in hospital.

Health promotion in this group of patients is paramount to prevent chronic non-healing. Holistic assessment of the patient, rather than considering only the wound in isolation, is the gold standard and will promote successful treatment. Consider referral to occupational therapy, social services, or hospital-at-home, in line with local policy, to provide added support.

Wound infection

Wound infection is a common presentation in the ED, and ENPs increasingly manage such patients autonomously. When assessing wounds and the cause of infection, the following approach is necessary.

- Consider that an FB may be present in the wound.
- Organic FBs (e.g. wood or cane) will never be tolerated and will always cause infection, if retained.
- X-ray for radio-opaque FBs, as appropriate (wood is not radio-opaque). If you are unable to locate an FB, consider referring the patient to orthopaedics for further exploration.
- Take a wound swab, and send for C&S.
- Record the patient's temperature and CBG, bearing in mind that patients who have diabetes are more prone to infection.
- Clean the wound thoroughly, and apply an appropriate dressing, according to local protocol.

Wounds that require antibiotic prophylaxis

- Human or animal bites.
- Lacerations involving joints.
- Compound fractures.
- Contaminated wounds.

Bites (animal and human)

- Assess for depth and extent of damage to the underlying tissue.
- Animal and human bites should not be sutured.
- Consider an X-ray if there is potential for bone involvement.
- Refer bites to the face or gaping wounds with deep structural involvement to the maxillofacial surgeon, as appropriate.
- Give antibiotics, as prescribed.
- Human bites will require hepatitis B vaccination, with an accelerated course if the patient does not already have immunity.

Superficial bites

- Clean well.
- Apply antiseptic dressing.
- Elevate or rest, according to the affected area.
- Check the patient's tetanus status, and consider tetanus Ig in unimmunized patients.
- Educate the patient about signs and symptoms of further infection, and emphasize the importance of review of the wound.
- Review all bites the following day.
- Consider the need for IV antibiotics and medical review if the patient is systemically unwell and if there are signs of cellulitis or lymphangitis.

Abscesses

An abscess is a collection of pus that has formed in the tissues. Abscesses can form in almost any part of the body and may be caused by infectious organisms, parasites, or FBs (e.g. splinters). Abscesses in the skin are easily identifiable, as they are red, raised, and painful. Abscesses in other areas of the body may not be obvious, but they may cause significant pain and organ damage.

Incision and drainage of abscesses
- Where there is clearly a collection of pus, incision and drainage are indicated.
- Small abscesses may be incised and drained in the ED, but some abscesses require specialist referral.
- The following are not suitable for treatment by the ENP and should be referred to the appropriate specialist:
  - breast;
  - perianal;
  - facial;
  - neck;
  - labial;
  - pulp and palmar.
- Always check for diabetes mellitus.

Adequate anaesthesia is essential for effective incision of an abscess. It can be achieved by injecting lidocaine circumferentially around the abscess and/or administering Entonox®, which is inhaled and exhaled for 2min prior to the incision.
- Make an incision.
- Express all the pus, and curette gently.
- Send a swab for C&S.
- Irrigate the cavity with saline, and then pack with a hydrogel compound.
- Re-dress the next day, and refer the patient back to their GP, as necessary.

Infected sebaceous cysts

Treat as described for abscesses.

Skin infections

Cellulitis is inflammation of the connective tissue under the skin, usually caused by a bacterial infection. It can be caused by the normal skin flora or by other bacteria when the skin integrity has been broken by cuts or insect bites, or at sites of IV cannula insertion. The commonest location for cellulitis is the lower limb, but it can occur in any part of the body. Cellulitis may be superficial, but it can spread to the lymph nodes and bloodstream, and the patient can be systemically unwell.

Early symptoms may include redness, swelling, and pain in the affected part, but, as the infection spreads, other symptoms can include pyrexia, nausea, and headaches. In advanced cases of cellulitis, lymphangitis (tracking) may be noted travelling up the affected area. The swelling can spread rapidly. Treatment is with the appropriate antibiotics, but many patients may require admission for elevation and IV antibiotics.

Bites and stings

Patients frequently present to the ED having been bitten or stung by an insect. They are often worried that the bite or sting is poisonous. Although the bites and stings of many insects can cause problems, those of other insects cause only itching and erythema (➲ see Box 9.2).

The difference between a bite and a sting is based on the nature of the bite or sting.

- Venomous insects, such as wasps, attack as a defence mechanism, injecting poisonous venom through their sting that can be extremely painful and can, in rare cases, cause an anaphylactic reaction.
- Non-venomous insects, such as mosquitoes, bite in order to feed on the blood. Although mosquitoes are not venomous, they are dangerous, because they transmit diseases such as yellow fever, malaria, filariasis, and dengue.

Box 9.2 Insect bites and stings

Venomous
- Wasps.
- Hornets.
- Bees.
- Ants.

Non-venomous
- Lice.
- Sandflies.
- Chiggers.
- Fleas.
- Ticks.
- Mosquitoes.
- Bugs.

Local irritation and allergic reactions can result from non-venomous bites. Severe reactions, such as anaphylactic shock, only result from venomous stings.

Bees leave the sting and venom sac attached after stinging the victim. Venom continues to be released, until the sting is removed. Bees die after they sting. However, wasps and hornets do not leave their stings behind and can sting repeatedly.

Treatment of bites
- Pruritus is usually the commonest symptom. Topical antihistamines provide some relief, as do anti-inflammatory gels.
- Systemic reaction with symptoms, such as facial and/or tongue swelling, wheezing, or SOB, will need urgent treatment and should be nursed in an appropriate high-observation area (➔ see Anaphylaxis, p. 284).

Treatment of stings
Remove the sting, and treat the patient with analgesia and antihistamines. Pain, swelling, and itching are the main complaints.

Removal of ticks
Ticks are notoriously difficult to remove intact. One method that works well is to place small forceps along the skin, with the ends on either side of the tick's head. Press down into the skin, and firmly grip the head of the tick. Apply even traction perpendicular to the skin, until the tick is finally removed. The aim is to remove the tick intact, and not leave any part behind. If this is not successful, it may be necessary to infiltrate the area with LA and excise the tick.

Needle-stick injuries

Needle-stick injuries are an occupational hazard that exposes health-care workers to a number of blood-borne pathogens that can result in serious or fatal infections. It is estimated that around 600 000–800 000 needle-stick injuries occur each year, half of which are not reported. Many infections can be transmitted via a needle-stick injury, but those that pose the greatest risk are:

- hepatitis B virus (HBV)—30%;
- hepatitis C virus (HCV)—3%;
- HIV, which is the virus that causes AIDS—0.3%.

HBV vaccination is recommended for all health-care workers (unless they are immune because of previous exposure). HBV vaccine has proved highly effective in preventing infection in workers exposed to HBV. However, no vaccine exists to prevent HCV or HIV infection. Taking precautions to prevent needle-stick injuries is the best protection. Health-care workers should avoid:

- recapping needles;
- transferring a body fluid between containers;
- failing to dispose of used needles properly in puncture-resistant sharps containers.

Management of needle-stick injuries

- Follow local guidelines, and report any injury to occupational health.
- Wash the wound thoroughly with soap and water, allowing it to bleed under the water. Do not suck the wound or apply pressure to cause bleeding. Wash mucous membranes with copious amounts of water.
- Take baseline blood for serology. If the source is possibly HIV-positive, take blood for FBC, U&E, LFTs, and amylase.
- If the source patient is known and also considered to be high-risk, discuss post-exposure treatment with the infectious diseases specialist on call. Prophylaxis is most effective if started 1h post-exposure but can be considered for up to 2wk afterwards.
- If the source is high-risk and prophylaxis is commenced, advise the patient to use barrier contraception and not to donate blood until seroconversion has been excluded.
- Organize counselling for the patient.
- Ensure HBV-accelerated vaccination.

Tetanus prophylaxis

Tetanus prophylaxis

Tetanus is an acute, and often fatal, disease, which is now rare in developed countries because of immunization. The disease is caused by tetanus toxin, which is released following infection by the bacterium *Clostridium tetani*, which is found in soil and animal manure. Typically, tetanus spores may be introduced into the body through a puncture wound, burn, or laceration. The wound may seem innocuous and not serious, and the infection mild, but the bacterium attacks the nervous system, and the condition is characterized by general rigidity and muscle spasm, which can involve the jaw and neck.

Although most patients born in Western countries are immunized, tetanus has not been eradicated and never will be, as the spores live in the soil. Anyone can contract tetanus, but farmers and those working with soil are at ↑ risk. It must also be borne in mind that people from developing countries may not have adequate immunity. Certainly children and young adult refugees from war zones may be particularly at risk because of interrupted vaccination programmes. More recent research also suggests that immunity declines with age, so older patients may well require a booster.

High-risk tetanus-prone wounds include:
- puncture-type wounds, especially where there has been contact with soil or manure;
- wounds or burns that show a degree of devitalized tissue;
- wounds containing FBs;
- compound fractures;
- wounds and burns in patients who are systemically septic;
- wounds and burns that require surgical intervention which is delayed for >6h.

Box 9.3 lists the indications for tetanus immunization.

Caution with regard to tetanus immunoglobulin

Tetanus Ig is given to patients who need to develop immediate immunity to tetanus after having certain wounds or burns.

It is important to take a full medical history before prescribing tetanus Ig, as it is not suitable for everyone. It should not be given if the patient:
- is allergic to, sensitive to, or has had a bad reaction to, blood transfusions or plasma derivatives in the past;
- is allergic to, sensitive to, or has had a bad reaction to, human Igs in the past;
- has bleeding problems;
- has IgA deficiency;
- has recently had a vaccination or will be having a vaccination soon.

Box 9.3 Indications for tetanus immunization

Patient fully immunized (five doses at appropriate intervals)
- Clean or tetanus-prone wound—vaccine not required.
- High-risk tetanus-prone wound—give human tetanus Ig.

1° immunization complete; boosters incomplete but up-to-date
- Clean or tetanus-prone wound—vaccine not required (unless next dose is due and it is convenient to give it now).
- High-risk tetanus-prone wound—give human tetanus Ig.

1° immunization incomplete or boosters not up-to-date
- Clean or tetanus-prone wounds—give a reinforcing dose of vaccine and further doses, as required, to complete the recommended schedule to ensure immunity.
- In addition, for tetanus-prone wounds, give one dose of human tetanus Ig at a different site.

Patient not immunized or immunization status unknown or uncertain
- Clean or tetanus-prone wound—give an immediate dose of vaccine, followed by, if records confirm the need, completion of a full five-dose course to ensure future immunity.
- In addition, for tetanus-prone wounds, give one dose of human tetanus Ig at a different site.

For further information, see ℘ http://www.gov.uk/government/uploads/system/uploads/attachment_data/file/148506/Green-Book-Chapter-30-dh_103982.pdf.

Gastrointestinal emergencies

Overview

GI problems are frequently encountered in emergency care areas, and patients can present with wide-ranging symptoms. Symptoms that suggest an underlying GI problem can include: abdominal pain; nausea; vomiting; diarrhoea; melaena; haematemesis; constipation; jaundice; and abdominal distension. Abdominal pain is a common ED presentation and can be the cause of a wide variety of GI problems. Pain is usually present when there is a disorder within the GI tract, but its severity is not a reliable indicator of the seriousness of the condition. However, the site and characteristics of the pain can often indicate the cause. Pain usually arises from an organ within the abdominal cavity that is either inflamed, distended, perforated, or ischaemic. Abdominal wall pain arises from irritation of the peritoneum and/or abdominal musculature from inflamed organs, free blood, or leaked gastric contents. Pain can also be referred from an organ outside the abdominal cavity, e.g. an inferior MI can present as epigastric pain.

The acute abdomen

The acute abdomen is a term given to sudden severe pain in the abdomen. This requires swift diagnosis, and treatment usually involves emergency surgery. Causes of acute abdomen may include: appendicitis; pancreatitis; peptic ulcer disease (PUD); gall bladder pathology; intestinal ischaemia; DKA; diverticulitis; intestinal obstruction; and ruptured ectopic pregnancy.

The gastrointestinal system

The abdomen (➲ see Fig. 10.1) contains the structures bordered by the diaphragm superiorly, the pelvis inferiorly, the vertebral column posteriorly, and the abdominal muscles anteriorly. The abdomen can be divided into three cavities: the peritoneum; pelvis; and retroperitoneum.

- The peritoneum contains the liver, spleen, stomach, gall bladder, small intestine, transverse colon, and sigmoid colon.
- The pelvis contains the rectum, bladder, uterus, ovaries, and iliac vessels.
- The retroperitoneum contains part of the duodenum, the ascending and descending colon, kidneys, pancreas, ureters, abdominal aorta, and inferior vena cava.

For purposes of examination, the abdomen is divided into four quadrants: right upper quadrant (RUQ); left upper quadrant (LUQ); right lower quadrant (RLQ); and left lower quadrant (LLQ).

- The *oesophagus* travels through the posterior of the mediastinum and passes through the diaphragm to join the stomach at the level of the T10 vertebrae.
- The *diaphragm* is a dome-shaped structure with three foramina (holes) at T8 for the vena cava, T10 for the oesophagus, and T12 for the aorta. The phrenic nerve passes through the thorax along both sides of the pericardium and divides into the anterior and posterior branches. Each phrenic nerve is the sole motor nerve to its own half of the diaphragm.
- The *stomach* is located in the LUQ and is divided into four parts: the cardia; fundus; body; and pylorus.
- The *liver* is the largest intra-abdominal organ and is extremely vascular. The liver tissue is very friable and is surrounded by a fibrous capsule. The liver lies at the level of the 6th–10th ribs on the right, and 7th–8th on the left. Circulation is via the hepatic artery and portal vein. Blood flow is ~30% of the CO. The liver has five main functions: detoxification; carbohydrate and fat metabolism; protein synthesis; and bile secretion.
- The *gall bladder* lies under the liver and stores 50mL of bile. Bile drains from the liver via the common hepatic, then cystic duct, into the gall bladder. Bile drains from the gall bladder via the common bile duct, meeting the pancreatic duct to drain into the duodenum.
- The *biliary system* (➲ see Fig. 10.2) is a collective term for the common hepatic duct, cystic duct, common bile duct, gall bladder, and pancreatic duct.
- The *spleen* is located in the LUQ and is in close proximity to the 7th–10th ribs. The splenic pulp is friable, and vascular supply is via the splenic artery. The splenic capsule is 1–2mm thick.
- The *pancreas* lies at the level of L1 against the posterior abdominal wall. The pancreatic juice is rich in digestive enzymes. The pancreas also produces insulin and several other hormones.
- The *kidneys* lie at the level of T12 to L3. The right kidney is slightly lower due to the liver.

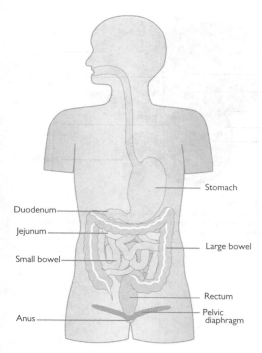

Fig. 10.1 The gastrointestinal tract.

(Reproduced from Norton, C., *et al.* (eds.) (2008). *Oxford Handbook of Gastrointestinal Nursing*, fig 1.1, p. 3. Oxford University Press, Oxford with permission from the Burdett Institute of Gastrointestinal Nursing, King's College, London.)

- The *small intestine* is 7m long. It is divided into three sections: the duodenum; jejunum; and ileum. Some of the duodenum is retroperitoneal. The small intestine is located in all four quadrants.
- The *appendix* is a 10cm, blind-ended tube connected to the caecum. It is a remnant of embryological development and is not known to have a function.
- The *large intestine* is 1.5m long and consists of the caecum; ascending, transverse, and descending colon; rectum; and anal canal.
- The *peritoneum* is a serous membrane that lines the abdominal cavity and covers the abdominal organs.
- The *bladder*, when empty, lies in the pelvic cavity; when full, it extends into the abdomen.

❶ The last six ribs overlie the abdominal structures. ∴ Injuries to this area can cause significant intra-abdominal pathology.

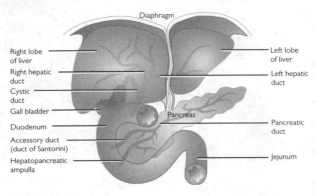

Fig. 10.2 The biliary tract.

(Reproduced from Norton, C., et al. (eds.) (2008). *Oxford Handbook of Gastrointestinal Nursing*, fig 13.1, p. 441. Oxford University Press, Oxford with permission from the Burdett Institute of Gastrointestinal Nursing, King's College, London.)

Nursing assessment: history

▶▶ Some patients with a GI problem will require immediate resuscitative interventions. ∴ A brief ABC assessment should always be undertaken (➔ see The handover of care, p. 17). The commonest life-threatening consequence of a GI problem is hypovolaemic shock. Severe pain also requires immediate intervention, usually with opiate analgesia.

It can sometimes be difficult to identify whether a patient's symptoms are GI in origin. The nurse should always be alert to the possibility that the symptoms may originate outside the GI system.

History

The presence of any of the following features is relevant and can help to direct further assessment and investigations:

- abdominal pain (➔ see Abdominal pain below);
- nausea (the feeling of wanting to vomit);
- vomiting; projectile suggests gastric outflow obstruction. Large volumes of faeculent fluid suggest intestinal obstruction. NB. Nausea and vomiting without abdominal pain may not be of GI origin.
- diarrhoea: duration; frequency; presence of blood; consistency;
- constipation. When were bowels last opened?
- melaena;
- haematemesis;
- coffee-ground vomit;
- fever and shivers may suggest sepsis;
- indigestion;
- weight loss;
- loss of appetite;
- dysphagia;
- LMP;
- dysuria;
- medications, particularly NSAIDs;
- alcohol intake;
- travel.

The PQRST mnemonic is a useful tool in the assessment of pain:
- *P*rovocation;
- *Q*uality;
- *R*adiation/relief;
- *S*ite/severity/other symptoms;
- *T*ime.

Abdominal pain Comprehensive assessment of abdominal pain can help indicate the source of pain, guides investigation, and enables the prescription of effective analgesia.
- Organ pain caused by stretching or inflammation. Often described as dull and not aggravated by movement, and tends to occur around the midline.
- Abdominal wall pain. Cause: activation of pain-sensitive fibres in the peritoneum. Well-localized pain aggravated by movement or stretching. Pain described as sharp and stabbing. Palpation is extremely painful and exacerbated when the palpating hand is removed (rebound tenderness).

Assessment of abdominal pain
- Where is the pain (site)?
  - Helps to localize an area/quadrant.
- What is the pain like (quality)?
  - Colicky pain comes and goes.
  - Spasmodic pain can be 'squeezing' in nature and suggests obstruction of a hollow structure.
  - Sharp pain is localized and suggests peritoneal irritation.
  - Dull pain is less localized and suggests an organ disorder.
- When did the pain start (time)?
  - Sudden onset suggests acute perforation or rupture.
- How long does the pain last (time)?
  - Is it intermittent or persistent?
- Where does the pain go (radiation)? (➲ See Table 10.1.)
- What makes the pain better or worse (relief and provocation)?
  - Eating can relieve pain in peptic ulcer disease (PUD), or make pain from pancreatitis or small bowel obstruction worse.
  - Breathing can aggravate pain if the disordered organ lies next to the diaphragm.
  - Movement that makes pain worse suggests peritonitis.
  - Position. Flexing the legs may relieve pain from peritonitis. Lying flat can ↑ pain from pancreatitis.
- What else is going on (other symptoms)?
- Nausea, vomiting, fever, diarrhoea, GU symptoms, LMP.

Table 10.1 Referred pain

Site of pain	Structure
RUQ, epigastric area, left shoulder tip pain, pain between shoulder blades	Gall bladder
LUQ, (left) shoulder tip pain (Kehr's sign)	Ruptured spleen
Lower anterior chest/epigastric region; mimics angina	Upper GI structures (oesophagus, duodenum, gall bladder, pancreas, biliary tree)
Epigastric radiating through to back	Pancreatitis; peptic ulcer
Throughout upper chest to back	Aortic aneurysm
Flank pain	Kidney
Loin to groin pain	Ureters (renal colic)
Periumbilical and shift to RLQ	Appendicitis
Testicles	Duodenal injury

Physical assessment, investigations, and nursing interventions

Physical assessment

Inspection

- Observe for abdominal distension, which can be caused by fat, flatus, faeces, fetus, or fluid.
- Ascites.
- Scars from previous surgery.
- Surface trauma to the abdomen or lower ribs: wounds; bruising; abrasions; impaled objects.
- Evisceration.
- Jaundice. Cholestatic jaundice is either directly related to a problem within the liver, e.g. cirrhosis, or due to extrahepatic causes, e.g. bile duct stone, pancreatitis, or carcinoma.

Palpation

Although not a skill routinely practised by ED nurses, palpation of the abdomen by the assessing clinician can identify the specific site of pain, pain patterns on examination, and the presence of any masses. In health, abdominal organs are not usually palpable, except in the very thin.

Pain patterns

- Tenderness. Pain may be localized to an abdominal organ or a quadrant on palpation.
- Guarding is the normal tendency to contract the abdominal muscles on examination. Guarding (↑ abdominal muscle tone), despite relaxing/ reassuring the patient, accompanies intra-abdominal disease.
- Rebound tenderness reveals deep-seated inflammation and is elicited on abrupt withdrawal of the palpating hand.
- Rigidity. Generalized 'board-like' rigidity implies peritonitis; the abdomen does not move on respiration.

Auscultation All four quadrants should be auscultated for bowel sounds. Absent bowel sounds are highly suggestive of intra-abdominal pathology. Tinkling bowel sounds suggest obstruction.

Percussion

- Dullness indicates fluid or an enlarged organ; hyper-resonance suggests air in the abdominal cavity.
- Percussion can be extremely painful, especially in the acute abdomen.

Investigations

Assessment of the patient with abdominal pain can be complex. Even those apparently well and triaged into a low-priority category *should* have a full set of vital signs. Even slight abnormalities, e.g. tachycardia, should not be dismissed. The elderly, critically ill, and immunocompromised may not develop a fever, even in the presence of overwhelming infection.

- Pulse.
- Temperature.

- RR.
- BP.
- Pain assessment and score.
- Urinalysis.
- ECG if pain is epigastric.

Not all patients will require all of the following investigations. Assessment and examination by the assessing clinician may be required to identify what, if any, investigations are indicated.

- FBC, U&E, β-HCG, amylase/lipase.
- Lactate in sepsis, and it is useful in helping to diagnose bowel ischaemia, especially in the elderly.
- CBG (DKA can present as an acute abdomen).
- Abdominal X-ray (AXR); erect CXR.
- ABG if the patient is shocked.
- USS, conducted by an experienced clinician, can be very useful in establishing a diagnosis or the detection of free fluid.
- CT: often provides the clinician with a definitive diagnosis, as is becoming the investigation of choice for most GI emergencies.

⚠ Every year, women still die of ruptured ectopic pregnancy, some having attended an ED with symptoms that were not fully explored. All ♀ of child-bearing age who present with abdominal pain should have an ectopic pregnancy actively ruled out as a cause of their pain. A pregnancy test should be done in the ED. *Beware*: ectopic pregnancies can present atypically as GU or GI upset, e.g. diarrhoea and vomiting, dysuria (➔ see Ectopic pregnancy, pp. 164–5).

General nursing interventions
- Analgesia. Opiate analgesia should be given IV, titrated to response. An anti-spasmodic can be useful in colicky pain.
- Anti-emetics.
- IV antibiotics. May be indicated in perforation and infection.
- IV fluids, fluid resuscitation if indicated. Patients who are dehydrated, NBM, vomiting, or shocked will require IV fluids.
- O$_2$ therapy if the patient is shocked.
- Psychological support. Patients will need support and explanation about procedures and treatment. During examination, the presence of the ED nurse is vital in maintaining the patient's privacy and dignity.
- Insertion of urinary catheter. In shock, this is essential; hourly urine measurements are required.
- Monitoring of fluid balance. An 'input/output' chart should be commenced.
- NG tube placement is indicated in bowel obstruction and perforation (➔ see Nasogastric tube insertion, pp. 722–3).

Epigastric pain

Epigastric pain is a very common presentation, both in 1° care and the ED. A wide variety of problems can present with epigastric pain, some relatively benign, e.g. indigestion, others much more serious, e.g. pancreatitis, inferior MI, PUD.

Nursing assessment

Nursing evaluation should take into account the need to assess for a range of problems and may need to include some, or all, of the following:
- vital signs;
- ECG;
- pain assessment and score;
- CXR/AXR;
- CBG;
- FBC, U&E, amylase/lipase, LFTs.

Nursing interventions
- Analgesia.
- Antacid.
- Anti-emetic.
- IV fluids.

Gastrointestinal bleeding

Bleeding can occur from any part of the GI system. Acute upper GI bleeding can present as haematemesis ± melaena. It is commonly caused by PUD (50%), oesophageal varices (10–20%), gastric erosions (15–20%), and Mallory–Weiss syndrome (5–10%). Chronic GI bleeding usually presents as anaemia. Iron deficiency anaemia in men and post-menopausal women is usually of GI origin, and investigations of the upper and lower GI tract may be necessary to identify the cause if it is not apparent from history and examination.

Massive acute lower GI bleeding is rare and most commonly seen in the elderly. A small amount of bleeding from haemorrhoids is much commoner and a frequent cause of anxiety that prompts an ED attendance. Massive lower GI bleeding is usually due to diverticular disease, inflammatory bowel disease (IBD), tumour, or ischaemic colitis. Patients require the same rapid assessment and resuscitation as those with upper GI bleeding.

▶ Patients who present with GI bleeding require an initial rapid assessment to identify those who are shocked and require resuscitation (for assessment of shock, ◐ see Shock, pp. 278–9).

Haematemesis Vomiting fresh blood or darker blood (sometimes called 'coffee grounds') occurs after bleeding in the oesophagus, stomach, or duodenum. Darker/coffee-ground vomit occurs, as blood is altered in the stomach over time by gastric acid.

Melaena is abnormally black, tarry stools with a distinctive offensive odour. The stools contain digested blood that has usually originated from an upper GI bleed that may be acute or chronic.

Mallory–Weiss syndrome is bleeding from a tear in the mucosa at the gastro-oesophageal junction. It is usually caused by protracted vomiting/retching and is often associated with the prolonged vomiting that results from excessive alcohol intake! Blood loss may be large, but, in most patients, it stops spontaneously. Diagnosis is by endoscopy, which then allows early discharge from hospital.

Massive gastrointestinal bleeding

▶▶ Bleeding from PUD or oesophageal varices accounts for up to 70% of upper GI haemorrhages. Urgent resuscitation is required prior to any in-depth assessment as to the cause.

Bleeding from ruptured varices can be phenomenal—like a hosepipe! Loss of >40% of blood volume is immediately life-threatening, and blood loss is often underestimated. Initiation of the massive haemorrhage protocol may be required. Early involvement and advice from a haematologist will guide blood replacement and help manage derangements in clotting that are often a consequence of massive transfusion (◐ see Blood transfusion, pp. 666–7).

- Airway protection. In patients with massive haemorrhage and a reduced level of consciousness, urgent intubation may be required to protect the airway (◐ see Endotracheal intubation, pp. 650–1).

- O_2 administration may be difficult if there is continued vomiting. Nasal prongs may be a useful way of administering low-flow O_2.
- IV access. × 2 large-bore cannulae (Ch 14 brown or Ch 16 grey) into large veins will allow rapid infusion of warmed fluids, blood, platelets, and FFP. Immediate central access may be indicated if the bleeding is significant.
- Bloods sent for FBC, U&E, LFTs, cross-match, clotting.
  - ❶ *Ensure* samples are labelled correctly, as mislabelling is the commonest transfusion risk. If resuscitation is prolonged with multiple interventions, these bloods will need to be repeated regularly.
- ABGs.
- IV fluids. Give warmed crystalloid or colloid, followed by blood. Blood transfusion is indicated when 30% of circulating volume is lost. O-negative blood can be given almost immediately, followed by type-specific, then fully cross-matched, blood.
- Replacement platelets/clotting factors. Platelets, FFP, and cryoprecipitate may need to be given in massive blood loss (usually when >100% blood volume has been lost). These replace essential clotting factors and can help prevent the development of DIC.
- Tranexamic acid may be indicated.
- CVP monitoring.
- Arterial line to enable continuous invasive monitoring.
- Urinary catheter. Aim for a urine output >30mL/h.
- NG tube.
- Keep the patient warm. Hypothermia ↑ the risk of serious complications, e.g. DIC.
- Further cardiovascular support may be needed with inotropes and vasopressors.

Monitoring of patients with massive blood loss
- Pulse.
- RR.
- SpO_2.
- BP (usually invasive).
- Skin colour.
- CVP.
- Urinary output, monitored hourly.
- GCS.
- Continuous cardiac monitoring.
- 12-lead ECG.
- CXR.
- Repeated bloods.
- Repeated ABGs.
- Record fluid balance meticulously.

Peptic ulcer disease

PUD is a collective term given to ulcers in the stomach (gastric ulcers) or the duodenum (duodenal ulcers; DU). The commonest cause of upper GI bleeding is peptic ulcers, accounting for about 50% of cases.

In health, a balance exists between peptic acid secretion and gastroduodenal mucosal defence. Inflammation and ulceration occur when the balance is disrupted. Factors, such as NSAIDs, *Helicobacter pylori* infection, and alcohol, can alter the mucosal defence by allowing acid to diffuse back and cause epithelial cell injury.

- Gastritis is superficial inflammation of the mucosa.
- In ulceration, there is a complete break in the mucosa down to the muscular layer.

Inflammation tends to respond well to antacids.

Signs and symptoms

- Epigastric pain—the patient may point directly to the epigastrium. Pain can be relieved by eating. Severe sudden pain may indicate perforation.
- Nocturnal pain—classically occurs with a DU.
- Nausea.
- Heartburn.
- Anorexia and weight loss.
- Melaena.
- Haematemesis.
- Shock in perforation.
- Fever in peritonitis.
- Rebound tenderness, rigidity in peritonitis.

For the management of massive GI bleeding, ➔ see Gastrointestinal bleeding, pp. 354–5.

⚠ Some patients may have been asymptomatic and present acutely with a perforation; this is more likely in the elderly or those on regular NSAIDs.

Peritonitis

Peritonitis is a common consequence of perforation of the GI tract and can be caused, for example, by a perforated ulcer, appendix, or diverticulum. Patients with peritonitis are often critically ill with septic shock.

Signs and symptoms of peritonitis

- Severe abdominal pain.
  - ⚠ In the elderly or those with underlying IBD, it may be more insidious.
- Rigid 'board-like' abdomen.
- Rebound tenderness.
- Absent bowel sounds.
- Hypovolaemic shock.
- Septic shock as time progresses.
- Fever.

- Vomiting.
- Tachycardia.
- Tachypnoea.

Nursing assessment

Patients with simple gastritis may require little more than antacids and GP follow-up. However, nursing assessment should be aimed at ensuring that all serious underlying problems are ruled out prior to discharge.

- Vital signs.
- Evaluate for signs of hypovolaemic or septic shock.
- Pain assessment and score.
- Bloods: FBC; U&E; amylase/lipase.
- ABG.
- Erect CXR. In 75% of patients with an acute perforation, free gas can be seen under the diaphragm.
- AXR.

Nursing intervention for patients with perforation

Patients with an acute perforation exhibit signs of peritonitis due to the leakage of gastric contents that irritate/infect and inflame the peritoneum.

- IV analgesia.
- Anti-emetic.
- IV access.
- O_2 therapy.
- Ensure bloods sent, and group and save.
- IV antibiotics.
- Fluid resuscitation.
- NG tube.
- Urinary catheter.
- Prepare for theatre.

Oesophageal varices

Acute bleeding from oesophageal varices is a fairly common ED presentation and accounts for 10–20% of acute upper GI bleeding. There is usually a history of alcohol abuse and cirrhosis. Ninety per cent of patients with alcoholic cirrhosis develop varices over a 10y period, during which they develop and enlarge. ∴ Patients with severe cirrhosis and large varices are most likely to bleed. Interestingly, the majority of patients with alcoholic cirrhosis who stop drinking have a reduction in the size of their varices—sometimes they disappear completely.

Varices develop, as necrosis of liver cells damages the structure and function of the liver. In patients with cirrhosis, all functions of the liver are disrupted, e.g. clotting is deranged as protein synthesis is affected. Because the structure of the liver is grossly abnormal, blood flow is affected. Portal hypertension develops, as blood can no longer drain freely from the GI tract via the portal vein into the liver. As the blood 'backflows' and portal pressure ↑, the venous system dilates, and a collateral circulation develops. The commonest site of this collateral circulation is at the gastro-oesophageal junction. Because these gastro-oesophageal veins are superficial, they tend to rupture. Fifty per cent of patients with portal hypertension will bleed from their varices.

- Mortality is extremely high—50% of patients die, following the first episode of bleeding.
- Patients may also have decompensated liver disease with encephalopathy.
- 1° prophylaxis tends to be with propranolol or surgery.
- Patients who present to the ED with massive upper GI bleeding, whatever the cause, require immediate airway protection and fluid resuscitation. For the management of massive GI bleeding, ➔ see Gastrointestinal bleeding, pp. 354–5.

Nursing interventions

⚠ Specific nursing interventions for oesophageal variceal haemorrhage depend on the availability of urgent endoscopy.

Urgent endoscopy available If endoscopy is urgently available, then the varices will be either ligated or subject to sclerotherapy (chemical injected into the vein to cause it to narrow/clot).

Urgent endoscopy not available
Several pharmacological interventions are available to control acute bleeding:
- vasopressin ± GTN infusion;
- somatostatin, octreotide.

Insertion of a 3-lumen Sengstaken tube can be used if endoscopy is not available and drug treatment is contraindicated or has failed. A Sengstaken tube is usually refrigerated, as it is stiffer and easier to insert when cold. The procedure is very unpleasant for the patient but can be lifesaving in the presence of severe haemorrhage. It stops bleeding in 90% of cases, although rebleeding occurs in 50% of patients on deflation of the tube (➜ see Sengstaken tube insertion, pp. 752–3).

Prophylactic antibiotics reduce mortality and morbidity.

Ruptured oesophagus

Although rare, this complication of vomiting or, even more rarely, blunt or penetrating trauma has significant morbidity and mortality.

Signs and symptoms
- Severe chest pain.
- Surgical emphysema in the neck.
- Normal ECG, which rules out cardiac causes of chest pain.
- Abnormal CXR: pneumomediastinum, pneumothorax.
- There may be a history of vomiting.
- Signs of shock.

Nursing interventions
- O$_2$.
- IV analgesia.
- IV fluids.
- IV antibiotics.
- Cardiothoracic opinion.

Appendicitis

Appendicitis is a common ED presentation in children (➋ see Appendicitis, pp. 136–7) and young adults. It is less common in patients >40y.

- Appendicitis is the commonest surgical emergency and should be considered as a cause of an acute abdomen in all patients if it has not been removed.
- The presentation can range from mild/moderate right iliac fossa (RIF) pain to generalized peritonitis with associated shock.
- Presentations are often atypical; symptoms vary, and up to 45% of appendices that are removed are normal. In sexually active women, acute salpingitis associated with sexually transmitted infections (STIs) is a common cause of RIF pain. Pain can be bilateral, and there is an associated vaginal discharge.

❶ The diagnosis of appendicitis is a clinical one, unless a CT scan has been performed and excludes it. ∴ Do not allow the surgeon to delay assessment by insisting on waiting until blood results are available.

Signs and symptoms

- Nausea.
- Vomiting.
- Abdominal pain. Classically, pain begins vaguely centrally/periumbilical and then localizes to the RIF.
- Fever.
- Diarrhoea occasionally occurs.

Nursing assessment

Accurate nursing assessment should enable differentiation between patients with localized pain in the RIF and those with more serious pathology, e.g. generalized peritonitis and shock. Assessment should also include investigations that may point to another cause.

- Vital signs.
- Pain assessment and score.
- Urinalysis.
- LMP; risk of pregnancy.
- FBC. The WCC may be raised, but not always.
- U&E.
- β-HCG.

Nursing interventions

- IV access.
- Analgesia.
- IV fluids if NBM or dehydrated.
- IV antibiotics reduce the risk of post-operative complications associated with infection.
- Prepare for admission.
- Preoperative preparation may be required if theatre is arranged imminently.

Biliary colic and acute cholecystitis

Gallstones are very common and are present in many people, often remaining asymptomatic throughout life.

- However, in some people, they move out of the gall bladder and cause severe pain when they become lodged in the gall bladder neck, common bile duct, or cystic duct. This is often termed biliary colic and is usually a temporary obstruction. The term 'colic' can be confusing when used in this context, as it usually does not 'come and go' but is constant and severe and ↑ in severity.
- Acute cholecystitis is the term given to inflammation of the gall bladder that results from a stone preventing the gall bladder from emptying. When the cystic duct is blocked, the gall bladder distends, becomes inflamed, and then may become infected and even distended by pus.

Signs and symptoms of biliary colic

Patients tend to be systemically well and can even be discharged home for GP follow-up and further investigation if their pain subsides, examination is normal, and blood results are not significantly abnormal.

- Pain is usually epigastric but can be localized to the RUQ. Pain may radiate to the right shoulder/through to the back.
- Pain may be related to eating food with a high fat content.
- Nausea and vomiting in more severe cases.

Signs and symptoms of cholecystitis

Initially, the signs and symptoms are similar to those of biliary colic. However, as time passes, severe pain localizes to the RUQ. There is overlying peritonitis due to inflammatory changes in the gall bladder. Patients tend to be systemically unwell and require admission. Occasionally, there can be septic shock, which requires resuscitation (❷ see Shock, pp. 278–9).

- Severe RUQ pain.
- RUQ guarding and rigidity.
- Fever.
- Mass in the RUQ. Occasionally, there is a palpable mass.

Nursing assessment

- Vital signs.
- Pain assessment and score.
- LMP. Ruptured ectopic can present with shoulder tip pain.
- ECG to rule out MI.
- FBC, U&E, LFTs, amylase/lipase.
- AXR. Stones may be visible.
- USS is the most useful investigation, as it can confirm cholecystitis.

Nursing interventions

- IV access.
- Analgesia, usually opiate.
- IV fluids if NBM, dehydrated.
- Fluid resuscitation if shocked.
- IV antibiotics if infection suspected.

Pancreatitis

Pancreatitis can be acute or chronic, and episodes can be recurrent. In the ED, the differentiation between an acute episode or one that develops on a background of chronic disease is difficult and probably unnecessary. Patients who have had previous episodes of pancreatitis are quick to recognize their symptoms and may present regularly to the ED, particularly those with chronic alcohol problems.

- The commonest causes of acute pancreatitis in the developed world are alcohol, gallstones, and trauma.
- Gallstones that obstruct the pancreatic duct can cause pancreatitis.
- ↑ alcohol intake is frequently associated with chronic pancreatitis.
- The severity of pancreatitis is wide-ranging; inflammation may be mild and self-limiting, but, in its severest form, it has a mortality of 40–50%.
- Consider a diagnosis of pancreatitis in all patients with epigastric pain.

Signs and symptoms

Mild disease may present with minimal signs and symptoms. Twenty-five per cent of all patients with pancreatitis will have severe disease; they will be critically ill, requiring resuscitation and intensive care. The earlier severe disease is identified, the sooner aggressive treatment can begin. However, in those with only mild symptoms, it is difficult to predict who will develop severe complications. The ED nurse needs to be vigilant in the ongoing assessment of the patient's physiological status. Predictive tools can be used to assess the severity of pancreatitis, but most are of limited value on presentation.

- Pain. Classically, it is epigastric and radiates through to the back.
- Nausea and vomiting.
- Tachycardia.
- Hypotensive.
- Septic.
- Oliguric.
- Widespread abdominal tenderness, guarding, rigidity.
- Absent bowel sounds.
- Jaundice if there is obstruction within the biliary tract or associated cirrhosis.

Nursing assessment

- Vital signs.
- Pain assessment and score.
- Urine output.
- FBC, U&E, LFTs, glucose, clotting, lactic acid, Ca^{2+}.
- Amylase.
- Lipase is sensitive and specific to pancreatitis, and can be more accurate in diagnosis than amylase, especially in chronic disease.
- ABG.
- Erect CXR. Excludes perforation, which can also cause a rise in amylase.
- ECG.

Patients with acute severe pancreatitis characterized by organ failure, abnormal observations, deranged biochemical markers, hypoxia, acidosis, alkalosis, and/or coma will require intensive care.

Nursing interventions
- O_2.
- IV access.
- IV fluids.
- IV antibiotics.
- Fluid resuscitation if shocked.
- Analgesia.
- Anti-emetic.
- NBM.
- NG tube.
- Urinary catheter.
- CVP monitoring in the critically ill, which can guide fluid resuscitation.
- Prepare for possible HDU/ICU transfer.

Alcoholic liver disease

The harmful effects of alcohol are wide-ranging, and the impact is social, psychological, and physical. Women are much more prone than men to the harmful physical effects of alcohol. Not everyone who has an ↑ alcohol intake develops alcoholic liver disease (ALD). ~30% of 'alcoholics' develop cirrhosis. Men drinking in excess of 8 units (4 pints) per day for 10y have a high risk of developing cirrhosis; for women, this is only 4 units.

Current recommended safe daily limits of alcohol for men and women are:

- men and women are advised not to regularly drink more than 14 units a week;
- drinking should be spread over 3 days or more if you drink as much as 14 units a week;
- a good way to cut down is to have several drink-free days each week (see ℘ http://www.nhs.uk/change4life/Pages/alcohol-lower-risk-guidelines-units.aspx).

ALD is a collective term given to a spectrum of diseases that result from excess alcohol intake.

- Fatty liver occurs with minimal amounts of alcohol. Fat is present in the liver, but there is no damage to the liver cells. The fat disappears when alcohol intake is stopped. There are often no symptoms.
- Alcoholic hepatitis is next in the continuum of ALD. As well as fatty changes, there is liver cell death. Symptoms may be mild; there may be general ill health, signs of chronic liver disease, and some jaundice. Abstinence from alcohol can reverse all the effects.
- If the patient continues to drink, then cirrhosis is likely. Alcoholic cirrhosis is the irreversible end-stage of ALD. The liver is grossly abnormal; there are problems with blood flow (portal hypertension), and liver function is deranged. General signs of chronic liver disease include fever and jaundice.
  - In compensated chronic liver disease, there is a range of signs that are present in the skin, abdomen, and endocrine system. People with compensated cirrhosis should lead a normal life.
  - When chronic liver disease becomes decompensated, ascites develops, and neurological function is markedly impaired.
  - Long-term survival from cirrhosis depends on complete alcohol abstinence. The 5y survival is 70% in those who abstain.

Signs and symptoms of chronic liver disease

- RUQ pain.
- Anorexia, weight loss.
- Ascites.
- Ankle oedema.
- Jaundice.
- GI bleeding (haematemesis, melaena, varices).
- Spider naevi.
- Palmar erythema.
- Dupuytren's contracture.

- Splenomegaly.
- Portal hypertension.
- Gynaecomastia.
- Disorientation, drowsiness progressing to coma (Wernicke's encephalopathy) (➔ see Alcohol misuse, pp. 602–4).

Nursing assessment

- Vital signs.
- AVPU/GCS.
- FBC, U&E, glucose, LFTs, clotting, ammonia level.

Nursing interventions

- IV access.
- IV fluids.
- IV thiamine (can cause anaphylaxis).
- Lactulose. Reduces the production of ammonia in the GI tract, which is the main cause of encephalopathy.

Intestinal obstruction

Intestinal obstruction is a common cause of acute abdomen and has different causes in the small and large bowel.

- Small bowel obstruction is very commonly caused by adhesions. Less common causes are strangulated hernias and intussusception.
- Obstruction of the colon is commonly caused by tumour, sigmoid volvulus, or diverticular disease.

The bowel becomes distended above the obstruction, inflamed, infiltrated by bacteria, and, in strangulation, ischaemic and gangrenous.

Signs and symptoms

Signs and symptoms are dependent, to some extent, on the site of the obstruction. If there has been previous abdominal surgery, adhesions are usually the cause. Obtaining hospital notes can be helpful.

- Abdominal pain. Severe pain suggests strangulation.
- Abdominal distension.
- Vomiting, especially in small bowel obstruction.
- Constipation.
- Signs of shock.
- Signs of peritonitis.
- Fever.
- Bowel sounds may be 'tinkling' or absent.

Nursing assessment

- Vital signs.
- Pain assessment and score.
- LMP.
- FBC, U&E, LFTs, amylase/lipase, group and save.
- ECG.
- CXR.
- AXR may reveal distended loops of bowel above the obstruction. Fluid levels may be seen.
- ABG.

Nursing interventions

- IV access.
- O_2.
- Analgesia.
- Anti-emetic
- IV fluids.
- Fluid resuscitation if shocked.
- IV antibiotics.
- NG tube.
- Urinary catheter.

Diverticulitis

Diverticulitis is a common GI disease, thought to be a result of ↑ pressure in the lumen of the colon associated with a lack of dietary fibre. ↑ luminal pressure contributes to the development of 'pouches' or diverticula on the outside of the colon. When these diverticula get blocked with food particles or faeces, they become infected. The severity of the symptoms depends on the extent of the infection and the development of any complications, e.g. peritonitis from perforation. Diverticulitis is commoner in the middle-aged and elderly. Older patients and the immunosuppressed may not mount a pyrexia or have obvious signs of peritonitis.

Signs and symptoms

- LLQ pain (usually the diverticula are in the sigmoid colon).
- Fever.
- Nausea.
- Constipation or diarrhoea.
- Peritonitis if the diverticula perforate.
- A tender palpable mass in the LLQ may indicate abscess formation.

Nursing assessment

- Vital signs.
- Pain assessment and score.
- LMP.
- FBC, U&E, group and save, blood cultures.
- Erect CXR may help to identify free gas in a perforation.
- AXR may help to identify perforation or obstruction.
- ABG.

Nursing interventions

- IV access.
- NBM.
- Analgesia.
- Anti-emetic.
- IV fluids.
- Fluid resuscitation if shocked.
- IV antibiotics.
- NG tube.
- Urinary catheter.

Complications

- Perforation.
- Intestinal obstruction.
- Massive PR bleeding.
- Fistula (small bowel, vaginal, bladder).

Inflammatory bowel disease

IBD covers two main diseases—ulcerative colitis and Crohn's disease. Ulcerative colitis affects the colon only, and Crohn's disease can affect any part of the GI tract from the mouth to the rectum. Patients with established IBD may present to the ED with a severe exacerbation of their disease. However, most patients remain relatively well and live a normal life when in remission. Patients may also present with their first episode and may require referral ± admission for assessment and diagnosis of their symptoms.

Signs and symptoms

- Diarrhoea. When the colon is affected, this is usually bloody. In ulcerative colitis, there is usually mucus.
- Abdominal pain.
- Weight loss.
- Malaise.
- Lethargy.
- Nausea.
- Vomiting.
- Fever.
- Signs of intestinal obstruction.
- Signs of shock.
- Anaemia.
- Tachycardia.

Nursing assessment

- Vital signs.
- Pain assessment and score.
- FBC, U&E, LFTs, amylase/lipase, CRP, ESR.
- AXR.

Nursing interventions

- IV access.
- IV fluids.
- Analgesia.
- Anti-emetic.
- IV antibiotics.
- NG tube.
- Urinary catheter if shocked.

Gastroenteritis

Gastroenteritis is a very common presentation in 1° care and the ED. Acute infection of the GI tract (gastroenteritis) may present with diarrhoea ± vomiting. The commonest cause in adults is bacterial infection, although viruses are increasingly common. Norwalk (Norovirus) virus is particularly virulent and is responsible for causing outbreaks of diarrhoea and vomiting on cruise ships, schools, hospitals, and nursing homes. Patients may have fever and abdominal pain. Children and the elderly are most vulnerable to the effects of gastroenteritis. The elderly can also present with diarrhoea when they have a UTI, constipation, or a chest infection.

Patients who present to the ED with diarrhoea ± vomiting where the cause is thought to be infectious should be asked to wash their hands if they are ambulatory and are remaining in the waiting room. Patients who require further nursing/medical assessment should be nursed in a cubicle, with strict infection control measures (➔ see Infection prevention, pp. 10–11).

Signs and symptoms

A careful history may reveal the cause of the gastroenteritis, duration of symptoms, drugs, travel, contacts, or contaminated food.

- Diarrhoea: frequency, consistency, watery, bloody, mucus.
- Vomiting.
- Abdominal pain.
- Fever.
- Dehydration (➔ see Box 10.1).
- Shock.

Nursing assessment

- Vital signs.
- Pain assessment and score.
- Assess degree of dehydration (➔ see Box 10.1).
- FBC, U&E if dehydrated.
- Stool for culture (not usually necessary) only if recent foreign travel, from residential/institutional care, severe illness.

Box 10.1　Dehydration

Identifying the presence and extent of dehydration is important, as it guides the approach to rehydration and the need for hospital admission. In children, it is commoner to classify dehydration as mild (<5%), moderate (5–10%), or severe (>10%). However, the following classification can also be used in adults:

- mild—thirst, dry lips/mouth, reduced urine output;
- moderate—lethargy, tachycardia, tachypnoea, postural hypotension;
- severe—hypotension, drowsiness, anuria.

Nursing interventions
- Strict infection control precautions.
- IV access.
- Oral rehydration if possible.
- IV fluids.
- Fluid resuscitation if shocked.

Admission

Patients with mild dehydration unable to tolerate oral fluids or those with moderate to severe dehydration require admission for IV fluids and monitoring of electrolyte balance.

Discharge

Patients with mild dehydration who are able to tolerate oral fluids can be discharged with advice about oral hydration and when to seek further medical assessment.

Rectal bleeding

The commonest cause of bleeding and/or melaena from the rectum is the passage of blood from acute upper GI bleeding. Only 20% of GI bleeding is from the lower GI tract. The passage of bright red blood from the rectum usually indicates lower GI tract bleeding. Diverticulitis, carcinoma, and IBD are the commonest causes. Patients with signs of hypovolaemic shock require urgent fluid resuscitation (⊃ see Shock, pp. 278–9).

Haemorrhoids

Haemorrhoids are the commonest cause of painless rectal bleeding that may prompt an ED attendance. ↑ pressure in anal veins causes them to bulge, protrude, and bleed. Blood from haemorrhoids is bright red, and is usually reported on toilet paper or on the outside of faeces; it is not mixed in the stool. Pregnancy, Crohn's disease, and ulcerative colitis are often associated with haemorrhoids.

Signs and symptoms
• PR bleeding, bright red.
• Pain.

Haemorrhoids can bleed, prolapse, or thrombose. Simple bleeding usually requires conservative management. Prolapsed or thrombosed haemorrhoids may require surgical referral to assess the need for surgery.

Nursing assessment involves identifying if the cause is likely to be haemorrhoids, i.e. painless, bright red blood not mixed with stools, or if the bleeding is likely to be from higher in the GI tract and requires further assessment/investigation.

Nursing interventions

• Analgesia.
• Advice about stool softeners.
• Surgical referral in some cases.

Pilonidal abscess

Patients can either present to the ED or GP with pain and swelling at the coccyx. It more commonly affects ♂ in late teens to early twenties and can cause acute embarrassment. Systemic illness as a consequence of the infection is rare.

Signs and symptoms
- Pain and tenderness.
- Swelling.
- Area of fluctuant pus.
- Discharge.
- Surrounding cellulitis.

Nursing assessment and interventions
- Pain assessment score and analgesia.
- Preparation for admission.

Genitourinary emergencies

Overview

Patients with a GU problem may present with relatively minor complaints or more significant problems. Management priorities include:

- analgesia and symptom control;
- information about investigations;
- health promotion prior to discharge or preparation for admission.

Few patients need resuscitation, unless they are shocked (e.g. sepsis, toxic shock, and rarely pyelonephritis).

However, although not usually life-threatening, it is important to recognize that sexual health issues may cause extreme embarrassment to the patient, and it is important that nurses respond sensitively in order to minimize any distress.

The field of GUM also offers the emergency nurse the challenge of recognizing and acting on subtle clues. Some patients may fall within the 'see and treat' category and be sent to another facility, but consideration needs to be given to the vulnerable patient.

Those with child protection issues, mental health issues, or post-sexual assault may see the ED as a place of safety or the first part of contact to access information, reassurance, or other services, particularly as most GUM services are closed at the weekend or out of hours.

If registration takes place before nurse triage, the real reason for presentation may not be revealed due to embarrassment, shame, and/or lack of privacy at reception. Sensitivity needs to be employed when obtaining a relevant patient history, along with the recognition that, whilst people are becoming sexually active at a younger age, elderly people have sex too and can become unwell. Cultural issues may also prevent patients from being frank about their presenting complaint, and language barriers may present additional challenges. Cultural competence on the part of the nurse is essential to be able to respond sensitively, but effectively, to patients who may be the victims of sexual assault, rape, and FGM. It is important to remember that, in some minority cultures, such assaults on women are not seen as criminal offences, and women may be both ashamed and reluctant to report such problems, out of a misplaced loyalty to their families and also for fear of retribution.

▶ Be vigilant and mindful. The patient labelled as an 'inappropriate attender' may need your professional awareness, understanding, and compassion.

Assessment

History taking

Discussing what are usually intimate and private details with a stranger (albeit a health professional) risks patient dignity, and requires privacy and sensitivity. Social norms have changed positively in recent years; information and reassurance can reduce perceived shame and embarrassment in relation to genital injury, sexual assault, and STIs. It is particularly important for health-care staff to be aware of cultural practices, such as FGM, and the harmful physical, social, and psychological consequences of these practices. Safeguarding policies should be followed for any patient assessed as being at risk of such practices (➋ see Chapter 5).

- Family/friend input into history taking can be useful, particularly if a patient is in pain.
- Caution needs to be employed with maintaining patient confidentiality in the ED.
- Patients who present with symptoms that necessitate sexual history taking or sexual health promotion advice require a professional and non-familial interpreting service.
- Allowing a minor to interpret for a parent should also be avoided, and again professional interpreting advice should be sought.

Physical examination

Rarely is a bimanual examination required for the ED GU assessment, unless there are signs or symptoms to suggest lower abdominal or pelvic pathology (➋ see Figs. 11.1 and 11.2). The nurse should be familiar with the indications for this, and they should sign their name in the notes if acting as a chaperone. The examination should preferably take place in a private room with a door, or screens if in the resuscitation room. Give the patient privacy to undress, and use blanket/drapes to maintain the patient's dignity. Do not assist the patient to undress, unless consent is obtained and it is clear the patient needs assistance.

Further reading

General Medical Council (2001). *GMC guidelines on intimate examinations.* General Medical Council, London.

Royal College of Nursing (2006). *Vaginal and pelvic examinations: guidance for nursing staff.* Royal College of Nursing, London. Available at: ℘ http://www.rcn.org.uk.

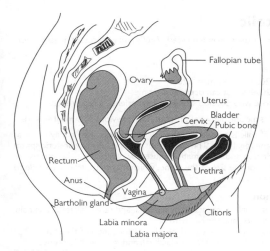

Fig. 11.1 Assessment of the genitourinary tract. Female genital anatomy.

(Reproduced with permission from Pattman, R., et al. (2010). *Oxford Handbook of Genitourinary Medicine, HIV, and Sexual Health*, 2nd edn, fig. 3.1, p. 55. Oxford University Press, Oxford.)

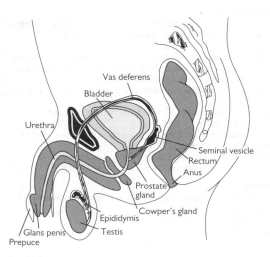

Fig. 11.2 Assessment of the genitourinary tract. Male genital anatomy.

(Reproduced with permission from Pattman, R., et al. (2010). *Oxford Handbook of Genitourinary Medicine, HIV, and Sexual Health*, 2nd edn, fig. 3.2, p. 57. Oxford University Press, Oxford.)

Renal colic

⚠ New-onset flank pain in the elderly (≥60y) may represent a leaking aortic aneurysm.

Prevalence

- In men 3:20, and in women 1:20.
- Peak age 20–40y, but can occur at any time.
- Half of those who develop stones will experience a recurrence.

Risk factors include dehydration, gout, UTI, previous or familial episodes.

Cause Renal colic is caused by calculi or blood clots, which may occur at any point in the renal tract. The pain is most often caused by ureteric spasm 2° to the irritation and inflammation caused by obstruction. Symptoms are not dependent on the size of the stone, which may range from a particle to a stone in the bladder.

Presentation

- The patient usually presents with unilateral, and rarely bilateral, loin pain from obstruction and/or haematuria.
- The location and type of pain depend on the location of the stone.
- Pain has been likened to that of childbirth and is acute. It is intense, constant, and dull, associated with excruciating colicky pain that can radiate to the abdomen or refer to the respective iliac fossa, testis, and tip of the penis or the labia.

Nursing assessment

- Family history or a past medical history of renal disease or GI problems.
- Patients are often unable to sit still, are restless with pain, and may be standing upright and pacing.
- The patient may be pale and sweaty, or experience intense nausea and/or vomiting as a result of acute renal capsule or ureteric distension and spasm with a sympathetic nervous system response.
- Frank haematuria. Microscopic haematuria is present in only 80% on dipstick.
- Dysuria and/or other signs of UTI with acute, intense pain and strangury suggest a urethral stone.
  - Symptoms usually resolve if the stone is passed or if the stone has caused complete obstruction.
  - The urinary flow is interrupted with a urethral stone, and, if large, acute urinary retention may occur.

Investigations

- Bilateral BP and femoral pulses. Examination for lower limb mottling may indicate AAA.
- Temperature, pulse, RR, BP, O_2 saturations.
- IV access, U&E, FBC.

Nursing interventions

▶▶ Ensure symptom control as soon as is possible.
- Diclofenac, usually PR/IM, is the analgesia of choice. It is effective with few side effects, but, as with all analgesia, its effect must be assessed. Sterile abscess incidence is 0.001% as a result of IM administration.
- An anti-emetic if nausea/vomiting are present.
- Start an IV infusion if persistent vomiting, and check postural BP and pulse.
- IV opioid analgesia.
- Anti-spasmodics and anticholinergics are of no benefit.
- Fever, if present, indicates a complicated renal colic. An antipyretic can also promote patient comfort.

Investigations *(continued)*

- Urinalysis for RBCs indicates renal tract trauma. A negative test does not exclude calculi.
- Sieving urine for passed stones and sending them for laboratory analysis is no longer practised in most areas. Check: urinalysis pH <5 suggests uric acid stones, and a pH >7.5 indicates co-infection.
- CT of the abdomen is the diagnostic gold standard, but usually a kidneys, urine, and bladder (KUB) X-ray film is done. This will identify 90–95% of renal calculi—75% are Ca^{2+} and radio-opaque.
- This is followed by an IV urogram (IVU). Two X-rays are taken at 20min and 1h post-contrast injection to examine the renal tract for the site and size/degree of the obstruction.
- Doppler/USS can be used in pregnant patients or those with renal disease.

Discharge

- Discharge, with renal outpatient follow-up, those who are symptom-free and whose IVU shows no obstruction.
  - Advise a fluid intake of 2–3L daily if no medical contraindications.
  - Nutritional advice for prevention is best provided by GP referral to a dietician.
- Prepare patients with infection, sepsis, renal impairment, or persistent pain for admission.

Urinary tract infection and cystitis (community-acquired)

Urinary tract infection/cystitis in women

- Twenty-five to 35% of women aged 20–40y have a history of UTI.
- This is not an STI, but coitus >4 times a month ↑ the risk of infection.
- Ninety per cent of UTIs are related to bacterial infection, particularly *Escherichia coli*, usually through self-transmission.
- One in 25 women will develop UTI in pregnancy.
- The use of spermicides with diaphragms can change the vaginal pH, ↑ susceptibility to *E. coli* infection.

Symptoms

- Symptoms of acute uncomplicated cystitis include dysuria, urinary frequency and urgency, lower back or suprapubic pain, cloudy or offensive urine, and haematuria.
- If loin pain, renal angle tenderness, fever, rigor, malaise, and vomiting are present, ascending infection/pyelonephritis is indicated, with the need for analgesia, antipyretics, IV antibiotics, and admission.

Investigations

- Urine dipstick: likely to be positive for nitrates and/or white cells and/or blood. Leucocytes/proteinuria is not indicative of infection.
- Midstream urine (MSU) should be taken and sent for laboratory analysis prior to starting antibiotics.

Health education

- Fluid intake may be reduced for the duration of oral antibiotic treatment to promote comfort, but thereafter ↑ to 2–3L daily if no medical contraindications.
- Advice that may reduce the risk of recurrence:
  - post-coital voiding (twice);
  - personal hygiene: wiping/washing genitals from front to back; no vaginal douching; wearing cotton pants; changing tampons more frequently.
- In those already experiencing recurrences, the above advice does not apply.
- There is no good clinical evidence that oral cranberry juice prevents UTIs. Anecdotally, patients are often advised to try cranberry juice to prevent UTIs.
- The use of oral probiotics is controversial.

Dysuria alone is suggestive of urethritis. Consider sexual history and the need for STI screening (➲ see Sexually transmitted infections, pp. 396–7).

Urinary tract infection/cystitis in men

Uncommon in ♂ under 50. Thereafter, it may ↑ 2° to incomplete bladder emptying and prostatitis.

Factors suggesting urinary tract infection

- Sexual history: long-standing stable sexual relationship/not sexually active.
- Age >50y (prostatism with UTI commoner).
- Symptoms: ↑ frequency, loin pain, pyrexia, and malaise.

Factors suggesting sexually acquired cause

- Presentation. ↑ likelihood if new sexual risk/suspicion about a partner. Urethritis arising within 4wk (usually).
- Age. Most commonly found in men from late teens to early 50s.
- Symptoms. Usually prominent dysuria and/or urethral discharge (may just be found on examination). ↑ urinary frequency and systemic symptoms unusual.

Investigations

- Urine dipstick: likely to be positive for nitrates and/or white cells and/or blood. Leucocytes/proteinuria is not indicative of infection.
- MSUs should be taken and sent for laboratory analysis prior to starting antibiotics.
- Fever indicates ascending infection.

Pyelonephritis and upper urinary tract infection

Cause Ascending renal tract infection/UTI.

Symptoms Loin pain, high fever, rigors, malaise, vomiting, and/or haematuria.

Management
- Baseline vital signs, symptom control, and fluid balance monitoring.
- Keep the patient comfortable, when shivering, with sheet/blankets, and remove them when rigoring has stopped.

Treatment Prepare for admission for IV antibiotics, symptom control, and observation.

Patient support and information
The National Kidney Federation. Tel: 0845 601 02 09. Available at: ℗ http://www.kidney.org.uk.

Acute retention of urine

In men, complaints are of suprapubic pain and a reduced or incomplete ability to pass urine. This may be 2° to a tumour or urethral stricture, or as a post-operative complication. Other causes seen in men and women are post-trauma, burns/scalds, uterine fibroids, infection, e.g. painful herpetic lesions, and blockage of long-term catheters.

Nursing assessment

History

- Last micturition, amounts of urine passed. Previous history.
- Consider a deliberate foreign body (➲ see Foreign bodies, p. 392) or a blocked indwelling catheter (IDC).
- Again provide privacy and a room with a door.
- Bladder decompression with an IDC is required if no contraindications, e.g. trauma or strictures.

Observation/inspection

- Obvious discomfort/distress. Exceptions are patients with chronic retention; this may be painless.
- Use a bladder scan to assess the size of the bladder.
- Abdominal percussion may reveal a distended bladder.
- Cloudy urine or pus with infection.
- Frank haematuria.
- Genital trauma, urethral bleeding in the unconscious patient.
- Palpation. Tender, enlarged bladder.
- Percussion:
  - suprapubic and above may be dull;
  - reduced or absent bowel sounds with constipation.
- Pyrexia indicates infection. Tachycardia due to this, pain, or haemorrhage 2° to infection, tumour, accidental or deliberate trauma.

Management

(➲ See Catheterization—female, pp. 676–7.)

- An IDC will provide pain relief. Insert, using an aseptic technique. Observe the urinary output for amount and frank haematuria.
- Document the catheter gauge and residual urine amount.
- Clamp after 1L has drained. Blood vessels previously compressed may now vasodilate with rebound hypotension.
- Remove the clamp after 30min.
- Confirm/exclude infection on urinary dipstick, and send an MSU specimen to the laboratory.

Bladder, urethral, and genital injury

- Be mindful of the mechanism of injury, and consider sexual assault in adults and NAI/abuse in children with genital injury.
- Cultural practices, such as ♀ circumcision, are illegal in the UK but may still be seen in diverse communities. It is important that nurses respond in a culturally competent way.[1]

Nursing assessment

Inspect

- Signs of FB, bleeding/trauma, and/or discharge.
- Inflammatory response 2° to scalds/burns. ►► Immediate referral to a specialist burns unit. Meanwhile, consider IDC, if appropriate, analgesia, and fluid replacement.
- IDC contraindicated post-blunt trauma resulting in anterior pelvic fracture with concomitant bladder/urethral trauma—blood visualized at urethral meatus.

Reference

1 Royal College of Nursing (2006). *Female genital mutilation: an educational resource for nursing and midwifery staff.* Available at: ℜ http://www.rcn.org.uk.

Priapism

Persistent painful erection not related to sexual desire.

Causes

In the ED, this may be:

- iatrogenic;
- related to spinal or perineal trauma;
- drugs, e.g. cocaine, cannabis, or phenothiazines;
- disease such as sickle cell, leukaemia, pelvic tumour, myeloma, renal dialysis.

Nursing assessment and interventions

- Apply ice packs, and give analgesia.
- If related to sickle cell, give O$_2$; this may resolve the priapism.

Management

- If the nursing interventions are unsuccessful or the patient presents >6h post-onset, this is an emergency.
- The nursing interventions just listed are not appropriate with priapism due to parasympathetic nervous system stimulation in spinal shock. Refer to the urology team, as aspiration of the corpora is needed. Rarely, surgery may be required.

Testicular torsion

- Testicular torsion is commoner in men <20y of age but can occur at any age.
- This is a paediatric/adolescent emergency.
- Presentation: acute onset of severe testicular pain ± vomiting. Pain from the testicles may be referred to the abdomen. Ask about (or examine a child for) red, tender, swollen testis.

Testicular torsion is seen mainly in neonates, children, and young men around puberty. In older ♀, it may be related to an undescended testicle.

- If not treated early, the testicle may need to be surgically removed, reducing future fertility and/or affecting body image.

Management

- Reassure the child or young person; give analgesia and/or anti-emetics, and give information to the patient or carer.
- ▶▶ An immediate surgical referral is required. This is a time-critical event and must be treated as such; the quicker the surgical intervention, the better the outcome.

Epididymo-orchitis

- In men <35y of age, epididymo-orchitis is usually related to bacterial STIs.
- In men >35y of age, it is most often related to bacteria that cause UTIs or viral mumps orchitis.
- Sexual health history in all cases is important.
- Non-infective causes can be seen in men with Behçet's disease or in relation to recent catheterization, other trauma, or high-dose amiodarone treatment.

Symptoms

- Unilateral scrotal pain and swelling (usually less severe and acute than torsion).
- If it is STI-related, symptoms of urethritis or a urethral discharge may be present but usually are not.
- Mumps orchitis: fever, myalgia, and malaise.
  - Parotiditis usually precedes the onset of orchitis by 3–5 days.
  - Incidence has reduced since introduction of measles, mumps, rubella (MMR) vaccination.

Investigations

- MSU for microscopy, culture, and sensitivity (M, C, & S).
- Doppler USS to exclude torsion of the spermatic cord.
- Referral to outpatient GUM clinic for STI screening, treatment, and partner notification, if appropriate.

Management and advice

- Bed rest, scrotal elevation, and ice packs to promote comfort.
- NSAIDs to provide analgesia and antipyretic benefits.
- Advise to avoid unprotected sexual intercourse (UPSI), until the patient and their partner have completed treatment and follow-up.
- The patient should return for reassessment if no improvement after 3 days of antibiotic treatment.
- Reassure the patient that full recovery is usual, complications are uncommon, and sterility is uncommon after acute epididymitis.

Bartholin's cyst or abscess

The Bartholin's glands lie at 4 and 8 o'clock within the vaginal vestibule. Damage or infection to the ostium of the gland ducts causes blockage, and a cyst occurs that may become infected. Found commonly in women aged 20–29, abscesses occur three times as often as cysts.

The onset is rapid over days or hours. Unilateral labial oedema precedes swelling and superficial dyspareunia, and painful swelling develops. The patient may have a wide-legged gait.

Staff should be cautious in attributing infective causes to *Neisseria gonorrhoeae/Chlamydia trachomatis*.

- STI screening can be arranged if sexual health history indicates.
- Nursing intervention should focus on prompt recognition and pain control.
- If STI screening is deemed necessary, reassure the patient that these infections are treatable with a short course of antibiotics.

Management

This depends on the size of the cyst.

- If small and no signs of infection, no action is taken; these cysts may rupture spontaneously.
- Marsupialization is considered as the best technique in preventing recurrence.
- More recently, the *Word* catheter technique is gaining in popularity in cyst management. This allows the cyst to heal naturally and reduces the incidence of the cyst re-forming.
- In women over 40, excision and histology to exclude malignancy are performed.

Foreign bodies

Genital FBs in adults can result from retained menstrual tampons, sexual practices, self-harm, or smuggling. These can include the following:
- Vaginal: tampons, contraceptive devices, and supportive pessaries;
- Vaginal/anal: condoms (after sex or containing drugs), sex toys;
- Urethra: self-harm, e.g. pens, paper clips.

Patients who are not compromised

The nurse's role with the well patient is to act as a chaperone and advocate, giving information and providing reassurance throughout the FB removal.
- Ask the patient to empty their bladder for removal of vaginal objects or to check for urethral obstruction.
- Check for haematuria if bladder injury is suspected.
- Consider Entonox® and/or other analgesia to promote a pain-free and speedy removal. Gather the equipment needed for this.
- Ensure privacy in a room with a lockable door.
- Reassure the patient that you will not be interrupted.
- Provide good lighting behind the practitioner removing the object.

Patients who are compromised

- The patient may be confused or unconscious, demonstrating signs of toxic shock.
- The effects of hidden, stored drugs would not be seen if they had not been orally ingested and passed through the GI system.
- Consider toxic shock syndrome if the patient is distressed, disorientated, confused, pyrexial, hypotensive (signs of shock), with a blanching generalized rash.
- Ask about LMP and retained tampons, and act as a chaperone and assist with a per vagina (PV) examination, which may find PV discharge, a forgotten pessary, or rarely a tumour.

Known drug users and/or attempting to avoid police arrest

- These patients may present with ↓ GCS and respiration, with pinned pupils (with no evidence of head injury).
- IV access, naloxone.
- The patient may return or be returned to police custody once medically cleared.

Self-harm and haemorrhage

- Measure baseline vital signs, and monitor level of consciousness and for signs of shock if bleeding is evident.
- Consider the patient's mental health needs if self-harming, and gain consent for mental health assessment.

Genital candidiasis

Thrush/moniliasis/candidosis is a fungal infection caused by a yeast, usually *Candida albicans* (80–90%). *Candida* commonly lives in small numbers around the genitals, especially the vagina, and is asymptomatic until it multiplies and penetrates the skin surface (➲ see Box 11.1).

Epidemiology

75% of women have at least one episode of genital candidiasis, with 40–50% having one or more recurrences. Men present with symptoms much less frequently.

Clinical features—women

- Symptoms.
  - Vulval pruritus and burning, with external dysuria and dyspareunia. These usually start/worsen from mid cycle and improve with menstruation (oestrogen level-related).
  - Twenty per cent have vaginal erythema, with a thick, white, curdy, adherent discharge in 20%, ↑ to 70% if pregnant. Discharge may be purulent or watery.
- Signs. Most commonly vulval erythema and oedema, with fissuring that can extend to the labia majora and/or perineum.
- In recurrent candidiasis (>4 times annually), vulval pruritus with burning is common. Signs are less common.

Clinical features—men

- In colonized men, the commonest symptom is post-coital itching/burning.
- It presents clinically as direct infection of the glans (balanitis) and/or prepuce (posthitis).
- Commoner in the uncircumcised, presenting as a glazed erythematous rash, sometimes with white papules/discharge, and, if severe, fissuring, oedema, and 2° phimosis.

Box 11.1 Transmission and predisposing factors—answering frequently asked questions

- Thrush is not usually sexually transmitted, particularly in women, although it is associated with recent cunnilingus.
- Partners do not need treatment, unless they have signs and symptoms themselves.
- Low (usual)-level oestrogen combined contraceptive pill does not ↑ the rate of thrush.
- Studies have shown that a yeast-free diet will not ↓ rate.
- The effectiveness of oral/topical yoghurt is controversial; PV use on a tampon may just soothe irritation.
- There is a small association with broad-spectrum antibiotics.

Vulvovaginitis

Vulvovaginitis in *children* arises in certain rare circumstances:
- insertion of FBs by the child herself;
- threadworm infestation;
- sexual interference.

▶ The possibility of NAI needs to be considered in any infection in children.

Sexually transmitted infections

Triage

- Whilst screening is not provided by the ED, post-exposure prophylaxis (PEP) for HIV/hepatitis B infection should be given priority at triage.
- Remain mindful and vigilant of *child protection issues in those underage*, and remember that ♀ and ♂ patients may present for STI screening *post-sexual assault/rape*. These patients are a triage priority. The patient may be distressed or aggressive, and de-escalation techniques may need to be employed.

Triage nurses need to be aware that, due to lack of privacy at reception, the patient may not have given their true reason for attending the ED.

- Taking a full sexual history is not appropriate at triage.
- The patient often realizes that they may need to attend elsewhere but needs reassurance that this is the case. ED staff awareness and input can demystify the GUM process for patients, reducing fear and misunderstanding, so that they access specialist services protecting their health and future fertility.

GUM clinic or ED?

STI prevalence in the young is ↑. Many infections are symptomless, with Chlamydia and gonorrhoea being predominant.

- Most GUM clinics now have a same-day, one-stop service with dedicated young person, ♂, and ♀ clinics.
- Over-the-counter Chlamydia urine screening is now available for 16–24y olds at some chemists, offering 70% sensitivity.
- Other patients may see the ED as an anonymous, safe place.
- Optimum screening time post-exposure/infection is usually within 10–14 days.
- Reassure patients regarding confidentiality in GUM practice, explaining that being known as only a number ensures privacy.

▶ Patients complaining of abdominal pain need to see a doctor.

Risk factors for sexually transmitted infections

- Age <25y. The highest rates of gonococcal and chlamydial infections occur in ♀ aged 16–19y and in ♂ aged 20–24y.
- Being single, separated, divorced, or not in a stable relationship (compared with marital, stable relationship, or widowed status) is associated with higher rates of STI.
- ≥2 partners in preceding 6 months.
- Use of non-barrier contraception.
- Residence in inner city.
- Symptoms in partner.
- History of previous STI.
- Ethnicity or migration. Prevalence of several infections, notably syphilis, gonorrhoea, and HIV infection, is higher in certain ethnic minority groups and immigrants.
- Sexual orientation. For example, syphilis, gonorrhoea, HIV, and HBV infections are more prevalent among homosexual men.

Genital herpes

- Patients may present with genital lesions and/or pain, itching ± vaginal or anal discharge.
- A vesicular swab must be taken, but treatment can be commenced on clinical grounds in the ED.
- GUM follow-up can be arranged for full STI screening, an internal examination, and long-term support.
- Codeine phosphate analgesia (with advice on its constipating effect), saline lavage, and micturition (if painful) in a warm bath can be advised to promote comfort.

Inspect/measure

- Pyrexia, tachycardia, hypotension. Consider sepsis 2° to PID.
- In other patients, a sexual health history may be important, and information about sexual practices may be a priority in order to prevent/minimize offence. For example, if there is an exudating, pustular sore throat or a painful, hot, swollen, non-traumatic joint in a sexually active person, consider gonorrhoea.

If treatment is started, patient details need to be taken, so that GUM referral can be made, facilitating patient follow-up regarding co-infection screening, treatment, surveillance, and partner notification.

Fraser guidelines

For under 16y olds, follow the Fraser guidelines (previously known as Gillick competence) in offering treatment/contraception.

Staff must respect their duty of confidentiality to a person under 16; this is as great as that owed to any other person. The guidelines exist to protect the practitioner and patient, ensuring best practice. If treatment is to be given to a person under 16, without the consent/knowledge of their parents, these guidelines must be followed.

- Maturity. The young person demonstrates understanding of the practitioner's advice.
- The practitioner has discussed the possibility of obtaining parental consent with the patient.
- The patient has begun, or is likely to begin/continue, having sexual intercourse.
- Unless the patient receives treatment/contraception, their physical/mental health is likely to suffer.
- Treatment/contraception is in the best interests of the patient.

Further reading

British Association for Sexual Health and HIV. Staff information. Available at: ℜ http://www.bashh. org.

Department of Health (2001). *The national strategy for sexual health and HIV.* Available at: ℜ http://webarchive.nationalarchives.gov.uk/20130107105354/http://www.dh.gov.uk/en/Publicationsandstatistics/Publications/PublicationsPolicyAndGuidance/DH_4003133.

Emergency contraception

Emergency contraception is used in coital exposure, whether from unprotected sex, condom breakages, omission or delay in taking/receiving contraception pills or depot injections, complete or partial expulsion of IUCD, and post-sexual assault/rape.

Oral progesterone-only emergency contraception

Oral progesterone-only emergency contraception (POEC) has replaced the combined emergency contraceptive. POEC is 99.6% effective and has reduced the rates of associated nausea and vomiting. Legally, POEC is a contraceptive, and not an abortifacient, as it prevents ovulation and/or implantation of a fertilized egg.

- The term 'morning-after pill' is discouraged, as POEC can be used up to <72h post-UPSI.
  - The earlier it is taken, the greater its effectiveness.
  - The risk of pregnancy ↑ by 50% for every 12h delay with POEC.
- POEC is available over the counter, but, if women present to the ED, consider age, vulnerability, socio-economic factors, and availability of participating pharmacies before sending the patient from the ED to the local pharmacy.
- Some patients who present saying pregnancy is their 'problem' are, in fact, asking for emergency contraception.
- POEC needs to be prescribed or given under PGD in the ED.
- Give POEC <72h after UPSI, but first ask and consider the following.
  - Was the sexual intercourse consensual?
  - When was the LMP? If within the last 4wk, a urine HCG is not required.
  - Ensure no previous UPSI or POEC in the last cycle. POEC may be used if clinically indicated.
  - Past medical history. A double dose is needed for patients taking enzyme-inducing drugs or antibiotics, e.g. St John's wort, anticonvulsant therapy, antiretrovirals, and some TB medication.
  - Warfarin users should have their INR checked within 3–4 days, as it may alter significantly or they may have an intrauterine device (IUD), instead of POEC.
  - Also consider alcohol and drug issues, and the need for referral to community drug or alcohol services.
  - <16y olds (➔ see Sexually transmitted infections, pp. 396–7). Consider child protection issues.
- Give 1.5mg levonorgestrel (now one tablet) as soon as possible. A PV examination is not required. A few discreet questions can establish whether the patient is in a safe, consensual sexual relationship.
- On discharge, tell the women to:
  - return for a repeat prescription if she vomits within 3h;
  - return if abdominal pain develops; consider the risk of ectopic pregnancy if the patient returns. If the next period is light or late, a pregnancy test should be taken.
- Before discharging, discuss safer sex, and raise awareness of local family planning services.

>72h post-unprotected sexual intercourse

Refer to a local family planning centre for a copper IUD within 5 days (120h) of:

- the first sexual exposure within a menstrual cycle; or
- the earliest calculated ovulation date. (Take the earliest next menstrual start date; subtract 14 days, and add 5—useful in cycles of 21–30 days.)

Post-exposure prophylaxis

Patients may present in an anxious state, following possible sexual exposure to HIV. It is thought that antiretrovirals may reduce dissemination and replication if initiated early post-exposure. These patients should be prioritized and assessed, and the decision to administer PEP should be based on the risk of HIV acquisition and the potential adverse effects of antiretroviral therapy. Follow local guidelines for PEP.

Skin emergencies

Overview

Skin problems are a frequent adult and paediatric presentation in emergency and urgent care settings, due to either the severity and acuteness of the condition (e.g. deep dermal burn) or its disruptive nature (e.g. itchy rash). A huge array of skin problems can present over the course of a shift. Some of these need urgent treatment and are covered in this chapter. Other less urgent, but common, presentations are also covered. However, many of the latter require follow-up by the GP for ongoing management or dermatology referral. Fig. 12.1 shows the structure of the skin.

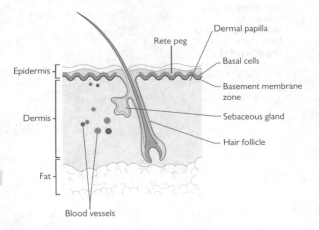

Fig. 12.1 Structure of the skin.

(Reproduced with permission from Burge, S. & Willis, D. (2011). *Oxford Handbook of Medical Dermatology*, p. 5. Oxford University Press, Oxford.)

The skin

The skin is composed of two layers. The epidermis is the superficial layer, and the dermis lies beneath it. Underneath these layers is the subcutaneous tissue, composed of adipose and connective tissue and blood vessels.

Epidermis

This does not contain blood vessels but receives its nutrients from the dermis. It is composed of five layers of cells. New cells are formed in the deepest layer (basal layer) and migrate upwards, until they are shed from the skin surface (horny layer). The entire epidermis is replaced every 3wk.

Dermis

This is composed of connective tissue, capillary loops, lymph vessels, nerve endings, temperature and touch receptors, sebaceous glands, sweat glands, and hair follicles. Fibroblasts produce collagen. It is a network of collagen and elastic fibres that give skin its strength and elasticity. Fibroblasts and macrophages move around within the dermal layers and are essential for wound healing.

Nursing assessment

> ❶ Occasionally, patients may present with a skin condition that is associated with a life-threatening problem that requires immediate ABC assessment and resuscitative intervention.

- A patient with a burn must be assessed for the presence or risk of a pulmonary injury, as this can develop rapidly, causing partial or complete airway obstruction.
- Upper airway swelling and laryngospasm associated with anaphylaxis may present initially as an urticarial rash.
- Purpuric or petechial rashes in an unwell patient should be treated as a potential presentation of septic shock, until proven otherwise.

History

The assessment and management of burns are dealt with separately in this chapter (❷ see Burns, pp. 406–8; Major burns, pp. 414–16; Minor burns, pp. 418–19). For other skin problems, the following features from the history will help to guide further assessment and management.

- Onset—this will indicate the acuteness of the condition. Rapid development can point to a more serious problem.
- Trauma—whether an injury preceded the problem.
- Main complaints—itching, weeping, oozing, crusting, burning, blistering, skin peeling, lesions, pain, swelling, bruising, petechiae, purpura.
- Site of skin problem—grouping, distribution, and extent of the spread.
- Relieving factors—any treatment that has improved the symptoms.
- Aggravating factors—any factor that has made the symptoms worse.
- Systemic upset—any systemic symptoms (e.g. fever).
- Contacts—consider whether it is possible that the skin problem is infectious.

Physical assessment

Inspection

Depending on the site and extent of the spread, the patient may need to be fully undressed to ensure that all affected areas are inspected. Careful inspection can identify the type of lesion(s) present (❷ see Box 12.1).

The exact site and shape or grouping of the lesion(s) should also be noted. Drawing the site of the lesion(s) can aid accurate description.

Palpation

Examination of the lesion or rash can identify whether it is solid, fluid-filled, painful, blanching, or oedematous.

Assessment and investigations

- A full set of vital signs should be obtained if infection is present or the patient is systemically unwell.
- Pain assessment and score.
- Wound swab of any exudate.

Nursing interventions

- Analgesia should be given, according to the patient's pain score.
- Wound dressing if appropriate.
- Antibiotics if infection is present.
- Antihistamine can help to relieve the itching and/or swelling associated with urticaria.

Box 12.1 Types of lesions

- *Macule.* Purely a colour change; flat and <1cm in diameter (e.g. freckle, petechiae).
- *Patch.* Macule >1cm in diameter (e.g. Mongolian blue spot).
- *Papule.* A solid elevated swelling <1cm in diameter (e.g. mole, wart).
- *Plaque.* Papules that merge to form a surface elevation (e.g. psoriasis).
- *Nodule.* Solid elevated hard or soft lump >1cm in diameter.
- *Tumour.* Soft or firm, deeper into the dermis, benign or malignant, >2cm in diameter (e.g. lipoma).
- *Wheal.* Superficial, raised, transient, and erythematous. Irregular in shape due to oedema (e.g. allergic reaction).
- *Hives.* Wheals that merge to form an extensive reaction. Intensely itchy.
- *Vesicle.* Elevated cavity containing clear fluid, <1cm in diameter (e.g. early chickenpox (varicella)).
- *Bulla or blister.* Fluid-filled elevated cavity >1cm in diameter, superficial in the epidermis, thin-walled and ruptures easily (e.g. burn blister).
- *Pustule.* Small pus-filled elevated cavity (e.g. acne).
- *Abscess.* Larger cavity containing pus.
- *Cyst.* Encapsulated fluid-filled cavity tensely elevating the skin (e.g. sebaceous cyst).
- *Ulcer.* Crater-like skin lesion, healing of which is often delayed (e.g. pressure ulcer, leg ulcer).
- *Crust.* Hard, dry exudate from vesicles or pustules that have burst (e.g. impetigo).
- *Scale.* Compact dry flakes of skin (e.g. psoriasis).

Burns

Burns are an extremely common presentation in urgent care settings and range from minor to life-threatening in nature. They can be acutely painful, painless, or limb-threatening. Some require no further assessment or management, whereas others require intensive resuscitation in the ED, followed by transfer to a tertiary regional burns centre that may be located many miles away.

Flame burns and scalds represent the majority of burns. Chemical and electrical burns account for only around 5%. Children under 5y of age often attend with contact burns or scalds sustained at home. In the summer months, patients can attend with burns from the sun or barbecues. In November, Bonfire Night can cause a rise in the number of patients attending with burns from fireworks or fires.

❶ As with any injury, always consider the possibility of NAI. Children and the elderly are most vulnerable. Around 10% of children with an NAI also have a wound or burn.

Nursing assessment of the patient with a burn

Rapid ABCDE assessment following the ATLS/ETC guidelines is required to identify individuals with any life- or limb-threatening problem. Subsequent assessment involves identifying the site, extent, and depth of the burn, and deciding how and where the burn should be managed until it has healed.

There are several life-threatening consequences of an acute burn injury that need to be anticipated in patients with all but the most minor burns. The ED team has to identify which, if any, are present or, more challengingly, which may develop over minutes or hours following the burn. The main pathophysiological effects are airway obstruction, pulmonary injury, and hypovolaemic shock.

Airway obstruction

Any patient who may have inhaled superheated air or smoke or toxic fumes is at high risk of upper airway burns and possible upper airway obstruction. Early intubation is key to successful management, as the oedema that accompanies airway burns develops rapidly and can make passage of an ETT impossible, if left too late.

Pulmonary injury

Damage to the lung tissue due to inhalation of the chemical by-products of combustion causes significant damage to the lower airways, resulting in atelectasis, reduced ciliary clearance, and loss of surfactant. This predisposes the patient to infection and sepsis. Carbon monoxide (CO) poisoning can result from inhalation injury, leading to severe hypoxia and brain injury. Pulmonary injury is associated with significant morbidity and mortality, and can be present in the absence of any burns to the skin. Intensive care treatment is required and is mainly supportive, aimed at preventing hypoxia, infection, and atelectasis.

Hypovolaemic shock

Major burns cause hypovolaemic shock some hours after injury, due to damaged capillaries leaking plasma and protein. Protein leakage causes more fluid to shift from the intravascular spaces to the interstitial spaces, and oedema develops. The rate of fluid loss is dependent on the size of the burn and the amount of time that has elapsed since the burn injury. The prevention of hypovolaemic shock begins in the ED with a fluid resuscitation regimen and continues for 24–48h.

History

- Time of burn. Has there been a delay in presentation?
- Type of burn—chemical, electrical, radiation, flame, scald, or contact.
- Where did the burn happen? Was it in an enclosed space? Is there a risk of inhalation of smoke, fumes, or heat?
- Other complaints. Does the patient have any other injuries or problems?
- Site. Are the face, mouth, or airways involved?
- First aid measures. Immediate application of cold water can reduce the depth and extent of the burn.
- NAI. Are there any features of the history that suggest the cause may be non-accidental?

Electrical burns

- Where did the electrical injury occur (i.e. was it domestic or industrial)?
- What was the path of the current?
- Are there entrance and exit wounds?

Electrical burns are almost always full thickness, but the extent of the tissue damage is rarely visible in the ED. Significant electrical burns can cause cardiac conduction abnormalities and myoglobinuria due to extensive tissue and muscle damage, which can cause renal failure. Significant or high-voltage electrical burns require aggressive fluid resuscitation. Most require referral to a regional burns centre, and advice will be given about a suitable fluid resuscitation regime.

Chemical burns

- What chemical was involved? Alkaline substances usually cause deeper burns.
- First aid. For how long was the burn irrigated prior to attending?

Chemical burns should be treated with copious irrigation for at least 20min. The regional poisons centre or ℘ https://www.toxbase.org/ can be contacted for specific advice about the chemical involved.

Cement burns

These are common and are not initially noticed, as cement falls inside a work boot and slowly erodes the skin surface. They can become full thickness, if not treated quickly with irrigation. Due to the nature of a chemical injury and the difficulty in completely removing the burn agent, the depth of a chemical burn can continue to ↑ over a period of several days. Patients should be warned about this, and early involvement of a regional burns centre is advised.

Pulmonary injury

A pulmonary or inhalation injury should be suspected if any of the following are present:
- history of being in an enclosed space where hot toxic fumes could have been inhaled;
- burns to the face, nose, lips, or palate;
- singed nasal hairs, eyebrows, or eyelashes;
- burns or erythema to the mouth or nose;
- hoarse voice;
- stridor.

Burn assessment

Extent of the burn

This is described as a percentage of the total body surface area (TBSA). In adults, the simple Wallace 'rule of nines' can be used to quickly estimate the percentage of the body that has been burnt. Each area of the body is awarded a multiple of nine (➔ see Fig. 12.2a).

Alternatively, the palmar surface of the patient's hand with the thumb adducted represents ~1% of their TBSA. This can be used in adults and children as an initial estimate of TBSA burnt.

Ideally, a burn assessment tool should be used to shade the areas of the body that have been burnt and allow an estimate of the percentage of the TBSA that has been burnt. The Lund and Browder chart offers an alternative tool and provides a more accurate assessment, as it makes allowances for the alteration in body shape with age. The extent of the burn as a percentage of the TBSA can be assessed using this method in the ED and regional burns centre (➔ see Fig. 12.2b).

> ❶ Major burns require immediate fluid resuscitation and referral to a regional burns centre from the ED.
> • A major burn in an adult is ≥15% of the TBSA.
> • A major burn in a child is ≥10% of the TBSA.

Inspection

Depth of the burn

The depth of a burn is dependent on the amount of heat applied and the duration of contact. Burns are commonly described as superficial, superficial partial thickness (SPT), deep dermal, or full thickness (➔ see Table 12.1). In fact, they are usually of mixed depth.

Accurate identification of the depth of the burn can be difficult, even for the experienced ED clinician. Due to continued damage to the microcirculation over the first 48h, burns can be deeper than first estimated. For this reason, all but the most superficial burns should be reviewed at 48–72h.

Site of burn

Identifying the exact site of the burn is important in all but superficial burns, as 'special areas' of the body may require management by a burns specialist, regardless of the size and depth of the burn. The following burn sites should be discussed with the regional burns centre:
• face;
• hands;
• feet;
• perineum;
• nipples;
• any flexure, especially the neck or axilla;
• circumferential burns.

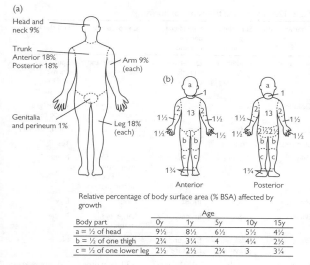

Relative percentage of body surface area (% BSA) affected by growth

Body part	Age				
	0y	1y	5y	10y	15y
a = ½ of head	9½	8½	6½	5½	4½
b = ½ of one thigh	2¾	3¼	4	4¼	2½
c = ½ of one lower leg	2½	2½	2¾	3	3¼

Fig. 12.2 (a) The Wallace 'rule of nines'. (b) The Lund and Browder chart.

Circumferential burns

Extremity burns that are circumferential can cause compartment syndrome. Patients with deep dermal or full-thickness burns are at greatest risk of a compartment syndrome that compromises perfusion to the limb. A significant compartment syndrome will require urgent escharotomy. This may have to be done in the ED, but more commonly the procedure is performed in theatre. Circumferential burns to the chest can significantly compromise ventilation and may also require urgent escharotomy, which, in some cases, may be palliative.

Palpation

Palpation of the burn (with sterile gloves) identifies texture, blanching, degree of pain, and ability to discriminate between blunt touch and pinprick.

Auscultation

Wheezing, stridor, and tachypnoea can indicate an inhalation injury.

Table 12.1 Estimating the depth of burns

Characteristic	Superficial (e.g. sunburn)	Superficial partial thickness	Deep dermal	Full thickness
Skin layer	Epidermis	Epidermis and superficial dermis	Epidermis and dermis	Epidermis, dermis, and deep structures
Colour	Red	Red	White, creamy, mottled	White, grey, black, brown
Texture	Soft	Soft	Soft	Hard, leathery
Skin loss	None	Yes	Yes	Yes
Pain	Painful	Very painful; sensitive to air and temperature	Slight; some insensate areas. Poor discrimination	None
Moisture	Dry	Moist	Moist	Dry
Blisters	None	Immediately	Large, easily liftable	None
Blanching	Brisk under pressure	Brisk under pressure	Delayed	None
Healing time	3–7 days	10–21 days if no infection is present	>30 days; may be preferable to skin graft	Will not heal without graft

Major burns

Following physical assessment of the patient, a decision has to be made about their subsequent management. This is based on whether the patient needs referral to a regional burns service (➜ see Box 12.2) or can continue to be managed by the ED. If an opinion about referral is sought from the regional burns service, further assessment and investigations are usually decided by them. The following assessment and investigations can act as a guide, even if a regional burns centre is involved.

Assessment and investigations

Assessment of ABCDE according to the ATLS/ECT guidelines is crucial for identifying individuals with potential or actual airway obstruction, pulmonary injury, and hypovolaemic shock. Assess patients who have been burnt during an explosion or who have jumped from a burning building for other injuries, using the standard ABCD approach (➜ see Major trauma: introduction, pp. 488–9). Perform the following assessments and investigations for patients with a suspected major burn:

- pulse, temperature, RR, and BP;
- pulse oximetry;
- GCS score—this may indicate developing cerebral hypoxia;
- cardiac monitoring;
- pain assessment and score;
- FBC, U&E, clotting, and cross-matching;
- CBG levels;
- CXR—will act as a baseline;
- ABG if the patient is shocked or inhalation is suspected;
- ECG if an electrical injury has occurred;
- tetanus status.

Box 12.2 Minimum threshold for referral to a regional burns service

- All burns ≥2% of the TBSA in children or ≥3% of the TBSA in adults.
- All full-thickness burns.
- All circumferential burns.
- Any burn that has not healed within 2wk.
- Any burn where there is suspicion of NAI should be referred to a regional burns service within 24h.

Factors that should prompt discussion with a regional burns service

- All burns to the hands, feet, face, perineum, or genitalia.
- Any chemical, electrical, or friction burn.
- Any cold injury.
- Any unwell or febrile child with a burn.
- Any concern about co-morbidities that may affect treatment or healing.

British Burn Association (2012). *National Burn Care Referral Guidance*. British Burn Association, London. Available at: ℘ http://www.britishburnassociation.org/downloads/National_Burn_Care_Referral_Guidance_-_5.2.12.pdf.

Nursing interventions

- Airway management. Suction may be required if the patient is unable to clear their own airway.
- Airway protection. Rapid endotracheal intubation will be required in patients with actual or potential airway or pulmonary burns. An ETT of small circumference (➔ see Ventilation: mechanical, pp. 764–5) is often needed if the airway is already oedematous. The ETT should not be cut, as a longer length will be required, as the airway and face swell over time.
- Administer O_2 to patients with suspected inhalation injury.
- Ventilation is required for patients with airway burns, pulmonary injury, or hypoxia.
- IV access. To allow administration of analgesia and IV fluids, patients with major burns will require two large-bore cannulae. Cannulae can be inserted into burnt tissue as a last resort. IO access can be used if venous access is difficult.
- Fluid replacement. Patients with a major burn require fluid resuscitation to prevent the development of hypovolaemic shock (➔ see Box 12.3). Hartmann's solution is most commonly used.
- Analgesia. Opiate analgesia should be given IV, titrated to response.
- Large doses of morphine (>30mg) may be required.
- Wound care. Initial cleansing can remove soot and debris to enable clearer assessment of the extent and depth. The burn should be covered as soon as possible. Large burns requiring transfer to the regional burns service can be covered in cling film. Smaller burns need non-adherent dressing in contact with the burn surface, and 2° dressing that is absorbent enough for the burn exudate over the first 48h.

Box 12.3 Fluid resuscitation for patients with major burns

The commonest fluid resuscitation formula is the Parkland (Baxter) formula.

A volume of 4mL/kg × % TBSA is given during the first 24h. Half is given in the first 8h after the burn injury occurs, and the remaining half is given over the next 16h.

❶ It is important to remember that the fluid resuscitation is calculated *from the time of injury*. For example, if the patient arrives in the ED 1h after injury, half of the fluid needs to be give over the next 7h.

Sample burn calculation

A 70kg man has a 35% TBSA burn, which he sustained in a house fire at 11 p.m. He arrives in the ED at 12 midnight. His fluid requirement is calculated as follows:

$$4 \times 70 \times 35 = 9800\text{mL over the first 24h}$$

A total of 4900mL are needed in the first 8h. Two hours have now elapsed since the burn, so 4900mL are required over 6h, which is equivalent to 817mL/h.

- Tetanus immunization. Burns are classified as tetanus-prone due to the degree of devitalized tissue. Patients who do not have adequate immunity require tetanus vaccination and Ig (➜ see Tetanus prophylaxis, p. 338).
- Maintain body temperature. Patients with major burns lose their ability to maintain their body temperature. This is compounded by the initial, and sometimes prolonged, cooling of the skin, infusion of cool IV fluids, and skin exposure in the ED. Infusion of warmed fluids, a warm environment, and keeping the patient covered can help to prevent hypothermia.

Minor burns

The commonest burn encountered in ED practice is the minor burn, which does not fulfil the criteria for urgent referral to a burns centre (➔ see Box 12.2). However, all but the most superficial burns require careful management to ensure optimal healing.

General management of the minor burn

- Analgesia should be given according to the patient's pain score.
- Cleansing to remove any debris, soot, or topical first aid treatments.
- Debridement, if appropriate.
- Dressing (➔ see Box 12.4).
- Tetanus immunization, if appropriate (➔ see Tetanus prophylaxis, p. 338).
- Discharge advice.
- Follow-up arrangements.

Debridement of burn blisters
There is still great controversy over the management of burn blisters. Research has highlighted the beneficial effects of leaving blisters intact, but equally there have been reports of the beneficial effects of removing them. Similarly, some studies suggest that leaving a blister intact is deleterious to wound healing, whereas other studies suggest that deroofing of blisters is just as harmful. Thus, the question of how to manage burn blisters is not an easy one to answer. However, application of the following principles can aid decision-making.

- Dead or devitalized tissue can act as a focus for infection and should therefore be removed.
- Total blister debridement can be painful.
- The depth of a burn cannot easily be assessed if there are intact blisters present, so these may need to be removed.
- Small blisters that do not restrict function can be left intact.
- Large blisters that restrict function may need to be removed.
- Burns that are allowed to dehydrate can become deeper. Therefore, if a blister is removed, an appropriate dressing is required.

Box 12.4 The ideal burn dressing

There is no one dressing that is ideal for all sites and types of burn and the stage of healing. Compromises will need to be made, and products changed as the burn heals. Ideally, a burn dressing should have as many of the following characteristics as possible.

- non-adherent;
- provides thermal insulation;
- provides a moist environment but does not create maceration;
- impermeable to bacteria;
- comfortable, conformable, and acceptable to the patient;
- hypoallergenic;
- absorbent (exudate is most prolific in the first 48–72h), but not likely to dry the burn;
- cost-effective and available in the right size;
- does not require frequent dressing changes.

Discharge advice

Patients (and, in the case of children, their parents) should be advised to:
- keep the burn clean and dry;
- attend a treatment room dressing service for a dressing change if the dressing leaks;
- elevate the burn if it is on a limb;
- attend any follow-up arrangement;
- return immediately if they become unwell.

A rare, but life-threatening, complication of a minor burn or wound (also sometimes associated with tampon use) is toxic shock syndrome (TSS). There are 15–20 recorded cases per year for all causes in the UK. Some of these will be from minor burns and result in the death of the patient. TSS is seen more commonly in children, as they have not yet developed immunity to the TSS toxins. Without alarming parents or patients, clear written and verbal advice needs to be given about the signs and symptoms of TSS and when to return to the ED.

▶▶ It is vital to return immediately to the ED if any of the following symptoms develop:
- high temperature;
- rash;
- loss of appetite;
- nausea or vomiting;
- abdominal pain or diarrhoea;
- sore throat;
- tiredness;
- muscle aches or pain;
- dizziness;
- confusion;
- fainting or feeling faint.

Follow-up for minor burns

All but the most minor burns require follow-up at 48–72h to confirm the depth and size of the burn. Dressings usually need to be changed at this stage, as they can be saturated with exudate.

Infected burns

Occasionally, burns can become infected and require investigation (wound swab) and treatment with antibiotics. Signs of a burn wound infection include:
- ↑ pain;
- cellulitis;
- erythematous wound margin;
- ↑ exudate;
- discoloration of the burn (e.g. dark brown or black);
- delayed healing;
- conversion of a partial-thickness burn to a full-thickness burn.

Treatment of an infected burn requires a course of antibiotics (according to local guidelines). Review at 48–72h, and give clear written and verbal advice about the need to return sooner if the patient becomes systemically unwell.

Skin infections

Skin infections and abscesses are commonly seen in emergency and urgent care settings, and most of them are easily diagnosed and treated. Local skin infections, such as paronychia, cellulitis, abscesses, wound infections, and bites and stings are covered in ➋ Wound infection, pp. 332–3 and Skin infections, pp. 334–5.

Erysipelas is a less common skin infection, worthy of mention due to its rapid onset and site of presentation. Necrotizing fasciitis is a rare, but life-threatening, tissue infection that requires rapid diagnosis and treatment.

Erysipelas

This is a streptococcal bacterial infection of the dermis that can spread rapidly, causing swelling, redness, and pain. Erythematous lesions enlarge rapidly and have raised well-demarcated edges (this is what distinguishes it from cellulitis), often described as having the texture of orange peel. There is usually rapid spread through the lymphatic vessels. Facial areas around the eyes, ears, and cheeks are susceptible, and facial swelling can be very dramatic. Treatment is with antibiotics, usually for a prolonged period, as recurrence can occur in one-third of patients.

Necrotizing fasciitis

This is a very rare, rapidly advancing soft tissue infection that causes wide-spread necrosis of the fascia and septicaemia. There may be gas formation in the tissues and gangrene. At first, the signs may be subtle, but they will progress rapidly. The skin is acutely painful, becoming swollen, blistered, red, and then purple. The patient is acutely unwell, with fever and signs of septic shock. Mortality can be as high as 70%. Treatment involves early antibiotics, surgical debridement and/or amputation of an affected limb, and intensive care.

Impetigo

Impetigo is a common skin infection, which is more often seen in children than in adults. It sometimes follows a recent URTI. It is a superficial infection involving the top layers of the skin, and is caused by *Streptococcus*, *Staphylococcus*, or both. Impetigo is contagious. The infection is carried in the fluid that oozes from the blisters.

Symptoms

- Skin lesions on the face or lips, or on the arms or legs, spreading to other parts of the body.
- It begins as a cluster of tiny blisters that burst, followed by oozing and the formation of a thick honey- or brown-coloured crust that is very tenacious.

Treatment

This consists of oral or topical antibiotics.

Rashes

A rash is any change in the appearance, colour, or texture of the skin. Adults and children with skin rashes frequently attend the ED and urgent care facilities, due to concerns that the rash is a sign of a serious illness (e.g. meningococcal septicaemia) or because it is causing significant irritation or discomfort.

In patients who present with a rash, it can be quite difficult to make an accurate diagnosis in an ED setting. ED assessment involves identifying any sign or symptom that requires immediate treatment (e.g. a purpuric rash or a skin infection that requires antibiotics). ED management involves the treatment of immediate symptoms, inpatient referral for continued management or further investigation, or outpatient treatment, usually with antihistamines, and referral back to primary care.

Skin infestations

There are several common skin and hair infestations that can present to emergency care areas. Most of them require only simple advice and over-the-counter treatment from a pharmacy.

Scabies

Scabies is a common mite infestation that produces tiny reddish papules and severe itching, as young mites hatch just beneath the skin. Scabies spreads easily from person to person via physical contact or shared objects. The mites are destroyed by normal laundering.

Signs and symptoms

- The commonest symptom of scabies is intense itching, which is usually worse at night.
- Thin lines with a lump at the end can sometimes be seen on the skin. These are the burrows of the young mites.
- Common sites are the webs between the fingers and toes, wrists, ankles, buttocks, and, in ♂, the genitals.
- Intense itching can lead to a bacterial skin infection.

Treatment

- Scabies can be cured by applying a topical cream containing an insecticide, which is left on the skin for 12–24h (depending on the preparation) and then washed off. One treatment is usually sufficient, although a second application 1wk later may be required.
- An antihistamine can help to relieve the itching, which can persist for several weeks.
- Any person who is in close physical contact with the patient should be treated as well.
- Clothing and bedding used during the preceding few days should be washed in hot water and dried in a hot dryer.

Head lice

Head lice can reach epidemic proportions in schools and are extremely common. Parents commonly detect lice in their children, or a letter may be sent from school informing parents of a recent outbreak.

Signs and symptoms

Severe itching is the commonest symptom, especially at night when the lice are feeding. Lice can be visible in the hair, and eggs are attached to the hair shaft close to the scalp.

Treatment

This involves the use of a topical solution and/or a metal 'nit' comb. The whole family will need treatment.

Threadworms

Threadworms are the commonest worm infestation in humans. They are 5–10mm long and resemble tiny pieces of white cotton. They most commonly infect children and are spread from person to person or via an object (e.g. toilet seat, towels). They are not caught from animals. The threadworm eggs are swallowed and hatch in the intestine. The ♀ threadworm migrates to the anus where thousands of eggs are laid.

Signs and symptoms

The main symptom is intense itching around the anus, especially at night. Itching can disturb sleep and may cause bed-wetting in children. The threadworms may be visible on faeces where they look like moving pieces of white cotton.

Treatment

- Over-the-counter treatments are available. Advice should be sought from a pharmacist as to which the most suitable is (e.g. for young children or pregnant women).
- General hygiene measures are vital to stop the spread or any re-infection (e.g. the use of separate towels, regular change of bedding washed on a hot cycle, strict hand hygiene).

Urticaria

An urticarial rash is the rapid appearance of erythematous, itchy swellings or wheals that are blotchy and vary in size and shape. It is usually transient and can disappear within hours. It can be caused by drugs, foods, infection, or emotional stress. Occasionally, angio-oedema around the lips and mouth can be present. If the tongue and upper airways are affected, this can be a life-threatening feature.

Urticarial rashes usually respond well to antihistamines. Patients who do not respond to antihistamines may benefit from a short course of systemic steroids. Treatment with adrenaline is indicated if angio-oedema threatens the airway.

Leg ulcers

A leg ulcer is defined as any break in the skin above the malleoli and below the patella that does not heal within 4wk. Leg ulcers are extremely common, and affect 1% of the adult population and 3.6% of people over 65y of age. They are debilitating and painful, and can significantly impair quality of life. The cost to the NHS is estimated to be around £400 million each year. About 90% of leg ulcers are caused by venous, arterial, or neuropathic disease.

Patients may attend the ED with a concern about an already established ulcer (e.g. infection), or they may simply attend requesting a dressing change. In addition, the ED nurse may coincidentally discover an untreated leg ulcer in a patient presenting with another problem. Another important consideration for the ED nurse is the identification of patients with an acute wound to the lower limb that is likely to undergo delayed healing and develop into an ulcer. In these situations, it is important to provide appropriate discharge advice and refer the patient to a community leg ulcer treatment facility.

Patients with an acute lower leg wound and any of the following features are predisposed to the development of a leg ulcer:
• previous leg ulcer;
• previous DVT;
• IV drug user;
• varicose veins;
• varicose eczema;
• venous flare;
• lower limb skin staining (haemosiderin pigmentation);
• lower limb pale areas (atrophie blanche);
• fibrotic areas on the lower limb (lipodermatosclerosis).

Management
• Leg ulcers of venous origin (the commonest aetiology) heal more rapidly with compression bandaging, as this aids venous return.
• Compression bandaging should only be started after a comprehensive assessment of the lower limb and exclusion of an arterial disease as the cause.
• Ulcer assessment and management are usually undertaken by specially trained community or tissue viability nurses and should not be attempted in the ED by a non-specialist.

ED management of a leg ulcer involves treating any infection, applying a temporary absorbent dressing, and referring the patient to the nearest leg ulcer service.

Leg ulcers

Management

Ophthalmological emergencies

Introduction

Eye problems are common presentations in emergency care areas. Adults and children frequently attend with minor injuries to the eye, visual problems, and other painful/red eye conditions. Assessment of patients with eye problems requires the clinician to have some basic eye assessment skills, e.g. lid eversion (➔ see Eyelid eversion, p. 702), and access to a slit lamp to enable a complete assessment of the eye/s to be made. If a slit lamp is not available or the clinician is not familiar with how to use it, the patient will need referral to a centre with comprehensive eye assessment facilities.

Assessment of the patient with eye problems

▶ Assessment of visual acuity (VA) is mandatory and should be under-taken at the point of triage for any patient presenting with an eye problem. A VA should be established before any other investigations or treatment (except irrigation or instillation of LA) are carried out. An accurate triage category cannot be assigned without an accurate VA and an assessment of whether this is normal for the patient.

History taking

An accurate history is important. Questions should include the following.
- How long have the symptoms been present?
- Are they getting better/worse/stable?
- How did the problem begin and over what period of time?
- The degree, type, and location of any pain?
- Whether vision is reduced and to what degree?
- Is there any discharge or watering?
- Is the patient photophobic?
- Has the patient had this, or a similar problem, before?
- Are there any concurrent systemic problems?

Examining the eye

It is very easy to assume a diagnosis from the history and miss less obvious problems. Eye examination, therefore, must be systematic, starting at the outside (eye position and surrounding structures) and working inwards to consider the globe itself. The clinician should consider the following points.

Eyes
- Position normal for the patient?
- Enophthalmos (may indicate orbital fractures) or exophthalmos (may indicate orbital bleeds in trauma, thyroid eye disease)?
- Restriction of movement or double vision in any of the eight gaze positions?

Lids
- Integrity. Lacerations of the lid and lid margin?
- Position. Entropion/ectropion?
- Lash line. Intact? Ingrowing lashes/infestation/crusting?
- Swelling. Whole or part of the lid/one or both lids?
- Puncta visible and correctly sited?

Conjunctiva
- Integrity.
- Structure. Smooth? Follicles or papillae?
- Other features. Conjunctival cysts, pingueculae, pterygia?
- Inflammation. Generalized or local?
- Subconjunctival haemorrhage?
- Discharge. Type, frequency?
- Fornices. Both lower and subtarsal areas. Concretions or FBs may be visible.

Cornea
- Integrity. Lacerations, abrasions, ulcers?
- Clarity?
- FBs?

Anterior chamber
- Depth. The distance between the curved cornea and the iris. Generally equal in both eyes.
- Contents, e.g. WBCs or RBCs; any cells are abnormal.

Iris and pupil
- Colour. Similar to the other eye?
- Position. Should be round and regular but may be slightly off centre (check both eyes).
- Integrity. Normal for patient? Previous surgery may change its appearance.
- Size and shape. Smaller or larger than the other eye; round or oval?
- Reaction to light and to near.

Always compare both eyes. What appears to be an abnormality may be bilateral and normal for the patient.

The injured eye

By far, the commonest ophthalmic problem to present to EDs and minor injury units is the injured eye. Adults and children frequently sustain minor injuries to the surface of their eye from FBs or 'poking'-type mechanisms. A carefully elicited history should enable the assessing clinician to determine if the injury is likely to be 'minor', and assessment can proceed without specialist intervention. Many minor eye injuries are successfully managed by ENPs. Obtaining a clear minor mechanism is key to ensuring that a potentially more serious injury is not missed.

History

It is crucial to identify and document the following.
- What actually happened, e.g. poke in the eye or felt FB go in the eye?
- Where did it happen—was the injury at work, home?
- Was any eye protection used?
- Was any first aid administered at the time?
- When did the injury occur?
- How was the injury sustained? Is there a risk of a penetrating eye injury?
- Past ophthalmic history. Has the patient any previous or current eye problems?

Blunt injuries to the eye, e.g. a punch to the face, can cause significant facial fractures, as well as eye injuries. The orbit tends to protect the eye from the force of larger objects. However, small balls, e.g. squash balls or golf balls, can cause significant globe trauma. Is there a history of a high-velocity injury? Hammer and chisel use typically causes small fragments to travel at high speed. Glass, knives, darts, and pencils are other causes of penetrating eye trauma and will require urgent ophthalmic referral.

- Common mechanisms for minor eye injuries include being poked in the eye with finger, hairbrush, plants, bushes, and twigs.
- Grinding injuries can be caused by metallic or brick FBs.
- Other common FBs are dust, grit, and flakes of metal/paint.

Symptoms

The following are the commonest symptoms of corneal injury or corneal FB.
- Pain. Injury to the cornea is acutely painful.
  - Large superficial abrasions are intensely painful (➲ see Fig. 13.1).
  - Deep lacerations with little epithelial loss are only mildly painful (➲ see Fig. 13.2).
- Visual disturbance.
- FB sensation.

Other symptoms include redness, watering, blurred vision, and discharge.

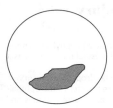

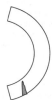

Fig. 13.1 Large superficial abrasions.

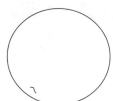

Fig. 13.2 Deep laceration.

Examination

- VA.
- Examine the eye systematically (➜ see Assessment of the patient with eye problems, pp. 430–1).
- Slit lamp examination to identify the depth of the injury and presence of any FB.
- Lid eversion to identify any subtarsal FBs.
- Fluorescein staining to reveal the extent of corneal injury.

Treatment of corneal injuries is based on the management of three areas: pain, prevention of infection, and optimization of healing.

Management of a corneal injury

Prevention of infection

Any corneal damage requires treatment with a topical prophylactic antibiotic (chloramphenicol or fusidic acid). Fusidic acid is useful for children, as it only requires a twice-daily application.

If perforation is suspected or confirmed, a single drop of unpreserved, single-dose chloramphenicol may be instilled before transfer to the ophthalmic unit. Both preservatives and ointment are toxic to ocular tissues and should not be used.

Pain

- Topical anaesthesia is for examination purposes only and obtaining an accurate VA assessment. Repeated instillation will result in dose-related toxicity and delay in epithelial healing.
- Cyclopentolate 1% will relieve ciliary spasm and associated pain.
- Topical NSAIDs four times daily (qds) also provide a significant degree of effective pain relief.

Padding

- Is for comfort only.
- There is no evidence that it aids healing.
- Pad those patients who have significant pain, advising that, if the pad makes the pain worse, they should remove it.

Double eye pad

A double eye pad should always be used, one pad folded over the closed lids and the other open on top of it. The whole is taped firmly to the face, so that the patient cannot open the eye underneath the pad. If comfortable, the pad should be left intact for 24h and then removed, and instillation of medication commenced. There is no need to pad the eye just because a topical anaesthetic has been instilled.

Optimization of healing

Reviewing simple corneal abrasions depends very much on the individual clinician. Large abrasions can be reviewed to ensure that healing is taking place and that there is no loose epithelium that needs debriding. Small abrasions heal very quickly.

At review, if there is any loose epithelium visible or any sign of infection, ↑ in pain, or reduction in VA, it is safer to refer the patient for an ophthalmic opinion.

Recurrent abrasion syndrome is common in those patients who have an animal- or vegetation-based cause for their abrasion (e.g. plants or fingernail). This can be prevented by using ointment at night before sleeping to keep the eye lubricated. 'Simple' or another lubricating ointment, or Lacri-Lube® (ointment based without drugs) should be used for a period of up to 3 months.

Referral of corneal injuries Each emergency care area will have guidelines about which types of corneal injuries should be referred for ophthalmic assessment and follow-up.

Foreign bodies

Conjunctival foreign body

These are usually superficial.

- Instil topical anaesthetic.
- Remove from the conjunctiva by wiping with a dampened cotton bud (any swab/cotton bud used on the eye should be pre-moistened with Saline Minims® or the residue of an anaesthetic Minims®—otherwise, epithelial tissue sticks to the swab, rather than the eye, and significant injury can result).
- Stain after the FB has been removed to identify the extent of damage.
  - If there is minimal stain, a single application of chloramphenicol ointment may be instilled.
  - If there is significant stain, chloramphenicol ointment should be prescribed qds until the eye feels back to normal.

Deeper FBs on the conjunctiva may be removed using a 21G hypodermic needle, often mounted on the end of a cotton bud to form a longer and more easily manipulated tool.

Corneal foreign body

- Assess depth using a slit lamp. The depth of the cornea may be seen within the slit lamp beam.
- If the FB is anything other than superficial, it should be referred to the local eye unit for further assessment and removal.

⚠ The cornea is only 1mm thick at its thickest. Accidental perforation does occur and can be devastating.

FB removal should always take place at a slit lamp to provide magnification and stability for the patient's head. If this is not possible, consideration should be given to referral to a more appropriate setting.

- Instil topical anaesthetic.
- Use a 21G needle; bore upwards to gently lift off the FB from the cornea.
- Metallic FBs may need slightly more forceful removal.
- Rust must be removed at some point. This can be facilitated by giving the patient chloramphenicol ointment or drops to use for 2 or 3 days, and then reviewing in the ED or in the eye unit. Rust is much easier to remove at this stage. Again, an antibiotic or ointment should be prescribed until the eye feels back to normal.

Once an FB is removed, treatment is the same as for a corneal abrasion and should be focused on preventing infection, relieving pain, and optimizing healing.

Superglue injuries

History

Superglue may be instilled into the eye, as its containers often resemble eye drop containers.

Signs and symptoms

- Pain.
- Eyelids stuck together.

As the eye is permanently wetted by the tear film, the glue does not generally stick to the tissues of the eye but hardens, forming a plaque inside the lids and abrading the cornea as the eye and lids move. The glue usually glues the eyelashes together and therefore holds the lids together.

Management

- Instil a topical anaesthetic to the lids, allowing it to drain between them to act on the cornea. This relieves pain and allows examination and treatment.
- Trim the eyelashes very close to the lid margin.
- Pick off the remaining glue to allow the lids to open. This must be done very carefully and may take some time. A very fine pair of scissors is required, and a laceration of the lid margin must be avoided. This may be a lengthy procedure, necessitating repeated topical anaesthetic and much patience.
- When the lids are open, remove the plaque of glue and all particles of glue.
- VAs.
- Treat resulting abrasions as corneal abrasions.

Children may be much less cooperative than adults and may need a general anaesthetic for this procedure. Referral to an ophthalmic unit should be considered.

⚠ Superglued eyelids will take a considerable time to open on their own, and practitioners should not be tempted to 'let nature take its course'. The abrasions are likely to be extremely painful, the glue plaque will abrade as long as it is in the eye, and the loss of corneal epithelium provides an entry point to the eye for pathogens.

Ultraviolet radiation injury (welder's flash, arc eye)

History
- Exposure to welding arcs.
- Exposure to ultraviolet (UV) 'sunlamps'.

The UV radiation is absorbed by the corneal epithelial cells, some of which are damaged or destroyed. There is a latent period before symptoms are experienced, which depends on the amount of exposure and explains the typical late-night presentation of these patients.

Signs and symptoms
- Gritty sensation to one or both eyes.
- Intensely painful eye(s).
- Photophobia.
- Watering and blurred vision.
- Lid swelling.
- Redness.

Examination
- Instil a topical anaesthetic.
- VA, and examine the eye systematically (➜ see Assessment of the patient with eye problems, pp. 430–1).
- Instil fluorescein.
  - Fluorescein reveals punctate staining on the surface of the cornea where some cells have been destroyed.

Management
- Treatment is as for a corneal abrasion.
- A mydriatic drop will provide comfort.
- Antibiotic ointment as prophylaxis and for comfort.
- Padding may help, but both eyes should not be padded simultaneously.
- Advise complete recovery is usually within 24–36h.

Chemical injury

History
It is almost irrelevant what chemical is splashed into the eye, and no time should be wasted in the ED trying to find out. Chemical splashes in the eye can result in devastating injury, and the time to irrigation is the most important factor in minimizing ocular problems.

Irrigation
The initial treatment of ocular chemical injuries involves irrigation to dilute the chemical and remove any solid debris (➲ see Eye irrigation, p. 701).

Examination
- VA.
- Examine the eye systematically (➲ see Assessment of the patient with eye problems, pp. 430–1).

Management
Superficial injury may be treated with chloramphenicol ointment qds until the eye feels back to normal.

- All but the most trivial chemical injuries should be referred to an ophthalmologist.
- Solvent injuries are generally much less damaging than those due to acid and alkaline chemicals.

Blunt trauma

Blunt trauma may result in disruption to any, or all, of the ocular tissues. Any patient presenting with blunt trauma to the eye or surrounding tissues with any reduction in vision should be referred to an ophthalmologist for specialist assessment.

Traumatic hyphaema

Signs and symptoms

- Blood in the anterior chamber, detected by slit lamp or visible with the naked eye, sometimes to the extent of filling the whole of the anterior chamber.
- ↓ VA.
- ↑ in intraocular pressure, as RBCs block the trabecular network.
- Severe pain.
- Irregular or sluggish pupil.

Management

- Urgent referral to an ophthalmologist is required.
- Sit the patient upright in order to allow the blood cells to settle and absorb away from the visual axis. This will reduce any staining of the corneal endothelium with haem pigment, which may affect vision.

Regular review is undertaken to monitor the intraocular pressure and treat any rise in pressure.

Traumatic uveitis

Is a common effect of blunt trauma and may be the only sign of trauma. Treatment is as for any uveitis, with pupil dilatation and topical steroids.

Iris and pupil abnormalities

Traumatic mydriasis or miosis may occur as a consequence of blunt trauma, and the pupil may be irregular, when compared with the fellow eye, due to partial or complete rupture of the iris sphincter.

Lens abnormalities

The impact of the iris on the lens, as the eye distorts and then moves back into shape, may leave a circle of iris pigment, which can be seen after dilatation (Vossius ring).

Traumatic rupture of the zonules holding the lens in place may occur, and luxation or subluxation of the lens may take place. ↑ intraocular pressure may occur if the lens blocks the pupil. Iridodonesis (iris tremble) may be visible.

▶ Urgent referral to an ophthalmic unit is required for any iris, pupil, or lens abnormalities, or if the patient reports any reduction in VA.

Major trauma

Orbital injury

Both facial and skull trauma can result in orbital injury.

Medial orbital fractures

The lacrimal secretory system (especially the nasolacrimal duct) may be damaged, and the medial rectus muscle may be trapped within the fracture.

Orbital floor fractures

Often referred to as blowout fractures, because they are produced by transmission of forces through the bones and soft tissues of the orbit by a non-penetrating object such as a fist or a ball. These fractures may be complicated by the entrapment of muscles and orbital fat, which limits ocular motility (➲ see Orbital floor fractures, p. 508).

Signs and symptoms

These include:

• diplopia;
• enophthalmos;
• infraorbital anaesthesia.

A classic presentation involves an injured patient, who perhaps would not have presented to the ED otherwise, blowing their nose and then attending because their eyelids have swollen alarmingly as air from the sinus has been driven into the tissues of the lid.

The patient should be given advice about the avoidance of the Valsalva manoeuvre such as blowing the nose or straining at stool.

> Any patient with an orbital fracture and any degree of double vision should be referred to an ophthalmic unit.

Orbital apex trauma

All clinicians in the ED must be alerted to the possibility of ocular involvement from indirect trauma, such as base of skull fractures, as well as from more direct trauma where the eyes themselves do not appear to be involved.

Fractures of the orbital apex may result from direct, non-penetrating blunt trauma or from penetrating trauma, e.g. with large orbital FBs. Orbital apex fractures present differently, depending on the degree of injury to the vascular and neural structures within the orbital apex, and a number of different presentations are possible.

• Optic nerve injury may occur, commonly due to traumatic optic neuropathy from indirect trauma (such as fractures of the base of the skull). A haematoma may compress the nerve, or it may be damaged by an FB or from a fracture, which can result in a spectrum of injuries from minor trauma to the nerve to complete transection.
• Injury to the cranial nerves present in the orbit (CN III, IV, and VI) may present as extraocular muscle palsy with double vision.
• Injury to the trigeminal nerve (CN V) presents as sensory disturbance to areas it supplies.

Collaboration of ophthalmic units with the ED is important in order to ensure that patients with this type of injury do not lose vision unnecessarily.

> ⚠ Patient complaints of loss of, or reduction in, vision must be taken very seriously. In order to quantify this, VA must be checked on arrival, as a baseline and then hourly. Ophthalmology opinion must be obtained immediately if vision is involved.

Retrobulbar haemorrhage

This may occur from direct or indirect trauma to the orbit and can progress rapidly.

Signs and symptoms
- Pain.
- Proptosis of the globe.
- Congested conjunctival vessels.
- Lid and conjunctival swelling.
- Subconjunctival haemorrhage may be dense and may extend beyond the visible conjunctiva.

Management
- Regular observation of the appearance of the eye patient with direct or indirect trauma to that orbit is required to minimize complications of the injury.
- VA should be measured as a baseline, and the patient should be encouraged to report new symptoms and any reduction in vision.
- ▶▶ If the globe begins to proptose after trauma, an ophthalmologist should be involved immediately. A CT or MRI scan may be required urgently, and the patient's VA should be checked very frequently (every 10min).

If VA reduces, emergency decompression by lateral canthotomy (a horizontal incision at the lateral canthus, through the skin and conjunctiva, and then through the lateral canthal tendon, under LA) will be required to relieve pressure on the optic nerve. Equipment for this procedure will not be needed very often but should be readily available in the ED, so that avoidable loss of vision may be prevented.

Open trauma

An open eye requires immediate assessment. No attempt should be made to remove any retained materials protruding from the globe.

Management

- Stabilize any protruding material as far as possible, perhaps by taping it to the cheek or by covering the whole area with a plastic shield or small receiver.
- No pressure should be put on to the eye, and an eye pad should only be used if absolutely no other method of covering the eye exists. The pad must be loose and taped well away from the globe—any pressure on the globe may result in further injury and/or loss of ocular contents.
- Manage pain and nausea. Vomiting with an open eye is likely to lead to loss of the ocular contents.
- Lie the patient flat or propped up at around a 30° angle. This can minimize any rise in intraocular pressure.
- Do not cover both eyes, unless they are both extensively damaged. A patient with one damaged eye is unlikely to be relaxed, comforted, or reassured by being unable to see anything or anyone around them.

▶▶ Immediate referral to an ophthalmologist is required.

Small penetrating injuries

Penetrating injuries and intraocular FBs may cause damage to the globe by:
- tissue disruption at the time of injury;
- formation of scar tissue causing long-term damage—retinal scars may contract and cause retinal detachment (RD); corneal scars will distort or disrupt vision;
- introduction of foreign material to which the eye reacts;
- allowing pathways for infection to enter the globe.

Large penetrating eye injuries are very obvious, but small perforations may be easily missed, as the eye may look completely intact. The wound may have self-sealed or may be obscured by the upper lid.

Examination

Must always include all aspects of the anterior part of the globe by asking the patient to look in each different direction, so that all segments may be examined. As the patient looks down, the upper lid should be retracted, so that the upper portion of the globe may be seen. All penetrations of the lid should lead to a high index of suspicion about the state of the globe.
- Corneal perforations always leave a full-thickness scar, even if very small.
- Scleral perforations may be masked by an overlying subconjunctival haemorrhage.
- A small hole in the iris may mark the passage of an FB.

▶ Analgesia and anti-emetics should be considered, as vomiting may lead to expulsion of the contents of a perforated globe.

▶▶ Patients with penetrating trauma should be referred urgently to an ophthalmologist.

The red eye

Another common eye problem that presents frequently to emergency care areas is the 'red eye'. Patients cannot identify any specific injury and can complain of varying symptoms, e.g. redness, pain, itch, watering, discharge, swelling, headache, and visual disturbance.

Allergies

Allergic conjunctivitis presents in several ways.

- Red eyes with itching and watering and an appearance of large bumps (papillae) on the subtarsal conjunctiva are particularly common during the 'hay fever season' and may therefore be associated with a runny nose, sneezing, and other allergic symptoms. Treatment is with systemic antihistamines and/or topical treatment such as emedastine or olopatadine. Sodium cromoglicate is of no value in allergic reaction. It is useful only when the allergic phase has been controlled, as a mast cell stabilizer.

- A more severe chronic atopic reaction, most often seen in children, is the appearance of 'cobblestone papillae'. The appearance of the subtarsal conjunctiva is of massive papillae arranged in a cobblestone fashion. This is intensely irritating and often requires complex management. Patients presenting in this way should be referred to an ophthalmologist urgently.

- An acute atopic reaction involves massive chemosis or swelling of the conjunctiva which the patient or parent often describes as 'jelly' on the eye. This is due to an allergen transferring directly to the eye on the fingers or by blowing in. This is completely self-limiting. It resolves quickly (over a period of hours), and reassurance and information are all that is required.

Conjunctivitis

Inflammation of the conjunctiva is by far the commonest cause of red eyes. Common organisms involved in infective conjunctivitis include viruses, bacteria, and Chlamydia (➐ see Table 13.1). Almost all conjunctivitis in adults is caused by a virus, often a type of adenovirus, and, unless there are large amounts of green/yellow discharge present all day, the infection should be presumed not to be bacterial. Conjunctivitis in children is more likely to be bacterial.

⚠ Eye pads should never be suggested for patients with conjunctivitis. The warm, damp atmosphere underneath an eye pad will allow further organism growth and exacerbate the condition.

Viral conjunctivitis

Signs and symptoms

- Gritty sensation to the eye/s.
- Profuse watering.
- Dry feeling to the eye/s.
- Stickiness often only in the morning when the watery discharge has dried and the lids are stuck together.
- Some types of adenovirus also cause URTI and general malaise.

Examination

- On lid eversion, the conjunctiva covering the lids will appear very bumpy, rather than smooth. This roughness of the conjunctiva is what makes the eye feel gritty and irritable.
- There may be punctate erosions (small staining areas) on the cornea when stained with fluorescein.

Management

- Symptom relief with artificial tears, and advice about very frequent use (hourly or even more frequently).
- Advice about the self-limiting nature of the condition. The patient should be aware that viral conjunctivitis may persist for 3–6wk, and the symptoms of dryness may last much longer. There is no point in prescribing antibiotic eye drops.

⚠ Adenovirus is highly infectious, and infection control is of paramount importance, both for the patient and the emergency care setting. Handwashing is vital to stop the spread of viral conjunctivitis. Major epidemics of viral conjunctivitis associated with ophthalmic units have been linked with poor handwashing. All equipment should also be cleaned between each patient. It is not necessary to take eye swabs for culture, and the patient should not be followed up.

Bacterial conjunctivitis

Signs and symptoms

- Redness.
- Irritable gritty eye.
- Profuse, purulent discharge; the lashes may be coated with discharge.

Management
A broad-spectrum antibiotic, such as chloramphenicol or fusidic acid, applied topically in the form of drops. The condition is self-limiting, and no investigations are required.

Chlamydial conjunctivitis

Signs and symptoms
- Unilateral.
- Chronic (the patient may have had a red and irritable eye for some time which has reached an irritating stage but not progressed to a severe viral infection).
- Large pearly follicles are present on lid eversion.

If Chlamydia is suspected from the clinical picture (➔ see Table 13.1), a chlamydial swab should be obtained from the eye. The patient's details should be checked to ensure that they are contactable, should the result be positive. Patients should be referred to sexual health services for treatment.

Table 13.1 Types of conjunctivitis

	Viral	Bacterial	Chlamydial
	Bilateral and acute	Rare, bilateral	Unilateral and chronic
Lids	May be swollen; follicles	May be swollen	Unlikely to be swollen
Conjunctiva	Injected	Injected	Injected
Cornea	May have keratitis (punctate staining of cornea)	No involvement	No involvement
Discharge	Watery, sticky in morning	Green/yellow discharge all day	Watery, stuck together in mornings
Vision	May be affected by corneal involvement	Unlikely to be affected	Unlikely to be affected
Pain	Gritty, dry; may be intensely irritating	Gritty and very sticky	Mild irritation
Investigation	None: clinical diagnosis only. Identification of organism does not change management	None: clinical diagnosis only. Identification of organism does not change management	If clinical appearance suggestive of Chlamydia, swab for Chlamydia
Treatment	Artificial tear regime; information; reassurance	Antibiotic drops	Artificial tear regime; on positive identification, appointment with sexual health services

Subconjunctival haemorrhage

Patients may present with a spontaneous subconjunctival haemorrhage with a deep red patch of blood under the conjunctiva, which may be quite small and circumscribed or may be severe enough for the conjunctiva to appear like a 'bag of blood'. Providing that there is no history of trauma, no treatment is needed, unless the haemorrhage is severe or the eye irritable, in which case artificial tears are useful to provide comfort and lubrication.

Subconjunctival haemorrhage may occasionally be associated with hypertension, so it might be useful to check the patient's BP. Patients with clotting disorders or those on anticoagulants may be prone to repeat episodes. Subconjunctival haemorrhages may take some weeks to resolve, and, because the conjunctiva is an elastic membrane, the blood may spread under it and the haemorrhage appears worse, before it begins to resolve.

Anterior uveitis (iritis, anterior cyclitis, or iridocyclitis)

Uveitis is an inflammatory condition, which may be associated with systemic disease or as a response to trauma, but is often idiopathic. It is unusual to encounter uveitis (especially as a 1° attack) in an elderly patient.

Signs and symptoms

(➲ see Box 13.1.)
- Photophobia.
- Pain (due to ciliary spasm).
- Conjunctival redness (injection), which may be more marked around the limbus.
- ↓ vision due to protein and WBCs in the anterior chamber.
- Small pupil that reacts sluggishly because of spasm and inflammation.

Examination

When the cornea is illuminated with a torch, the reflection will be bright, and there will be no staining with fluorescein.

Treatment

The patient must be referred on to an ophthalmic unit for investigation and treatment.

Box 13.1 Characteristics of uveitis

- Lids normal.
- Conjunctiva injected.
- Cornea normal.
- Anterior chamber deep.
- Iris may look 'muddy'.
- Pupil: slight miosis (compared with fellow pupil); sluggish.
- Pain: deep pain in eye.
- Discharge: may water.
- Photophobia.
- Systemically well.

Corneal ulcers

There are three main types of corneal ulcer that are likely to be seen in the emergency care settings. All should be referred to an ophthalmologist urgently. Differentiation between the different types of corneal ulcer is sometimes difficult, and the treatment is completely different.

A careful history will usually identify symptoms of a 'red eye': pain; redness; visual disturbance; and no history of injury. Ulcers are seen in contact lens wearers, and the clinician should always be alert to the possibility of a corneal ulcer if there has been a history of lens wearing. On staining, a defect is seen on the cornea, which may have a characteristic shape.

▶ Any corneal defect that cannot be explained by a history of injury should be discussed with an ophthalmologist.

Bacterial ulcers

On staining, bacterial ulcers occur as 'fluffy', white demarcated areas. They are caused by a number of organisms, e.g. *Pseudomonas*, which is very difficult to treat, and are most commonly, but by no means exclusively, seen in contact lens wearers. The patient should be urged to leave their contact lens out of their eye, whilst waiting to be seen in the ophthalmic unit, but should keep it with them, as it is likely to be sent for culture.

▶▶ Delay in treatment of infected corneal ulcers can result in a devastating intraocular infection.

Viral ulcers (dendritic ulcers)

These are caused by the herpes simplex virus. They are known as 'dendritic' ulcers because of their branching, tree-like shape when stained with fluorescein. They are treated with aciclovir eye ointment, and should be referred to an ophthalmologist for treatment and follow-up.

Marginal ulcers

Appear as ulcerated areas that stain with fluorescein and are usually close to the limbus. They are part of a hypersensitivity response by the eye to staphylococcal exotoxins and are treated with steroidal or nonsteroidal anti-inflammatory eye drops by an ophthalmologist.

Glaucoma

Glaucoma describes a rise in the pressure inside the eye, causing damage to the neural tissue that makes up the retina and resulting in permanent reduction in the field of vision.

There are two main types of glaucoma:

- chronic, open-angle glaucoma where the rise in pressure is small, damage is done to the retina over a large period of time, and visual field loss is insidious;
- acute, closed-angle glaucoma, which is an ophthalmic emergency.

Chronic open-angle glaucoma

This type of glaucoma is only likely to be encountered in the ED if the patient has run out of eye drops or as an incidental part of history taking.

Although it cannot be recommended that patients manage without the appropriate medication for their condition, it cannot be considered an emergency in the same way as perhaps a diabetic without insulin. The patient should be referred to their own ophthalmic clinic or GP at the earliest opportunity.

There is no danger associated with dilating the eye of a patient who has chronic, open-angle glaucoma. Indeed, on each visit to the ophthalmic outpatient department, this procedure will be undertaken to evaluate the optic disc.

Acute glaucoma (angle-closure glaucoma)

In acute glaucoma, the outflow of aqueous in the eye is obstructed by the peripheral iris covering the trabecular meshwork at the drainage angle in the anterior chamber. As aqueous continues to be produced, the pressure inside the eye ↑ rapidly. Patients are usually elderly.

A key thing to remember is that patients with acute glaucoma often present with a 1° complaint other than their eye. Severe abdominal pain is often the presenting symptom. Nausea and vomiting may also be the main presenting feature.

Any red eye that is noticed may be assumed to be a 2° and unimportant issue, unless the clinician keeps a high index of suspicion. Dealing with the eye problem will cure the abdominal pain/nausea/vomiting. Ignoring the eye problems will result in irreversible (and preventable) visual loss.

Signs and symptoms
(➲ See Box 13.2.)
- Severe pain (due to ↑ intraocular pressure).
- Blurred vision (due to corneal oedema).
- Haloes seen around lights.
- Headache.
- Nausea and vomiting, and abdominal pain.

Examination
- Red eye.
- Reflection of light from the cornea will be very diffuse—showing that the cornea is oedematous.
- Semi-dilated oval pupil that responds to light sluggishly, if at all.

▶▶ Acute glaucoma is an ophthalmic emergency, and the patient should be referred to an ophthalmologist urgently, including emergency ambulance transportation, if necessary.

Initial treatment—in emergency care
- Analgesia and anti-emetics may be required.
- Treatment of dehydration if vomiting has been prolonged.
- Reassurance and careful explanation are needed by these ill, and often terrified, patients.

Box 13.2 Characteristics of acute glaucoma
- Lids normal.
- Conjunctiva injected.
- Cornea very hazy.
- Anterior chamber shallow or flat.
- Iris may be difficult to see.
- Pupil fixed, oval, semi-dilated.
- Pain: severe pain in and around eye and head.
- Discharge: none.
- Photophobia: none.
- Systemically:
  - nausea and vomiting;
  - severe abdominal pain;
  - dehydration.

Loss of vision: history

An accurate history of visual loss is crucial to the identification of possible causes. This is especially the case in the emergency setting where specialist examination may not be immediately available.

History—important features

- Are there patches or areas of absolute vision loss, or is the vision blurred?
- Sudden or gradual loss? If sudden, is it possible that it has been there for a while but has only just been noticed? If the loss was gradual, over what period of time has it occurred (days, weeks, or even months)?
- Does the loss of vision involve some, or all, of the vision? Are there sectors of the field of vision that are missing? Is the loss worse centrally or peripherally?
- Was the loss transient—has it come back now or is it recovering (for how long was vision affected), or does it seem to be permanent?
- Is the vision now getting better or worse, or is it staying the same?
- Are there any other symptoms that the patient is experiencing (such as headache, weakness, or pain elsewhere)?

Monocular versus binocular loss of vision

Ocular pathology, or optic nerve problems, will cause monocular loss of vision. A problem at, or posterior to, the optic chiasma in the brain will cause binocular loss of vision. Conditions include migraine (with visual symptoms, such as fortification spectra, hemianopia, and blurring, that may not be accompanied by headache), vascular lesions, tumour, and stroke.

A generalization, but one that works in practice, is that, if a patient complains of binocular loss of vision, the problem is likely to be of neurological, rather than ophthalmic, origin, and a neurological opinion should be sought. Two rare exceptions to this are bilateral blurring of vision that has appeared over a small number of days—this is characteristic of papilloedema and can be discovered by eye examination.

Bilateral transient blurring may be caused by a rise in blood glucose (causing an oedematous lens) in diabetes (known or unknown).

Profound monocular loss of vision

This is defined as complete or severely diminished vision affecting the whole of the visual field that may occur suddenly or gradually over a period of days. Sudden, profound loss of vision suggests a vascular cause, and the most likely of these are central retinal artery occlusion and vitreous haemorrhage.

Vitreous haemorrhage

Is the most likely cause if there is an associated history of diabetes.

Signs and symptoms
- The patient may be aware of the haemorrhaging.
- Floaters can be seen by the patient, becoming denser over a short period and resulting in a profound loss of vision.

Any attempt by the clinician to visualize the back of the eye will be unsuccessful due to haemorrhage between the clinician and the retina.

Management
The patient should be referred to an ophthalmologist, although it is unlikely that treatment (LASER) will take place until the haemorrhage has cleared sufficiently for the retina to be visualized.

Central retinal artery occlusion

The patient may describe the vision disappearing 'like someone switching the light off'. The loss may be absolute.

Examination
- The retina is likely to be pale due to swelling, and the macular area is seen as a 'cherry red spot'.
- An embolus in the central retinal artery may be seen.

▶▶ This condition is an ophthalmic emergency, and immediate treatment must start in the emergency setting.

Investigations
- ESR, CRP.
- FBC, lipid, and clotting profile.
- USS of coronary arteries and ECG—to identify the site of embolus.

Treatment
- IV acetazolamide 500mg ↑ perfusion of the retina by reducing the intraocular pressure.
- Ocular massage to encourage the outflow of aqueous.
- Rebreathing exhaled air by breathing into a paper bag. This ↑ the CO_2 concentration in the body, dilating blood vessels, and perhaps allowing the embolus to move further into the retinal circulation. If the latter occurs, a sector of visual loss, rather than profound loss, may be a good outcome for the patient.

An anoxic retina is irreversibly damaged in 90min, and the visual outcome of this condition is often poor.

Segmental loss of vision and loss of central vision

Segmental loss of vision

The most likely causes of the loss of an area of the visual field in one eye are vascular causes such as occlusions of branches of the retinal artery or vein (branch retinal artery or vein occlusions) or RD.

- If onset is sudden and the loss stable, the cause is likely to be vascular.
- If the area of visual loss changes over time, the cause is more likely to be an RD.

Branch retinal artery and vein occlusions

These may be seen with an ophthalmoscope.

- A branch retinal artery occlusion will lead to a segment of the retina being paler than the rest; all the vessels appear in the correct location, and an embolus may be seen in one of the vessels.
- There may be multiple retinal haemorrhages if the cause of the loss of vision is a branch retinal vein occlusion. The haemorrhages will be in the area of the retina that is served by the blocked vein. Retinal oedema may be seen, and an occlusion may be visible.

There is no immediate treatment for either of these conditions, although follow-up by an ophthalmologist will be necessary.

Retinal detachment

Spontaneous RD affects 1 in 10 000 of the population each year and is commoner in ♂ and in short-sighted (myopic) eyes. It most commonly occurs due to collapse of the vitreous gel in middle age, resulting in traction on a weak area of the retina causing a hole to form. Serous fluid may get between the retina and its basement membrane, pushing them apart and resulting in an RD.

Signs and symptoms

- Flashing lights. The only way that the brain can interpret movement of the retina is in terms of light, so, as the retina moves, the brain interprets and the patient 'sees' flashes of light.
- Floaters. The appearance of a large circular floater is due to the detachment of the vitreous gel from its ring-shaped adhesion to the optic disc. A shower of tiny floaters is due to haemorrhage into the vitreous, as a small retinal blood vessel is damaged.
- A sector of loss of vision that tends to enlarge over a period of hours or days may be noticed. The patient may complain of seeing a 'shadow' that tends to move or a 'curtain' descending over the eye.
- Central vision may be lost due to macular detachment.

The detached retina will appear grey and may seem slightly wrinkled.

▶▶ Patients with RD need an urgent ophthalmic opinion. Surgery may be almost immediate in order to preserve macular function.

Loss of central vision

Common causes of loss of central vision include age-related macular degeneration (AMD), optic neuritis, central serous retinopathy (CSR), and macular burns.

Age-related macular degeneration

Refers to a degeneration of the macula. It is the commonest cause of visual loss in the over 75s and affects ~20% of individuals. There is usually a very gradual loss of central vision, although different types of AMD may proceed at different speeds, and marked, sudden reduction in central vision should be referred urgently, as effective treatments to preserve, and even retrieve, vision are readily available.

Optic neuritis

Is inflammation of the optic nerve. Episodes are usually monocular, and it is commonest in ♀ aged 20–40y. It is strongly associated with multiple sclerosis (MS) and is the presenting problem in 25% of cases.

The patient is likely to present with loss of central vision that may progress to a generalized loss of vision and can become severe. Other symptoms include pain that is worse on ocular movement (due to the inflamed optic nerve moving as the eye moves) and altered colour perception. The pupil reactions will be abnormal, and the optic nerve head may be swollen. Referral to a neurologist or neuro-ophthalmologist for further assessment is required.

Central serous retinopathy

Usually occurs in young adult ♂. The cause is unknown. Symptoms usually include a unilateral blurring of central vision and a generalized darkening of the visual field with some distortion. VA is usually only mildly reduced. Referral to an ophthalmologist is necessary, although most episodes of CSR resolve spontaneously within 3–6 months.

Macular burns

May be caused by MIG (metal inert gas) welding equipment, which produces high-intensity white light that the eye transmits, rather than absorbs. It can cause macular burns, resulting in loss of central vision. The patient may notice a black mark in the centre of the visual field that stays in the same place when they move the eye. Macular burns may be caused by the patient looking at the sun without adequate eye protection.

Blurring of vision and transient loss of vision

Blurring of vision

Blurring of vision may be due to problems anywhere in the visual pathway, between the cornea and visual cortex. Many patients will have problems in differentiating between generalized blurring and loss of central vision—therefore, careful questioning is required. Some causes of blurring (vitreous haemorrhage, CSR, optic neuritis, vessel occlusion) have already been described.

- Patients with papilloedema often present with blurring of vision. This may be worse in one eye and may be exacerbated by a change in position (lying to standing). Patients with bilateral swollen optic discs need urgent neurological referral.
- Opacities in any of the clear structures of the eye will result in blurring of vision, as less light reaches the retina.
  - The commonest opacity is a cataract—lens opacity. Cataract causes glare and reduction in vision, and lens opacities may be seen on examination with a slit lamp or, if severe, with a pen torch. Reassurance and referral to an optometrist (for optimization of vision) and GP for referral to an ophthalmologist are appropriate. If the lens opacity has occurred after trauma or is in a younger person, more urgent referral to an ophthalmologist should be considered.
  - ▶▶ Corneal opacities or irregularities resulting in blurring should be referred to an ophthalmologist urgently.

Transient loss of vision

The commonest causes of transient visual loss are vascular, and not ophthalmic. Carotid artery disease and giant cell arteritis require referral to a physician.

If transient loss of vision is accompanied by pain in an elderly person, particularly when light levels are low and especially if accompanied by a red eye, intermittent angle-closure glaucoma may be suspected, and urgent referral to an ophthalmologist is required.

ENT emergencies

Overview

Most EDs see a fair proportion of patients who could be treated in a primary care setting. The proliferation of walk-in centres in recent years, which are mainly nurse-led, means that many patients presenting with ENT primary care conditions will be treated by an ENP. This chapter reflects this development and offers advice on when and what to refer on to the GP or the local doctor.

Acute sore throat: assessment

History

Acute sore throat: assessment

Sore throat is a common presenting complaint and mostly viral in origin. An estimated 30% are caused by bacteria where group A β-haemolytic streptococci (GABHS) are, most frequently, the causative organisms. Regardless of the cause, symptoms will resolve spontaneously in the majority of cases within 1wk of onset. However, a full history is required to exclude other important causes of an acute sore throat.

▶ Any patient having difficulty with breathing or unable to swallow should be referred on to an ENT specialist.

History

Signs and symptoms
- Onset and duration.
- Severity of pain/soreness.
- Ear pain—may be referred.
- Coryzal symptoms.
- Cough.
- Dysphagia.
- Trismus (spasm of pterygoid muscles preventing opening of the mouth).
- Rash.
- Abdominal symptoms.
- Headache.
- Fatigue.

Past medical history
- Diabetes.
- Rheumatic fever.
- Disease causing immunosuppression.
- Asthma—may be relevant if NSAIDs or aspirin gargles are indicated to treat symptoms.
- Immunization history.

Medication
- Combined oral contraceptive pill (OCP)—may be relevant if treatment with antibiotics is indicated.
- Drugs known to cause neutropenia, e.g. methotrexate, azathioprine, sulfonamides, carbimazole, and sulfasalazine (a sore throat may be the first sign of neutropenia).
- Steroids: oral or inhaled.
- Recent antibiotic use.
- Over-the-counter medications used to treat symptoms, e.g. use of analgesia (what and when last given).

Ask about allergies with specific reference to:
- antibiotics;
- NSAIDs;
- aspirin.

Examination

- Temperature.
- Pulse.
- Inspect and palpate the cervical lymph glands.
- Inspect the external auditory canal and the TM.
- Inspect the oral cavity, buccal mucosa, and oropharynx. Look for exudates or slough, peritonsillar swelling, the position of the uvula, petechiae on the soft palate, and a strawberry tongue.
- Check for trismus.
- Inspect the skin for colour and rash and circumoral pallor.

⚠ Do *not* attempt to examine the throat of an individual who has drooling, stridor, or breathing difficulties. They may have epiglottitis.

Pharyngitis and tonsillitis

- Pharyngitis: inflammation of the pharynx and surrounding lymph tissues.
- Tonsillitis: acute inflammation of the tonsils.

Both of these conditions commonly present as an acute sore throat and can be either viral or bacterial in origin. Realistically, it is difficult to determine whether an acute sore throat is viral or bacterial in origin. For most patients, antibiotics have little effect on the extent and duration of symptoms. ∴ Management is principally focused on advice regarding symptom management. Antibiotics are reserved for those who are most likely to benefit from them.

Viral causes

Caused by adenoviruses, rhinoviruses, and parainfluenzae viruses.

Clinical characteristics
- Sore throat that is reported to be worse on swallowing.
- May be accompanied by fever.
- Possible tender cervical lymphadenopathy.
- Headache and malaise.
- Cough and coryzal symptoms are common.

Bacterial causes

Caused by GABHS. Commonest in children of school age; less so in adults and children <3y.

Clinical characteristics
- Sore throat that is reported to be worse on swallowing.
- Fever.
- Tender cervical lymphadenopathy (particularly anterior cervical) and slough on inflamed tonsils.
- Headache, malaise, abdominal pain, and vomiting may all occur.

Management

Pain relief and fever management
- Paracetamol and/or ibuprofen should be recommended/prescribed. In children, if both preparations are used, they should be given simultaneously, and not staggered.
- Soluble aspirin gargles.
  - ⚠ For children >16y of age only.
  - Anecdotally, gargling with aspirin is reported to relieve pain in some people.
  - Soluble aspirin, if used, should not be advised in conjunction with ibuprofen.
- Benzydamine gargles: there is some limited evidence to support use. Can be prescribed or obtained over the counter.

Treatment with antibiotics

NICE[1] advises that antibiotics should be reserved for those with one or more of the following criteria:

• features of marked systemic upset 2° to the acute sore throat;
• unilateral peritonsillitis;
• history of rheumatic fever;
• ↑ risk from acute infection (such as those with diabetes mellitus or immunodeficiency).

(➲ See Box 4.3.)

When indicated, antibiotics should be prescribed, or alternatively supplied, using a PGD:

• phenoxymethylpenicillin (penicillin V);
• erythromycin (if allergic to penicillin).

► Women taking the combined OCP should be advised that additional contraceptive precautions should be taken whilst taking a short course of an antibacterial and for 7 days after stopping. If these 7 days run beyond the end of a packet of OCPs, the next packet should be started immediately without a break (in the case of ED (everyday) tablets, the inactive ones should be omitted).[1]

Other advice

Provide information to the patient about the following.

• Prevention of dehydration. Children particularly may be reluctant to drink. Ensure patients or parents understand the importance of maintaining a high fluid intake. Ice lollies can be a useful source of extra fluid for a reluctant child. Adults may find sucking on ice soothing.
• The expected pattern of recovery and duration of symptoms.
• The rationale for providing/not providing antibiotics.
• Signs or symptoms requiring further assessment by a health professional.

Follow-up No specific follow-up required in most cases. Patients should be advised to seek further advice from a primary health-care professional if they experience: any deterioration in their condition, new symptoms, or if presenting symptoms do not resolve in 5–7 days from onset.

Reference

1 National Institute for Health and Care Excellence (2001). *Referral advice. A guide to appropriate referral from general to specialist services: acne, acute low back pain, atopic eczema in children, menorrhagia, osteoarthritis of the hip, osteoarthritis of the knee, persistent otitis media with effusion (glue ear) in children, psoriasis, recurrent episodes of acute sore throat in children aged up to 15 years, urinary tract 'outflow' symptoms ('prostatism') in men, and varicose veins.* National Institute for Health and Care Excellence, London.

Scarlet fever

Scarlet fever is caused by GABHS.

Clinical characteristics

As in bacterial pharyngitis/tonsillitis (⊃ see Pharyngitis and tonsillitis, pp. 462–3), plus:
• a 'strawberry' tongue;
• an erythematous 'sandpaper' rash on the trunk and limbs;
• on occasion, Pastia's lines (petechiae in flexor skin creases of joints).

Management

(⊃ See also Pharyngitis and tonsillitis, pp. 462–3.)
• Management and follow-up are as for pharyngitis/tonsillitis.
• Antibiotics are indicated and should be provided as for pharyngitis/tonsillitis, but for a duration of 10 days.
• Scarlet fever is a notifiable disease, and, as such, the proper officer of the local authority (usually the consultant in communicable disease control) should be notified.
• Children should be excluded from school for 5 days from the start of antibiotic treatment.

Glandular fever (infectious mononucleosis)

Glandular fever is caused by the Epstein–Barr virus. It commonly affects those aged 15–25y of age. In the early stages, it may be difficult to differentiate from bacterial pharyngitis.

Clinical characteristics

- Fetor (bad breath).
- Plummy speech.
- Slough on inflamed tonsils.
- Palatal petechiae.
- Fever.
- Lymphadenopathy (particularly posterior cervical) and general malaise.
- Mild hepatosplenomegaly.

Management

- Pain relief and general advice should be given as for pharyngitis/ tonsillitis (→ see Pharyngitis and tonsillitis, pp. 462–3).
- Antibiotics are not indicated but, in reality, may be given due to the difficulty in differentiating glandular fever from other causes of sore throat.

Follow-up The symptoms of glandular fever can persist for some time, causing long absences from school/college or university. It is therefore important to advise the child or their parents to see a primary care clinician if the symptoms are not resolving within ~7 days, so that an FBC and film and a Paul Bunnell or Monospot test can be performed to confirm the diagnosis.

In confirmed glandular fever, advice should be given to avoid contact sports for 3 months.

Coxsackie virus (hand, foot, and mouth disease)

Hand, foot, and mouth disease occurs in children aged 3–10y.

Clinical characteristics
- Sore throat.
- Vesicles on the oral cavity, buccal mucosa, tongue, hands, feet, and sometimes buttocks.
- Fever.

Management and follow-up is as for pharyngitis/tonsillitis (➔ see Pharyngitis and tonsillitis, pp. 462–3).

Diphtheria

Diphtheria is caused by *Corynebacterium diphtheriae*. It is uncommon in the UK, but quite common in South Africa, Russia, and the developing world.

Clinical characteristics
- Grey adherent membrane on the tonsils, uvula, and pharynx. Bleeding occurs when the membrane is removed.
- Fever.
- Severe sore throat.
- Malaise.
- Restlessness.
- Weakness and a thready pulse should raise suspicion when present in an unimmunized individual.

Management These patients require urgent medical management, including airway management and intensive care support.

Thrush (candidiasis)

Thrush is usually caused by *Candida albicans*. Individuals are likely to have a history of antibiotic or inhaled steroid use, or be immunosuppressed.

Clinical characteristics
- Thin, diffuse, or patchy exudates on mucous membranes.
- Afebrile.

Management
- If immunosuppressed, refer to a medical practitioner.
- Normal immune state. Prescribe nystatin.
- Advise those using inhaled steroids to rinse their mouth after inhalation to avoid future problems.

Follow-up No specific follow-up will be required in most cases. Patients should be advised to seek further advice from a primary health-care professional if they experience: any deterioration in their condition, new symptoms, or their presenting symptoms are not resolving in 5–7 days from onset.

Peritonsillar abscess (quinsy)

Commonest in older children and adults.

Clinical characteristics
- Fever.
- Worsening pharyngitis.
- ↑ unilateral throat and ear pain.
- Dysphagia, drooling, and trismus are common.
- Unilateral peritonsillar swelling and inflammation.
- The uvula may be displaced away from the affected side.

Management
- The airway may become compromised, so vigilance is essential.
- IV cannulation and benzylpenicillin may be indicated.
- Refer to an ENT surgeon for incision and drainage.

Epiglottitis

Usually caused by *Haemophilus influenzae*. Commonest in children aged 2–8y, but incidence has diminished since the introduction of Hib immunization. Occurs uncommonly in adults (➲ see Meningococcal septicaemia, p. 106).

Clinical characteristics

- Abrupt onset of severe sore throat, fever, and toxicity.
- Usual appearance is a child in a sitting position, leaning forward, head extended, jaw thrust forward, mouth open, tongue protruding, and drooling.
- Voice is muffled.
- Stridor may be present.
- In adults, the onset may be slower, and severe pain on swallowing may be the only symptom.

Management

  ❶ Do *not* examine the throat, as it may cause spasm and obstruction.

▶▶ Seek urgent assistance from an anaesthetist and an ED medical practitioner.

Mumps (epidemic parotitis)

Mumps is an acute, generalized infection caused by the paramyxovirus. It can infect any organ, including salivary glands, pancreas, testis, ovary, brain, mammary gland, liver, kidney, joints, and heart. It is highly infectious and spread through respiratory droplets, saliva, and possibly urine. The incubation period is 15–24 days, with the period of infectivity extending from about 2–6 days before symptoms appear and for up to 4 days afterwards. Symptoms usually resolve within 7–10 days. There has been a recent ↑ incidence in older children and young adults who have not received an MMR booster preschool.

Clinical characteristics

- Non-specific flu-like symptoms, followed by the development of parotitis.
- Pain near to the angle of the jaw.
- Fever (40–40.5°C).
- Swelling, often bilateral, that causes distortion of the face and neck. The area over the glands may appear hot and flushed.
- In severe swelling, the mouth cannot be opened and is dry through blockage of saliva.
- Discomfort usually lasts for 3–4 days.
- May be accompanied by abdominal pain, headache, mild mastitis, and oophoritis in women.

Management

- Management is mainly aimed at pain and fever management.
- Local heat to the inflamed glands may provide some relief.
- Foods and drinks that stimulate saliva production may ↑ pain and should therefore probably be avoided.
- Mumps is a notifiable disease. The proper officer of the local authority (usually a consultant in communicable disease control) should be notified.
- Patients or carers should be informed about the period of infectivity, that mumps is highly infectious, and that contact with those who are most at risk of complications, should they contract mumps (see ⮞ Complications below), should be avoided.
- It is recommended that those who have contracted mumps, but not yet been immunized, should still have the vaccine.

Complications

Orchitis

Orchitis is unusual before puberty but occurs in ~1 in five cases of mumps in adolescent ♂. Symptoms usually develop 4–5 days after the start of parotitis. Some degree of atrophy of the testicle is seen in 1/3 of cases, but sterility is not as common as often feared.

Clinical characteristics
- Severe, usually unilateral, localized testicular pain and tenderness (the second testicle may develop symptoms, as symptoms in the first resolve, usually after a few days).
- Swollen, oedematous scrotum with impalpable testicles.
- Fever and sweats.
- Headache and backache.

Management
- Management is mainly aimed at pain and fever management.
- Prednisolone has been suggested for 2–3 days for severe parotitis or orchitis. It may provide good pain relief but does not reduce swelling.
- Reassurance regarding future problems about infertility may be required.
- Patients/carers can be directed to the Patient website for comprehensive evidence-based information.[2]

Meningitis and encephalitis generally occur without symptoms of parotitis. Patients exhibiting symptoms suggestive of meningitis or encephalitis should be referred to a medical practitioner or the ED (➔ see Meningitis, pp. 188–9, and Encephalitis, p. 190).

Deafness is a rare complication occurring only in around 1:15 000. Individuals with symptoms of hearing loss should be followed up by their GP.

Miscarriage The risk of miscarriage may be ↑ if mumps is contracted in the first trimester of pregnancy (the first 12–16wk). Mumps is not, however, thought to ↑ the risk of fetal abnormalities.

Reference

2 Patient. Available at: ℜ http://www.patient.info.

Earache or ear pain (otalgia): assessment

Earache is a common presenting problem. It is estimated that, in 50% of cases, pain or discomfort can be attributed to some pathology within the ear. In the other 50%, pain is referred from other structures. The history and examination should be sufficiently comprehensive to ensure that the differential diagnoses of ear pain are considered and that those individuals at risk of developing complications are identified and referred urgently to a doctor or the ED. Fig. 14.1 shows the structure of the ear.

History

Enquire about the following signs and symptoms:
- onset and duration;
- location of pain (deep or superficial, radiation);
- itching;
- severity of pain/soreness;
- fever or irritability;
- ear discharge and quality;
- dizziness, vertigo, or tinnitus;
- trauma (includes barotrauma, minor localized trauma with, e.g. a cotton bud in the ear, trauma inflicted by another individual, e.g. a slap or punch to the ear);
- possible presence of FB;
- hearing loss;
- sore throat—pain may be referred;
- coryzal symptoms (Eustachian tube blockage/dysfunction causes earache);
- dental pain or recent dental treatment (referred pain causes earache);
- facial numbness or paralysis;
- nausea or vomiting;
- previous episodes;
- recent ear syringing (disturbance of normal environment may precipitate otitis externa (OE));
- recent ↑ frequency of boils, thrush, or other infections (may be suggestive of diabetes).

Enquire about past medical history:
- ear surgery or grommets;
- congenital disorders such as cleft palate;
- diabetes;
- immunosuppression;
- cerumen build-up;
- chronic skin disease, e.g. eczema, psoriasis, seborrhoeic dermatitis.

Enquire about social history:
- location and frequency of swimming (↑ incidence of OE with frequent swimming);
- use of a soother/dummy by infants (whether breast- or bottle-feeding) leads to an ↑ risk in acute otitis media (AOM);
- passive smoking (↑ risk of ↑ episodes of otitis media);
- recent use of different hair or facial products (can cause OE).

Specific enquiry should be made about the following medications:
- combined OCP—may be relevant if treatment with antibiotics is indicated;

- recent antibiotic use: topical and systemic;
- over-the-counter medications used to treat symptoms, e.g. use of analgesia (what and when last given);
- hypoglycaemic drugs;
- steroids, both topical and systemic.

Enquire about allergies with specific reference to antibiotics and NSAIDs.

Examination

- Temperature and pulse.
- Inspect and palpate the auricular and cervical lymph glands.
- Examine the temporomandibular joint (temporomandibular joint syndrome/pain refers to the ear).
- Inspect and gently move the pinna and tragus.
- Inspect the external auditory canal for inflammation, swelling, discharge, and cerumen.
- Thoroughly inspect the TM, taking care to identify the following landmarks:
  - the location of the light reflex;
  - the umbo;
  - the annulus.
- Carefully note the position of any perforation.
- Inspect the oral cavity, buccal mucosa, and oropharynx.
- Inspect dentition.

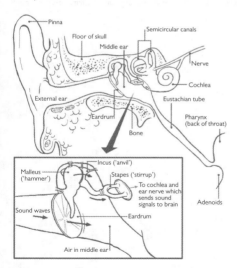

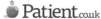

Fig. 14.1 Structure of the ear.

(Diagram with permission from Patient.co.uk available at http://www.patient.co.uk/health/the-ears-hearing-and-balance © 2014, Egton Medical Information Systems Limited. All Rights Reserved.)

Otitis externa

The term otitis externa (OE) is used to describe any inflammatory condition of the auricle, external ear canal, or outer surface of the eardrum. OE can be classified as localized or diffuse.

- Localized OE is used to describe a furuncle (boil) in the ear.
- Diffuse OE can be acute or chronic, and is caused by infections, allergies, irritants, or inflammatory conditions.[3]
- *Staphylococcus aureus* is the causative organism in the vast majority of cases of localized OE. *S. aureus* and *Pseudomonas aeruginosa* are the bacteria most commonly implicated in cases of diffuse OE. Fungal infection is estimated to be the cause in only 10% of cases of diffuse OE. OE is common in all ages, with the exception of those under 2y. It is commoner in ♀ than ♂, except in the elderly. There is an ↑ in incidence at the end of the summer months.
- Chronic OE describes frequent episodes of OE due to long-term damage to the normal ear canal through trauma, chronic skin conditions, or infection. If seen during an acute episode, it should be managed as acute OE, but an ear swab should ideally be taken before treatment is instigated.

Reference

3 Clinical Knowledge Summaries. *Otitis externa*. Available at: ◌ http://cks.nice.org.uk/otitis-externa.

Localized otitis externa

Clinical characteristics
- Earache/pain, sometimes severe.
- May report pain on touching, or lying on, the ear.
- The post-auricular node may be enlarged and tender.
- Pain is experienced on movement of the pinna and tragus.
- Otoscopic examination may be extremely painful.
- A localized area of inflammation and swelling is visualized.
- Little, if any, discharge is present.
- The TM, if visualized, appears normal.
- Pre-auricular and/or post-auricular lymphadenopathy may be present.
- Mild fever <38°C.

Management
Pain relief
▶ Refer to the *BNF* for advice on dose, contraindications, and interactions of the following medicines before advising them to patients.
- Paracetamol and/or ibuprofen should be recommended/prescribed. In children, if both preparations are used, they should be given simultaneously, and not staggered.
- Codeine is the second-line analgesia of choice.
- A combination of codeine, paracetamol, and an NSAID may be required to control severe pain.
- Local heat may be soothing.

Antibiotics
Flucloxacillin (or erythromycin if penicillin-allergic) are the antibiotics of choice. Dose and regimen are as follows:
- flucloxacillin;
- erythromycin (if allergic to penicillin).

▶ Advise women taking the combined OCP that additional contraceptive precautions should be taken (➲ see Pharyngitis and tonsillitis, pp. 462–3).[4]

Other interventions Consider testing the urine or capillary blood for abnormal glucose levels.

Referral criteria
Patients who are significantly systemically unwell require assessment by a medical practitioner.

Follow-up
- No specific follow-up will be required in most cases.
- Patients should be advised to seek further advice from a primary health-care professional if they experience: any deterioration in their condition, new symptoms, or their presenting symptoms are not resolving in 5–7 days from onset.
- Infrequently, furuncles in the ear may require referral to ENT specialists for incision and drainage.
- Patient information provided by Patient is an excellent lay resource.[5]

References
4 *British National Formulary*. Available at: ℜ http://www.bnf.org.
5 Patient. Available at: ℜ http://www.patient.info.

Diffuse otitis externa: acute uncomplicated

Clinical characteristics

- There may be a recent history of swimming or visit to a country where the climate is hot and/or humid.
- Low-grade fever <38°C.
- Rapid onset (generally within 48h) of ear pain.
- Itch.
- Discharge (usually scant white, but occasionally thick).
- Hearing loss (conductive if inflammation occludes the canal).
- Pre- and/or post-auricular lymphadenopathy.
- Pain on movement of the tragus, pinna, and jaw.
- The TM may be inflamed.

Management

Management is focused on pain control, restoration of the normal pH of the ear, and treating the most likely cause, i.e. bacterial infection.

- Topical preparations are recommended for first-line treatment, unless there is evidence of spreading infection or the individual is systemically unwell.
- If discharge is profuse, topical preparations are unlikely to reach the affected tissue. Under such circumstances, referral to the ENT team for microsuction and aural toilet should be considered.
- ▶ Ear syringing should be avoided.

Pain relief

- Paracetamol and/or ibuprofen should be recommended and prescribed/supplied using a PGD.
- The addition of codeine may be required and can be provided as described earlier.

Topical antibacterials and steroids

The choice of topical agents is based on probable causative organisms. However, infection is often 2°, and dampening down of the inflammatory response may be all that is required. Optimal first-line treatment is a combined antibacterial/steroid preparation. There is little evidence to demonstrate ↑ efficacy of one preparation over another. The Clinical Knowledge Summaries provide pragmatic advice on selection of treatment.[6] Suggested first-line options are as follows:

- flumetasone 0.02% + clioquinol 1% ear drops;
- betamethasone 0.1% + neomycin 0.5% ear drops;
- prednisolone 0.5% + neomycin 0.5% ear drops.

The following should be reserved for use when first-line treatment has failed:

- hydrocortisone 1% + gentamicin 0.3% ear drops.

Systemic antibiotics

Reserve oral antibiotics for treating those with evidence of spreading infection or cellulitis. Use in conjunction with a topical preparation.

- Flucloxacillin (or erythromycin if penicillin-allergic) are the antibiotics of choice.

▶ Advise women taking the combined OCP that additional contraceptive precautions should be taken (➲ see Pharyngitis and tonsillitis, pp. 462–3).[7]

Patient advice

Patients should be advised about the following.

- Application of ear drops.
  - Lie down with the affected ear upwards.
  - Put the prescribed number of drops into the affected ear, and remain lying for a few minutes.
  - Depress the tragus a few times to allow the drops to seep into the ear canal.
- Avoid using cotton buds to clean the ears.
- Avoid soaps, shampoos, and chemicals running into the ear. Do this by using cotton wool with petroleum jelly in the ears when bathing.
- Use a swim cap or earplugs when swimming or diving.

Prevention

Prevent OE by avoiding water and moisture build-up in the ear canal and maintaining a normal canal environment. Achieve this by:

- using acidifying ear drops (acetic acid) before and after swimming;
- using a hairdryer to dry the ear canal;
- using earplugs when swimming;
- avoidance of ear trauma such as that from use of cotton buds.

Follow-up

No specific follow-up required. Patients should be advised to seek further advice/assessment from their primary care practitioner if symptoms fail to resolve within 5–7 days, or before then if they should experience any ↑ in symptoms.

References

6 National Institute for Health and Care Excellence, Clinical Knowledge Summaries (2015). *Otitis externa*. Available at: ℘ http://cks.nice.org.uk/otitis-externa.

7 *British National Formulary*. Available at: ℘ http://www.bnf.org.

⚠ If there is suspicion of eardrum perforation, the Committee on Safety of Medicines (CSM) has stated that drops containing aminoglycosides (neomycin and gentamicin) are contraindicated due to the risk of ototoxicity.

Cholesteatoma

A cholesteatoma is a cyst-like tumour made up of a collection of epithelial debris. It usually originates in the attic region. It has erosive properties and requires urgent referral to an ENT specialist. Onset tends to be more gradual than in OE.

Clinical characteristics
- Earache and headache.
- Malodorous (faecal) discharge.
- An attic TM perforation may be visible.
- A history of treatment failure for OE.
- Collection of abnormal tissue may be visible, typically in the attic region.

Management Refer to an ENT specialist for further assessment.

Malignant (necrotizing) otitis externa

This is a rare condition that occurs mainly in the elderly, the immunosuppressed, or those with diabetes. Infection extends into the bone surrounding the ear canal (i.e. mastoid and temporal bones).

Clinical characteristics
- Severe pain.
- Headache.
- Discharge.
- Intensely inflamed ear canal.
- Cellulitis of the pinna and surrounding tissue.
- There may be unilateral facial palsy.

▶ This may be difficult to differentiate from a severe OE. If in doubt, refer.

Management ▶▶ Refer urgently to a medical practitioner or an ENT specialist.

Ramsay Hunt syndrome

Ramsay Hunt syndrome is often used to describe herpes zoster infection of the facial nerve.

Clinical characteristics

- Ear and mastoid region pain.
- Phonophobia.
- Loss of taste.
- Facial paralysis (Bell's palsy).
- Vesicular eruption around the external auditory meatus.
- Vertigo.
- Deafness.

Risk groups The elderly and immunosuppressed are at greater risk of complications.

Management Refer to a medical practitioner for further assessment. Aciclovir is the drug of choice.

Acute otitis media

AOM describes fluid in the middle ear in association with signs and symptoms of acute infection. It is one of the most frequent diseases in early infancy and childhood. Peak incidence is 6 months to 3y. Most cases resolve without antibiotic treatment. ∴ 'Watchful waiting' with fever and pain control are the treatment of choice for the first 72h in most cases. A lower threshold for providing antibiotics is necessary when the child is <2y or if there is perforation with otorrhoea, bilateral AOM, or systemic symptoms, including high temperature (>38.5°C) or vomiting.

Clinical characteristics

- Earache/pain.
- May be worse on swallowing.
- Preceding or current URTI.
- Fever often >38.5°C.
- Nausea and/or vomiting.
- Distorted TM and light reflection.
- Handle of malleus flush.
- Bulging TM with loss of landmarks.
- Changes in membrane colour (typically red or yellow).
- Perforated TM with discharge of pus (which may alleviate symptoms); the TM may not be visible.

Management First-line management largely aimed at fever/pain control.

Pain relief and fever management

- Paracetamol and/or ibuprofen should be recommended/prescribed.
- When prescribed or provided together, they should be given at the same time, rather than staggered.[8]
- Fluid intake should be encouraged.
- Advice regarding management and prevention of febrile convulsions should be provided. The Clinical Knowledge Summaries website provides comprehensive advice for parents on the prevention and management of febrile convulsions (see ☞ http://cks.nice.org.uk).

Antibiotics

- Amoxicillin (or azithromycin if penicillin-allergic) are antibiotics of choice.

► For advice for women taking the combined OCP, ➜ see Pharyngitis and tonsillitis, pp. 462–3.

Follow-up

- Further assessment is indicated if pain has not resolved in 72h from first consultation. Antibiotic treatment is then required.
- Advise those with discharging ears to seek further assessment if the discharge has not resolved in 7 days. If so, consider antibiotic treatment.

Advice Smoking, bottle-feeding, and use of dummies or soothers are risk factors for ↑ episodes of AOM. Parents of children who use soothers or dummies should *not* be advised to stop use until the child reaches the age of 1y.

Acute otitis media with perforation Care should be taken to ensure that the perforation has been caused by AOM. Consider and exclude other causes of discharging ears or perforation such as:

- trauma (► if the suspected cause of TM perforation is trauma and the patient is a child, consider issues of child protection);
- barotrauma;
- OE;
- cholesteatoma.

Follow-up
- The patient or child's parents should be advised that the TM should be reassessed 2wk after the acute episode.
- Persistence of discharge for >7 days also requires further evaluation.

Complications of acute otitis media with or without perforation

Mastoiditis
- Fever.
- Tenderness over the mastoid antrum.
- Displacement of the pinna down and forward due to post-auricular swelling.
- Inflamed, bulging, or perforated TM.
- Signs of conductive deafness.

Management Urgent referral to an ENT specialist.

Meningitis Urgent referral to an emergency medical practitioner.

Conductive deafness due to perforation or debris in the middle ear not uncommon. Should resolve after the acute episode resolves. Prolonged deafness for >2wk after the initial episode needs evaluation by the GP.

Reference
8 National Institute for Health and Care Excellence, Clinical Knowledge Summaries (2015). *Otitis media—acute*. Available at: ℘ http://cks.nice.org.uk/otitis-media-acute.

Epistaxis

Epistaxis is common inasmuch as most people will have had a nosebleed at some time. However, it is an unpleasant and worrying experience and, as such, a fairly common presentation in the ED. Epistaxis is classified as anterior or posterior, depending upon the source of bleeding.
- Anterior haemorrhage. The source of bleeding is from the nasal septum (Little's area).
- Posterior haemorrhage. Bleeding is from deeper structures of the nose; commoner in older people.

Causes

Often there is no cause, but consider:
- trauma to the nose;
- nose-picking;
- vigorous nose blowing;
- platelet disorders;
- drugs: aspirin and anticoagulants;
- abnormalities of blood vessels (especially in the elderly);
- cocaine use: the drug can lead to destruction of the nasal septum;

Most nosebleeds stop spontaneously, and patients can be discharged if there is no further active bleeding. They should be given an advice leaflet.

Management of severe epistaxis

⚠ Remember that patients can die from an epistaxis. If concerned, get specialist help.

- Ask the patient to sit upright and forward, and to squeeze the nostrils. Offer constant reassurance, as patients find this very distressing.
- Give the patient a bowl, and encourage them to breathe through the mouth.
- Monitor pulse and BP.
- Monitor for signs of hypovolaemia.
- Establish IV access, and collect blood for FBC, group and save, and clotting if the patient is on anticoagulants.

If bleeding continues, prepare for packing.
- Use a nasal tampon. These are easy to insert and comfortable for the patient. Use Naseptin® cream to lubricate the tampon.
- Pack both sides. Packs are usually left in place for 24h. Use BIPP (bismuth subnitrate and iodoform paraffin paste) or 1cm of ribbon gauze impregnated with petroleum jelly if nasal tampons are not available. Posterior bleeds, which are much less common (~5%), require packing and a balloon catheter to arrest bleeding.
- Patients with posterior packs require admission and are usually commenced on antibiotics.

Nasal foreign bodies

Nasal FBs are commonest in children aged 1–5y where anything that can be inserted into the nostril may be there! Common FBs are stones, tissue, and beads. Some may have been *in situ* for a long period of time. If a child presents with a foul-smelling nasal discharge, always suspect an FB. It is important to remove nasal FBs, as those left *in situ* are at risk of pulmonary aspiration.

Management

The challenge is obtaining the cooperation of the younger child. Usually, you only get one attempt, before the child will be less cooperative.

- *Do not* attempt removal with a struggling/uncooperative child. Refer to ENT.
- *Do not* attempt removal if you have not got the right equipment. Refer to ENT.
- *Do not* attempt removal if you do not feel you have a reasonable chance of success. Refer to ENT.

If the FB is visible, suction can be applied with a rigid suction catheter and can be successful. Depending on the shape, size, and texture of the FB, different equipment is needed.

- Soft FBs (tissue/peas): use crocodile forceps to gently grasp the FB.
- Round, hard FBs (beads/stones): a blunt-ended probe, which is slightly bent into a hook shape, needs to be inserted behind the FB to 'hook it' out.

- Once removed, the nostril should be checked for any further FB or signs of trauma.
- Always check the other nostril for an FB.
- Failure to remove requires referral to ENT.

Ear (auricular) foreign bodies

These are common in children, and, as with nasal FBs, anything can be inserted into the ear. In adults, cotton wool is the commonest FB.

The same principles and techniques for removal that are used for nasal FBs can be applied to auricular FBs. However, failure to remove does not require urgent ENT referral, and an ENT outpatient clinic appointment can be made.

Following removal, the ear should be examined. Signs of trauma to the canal or perforation to the drum should be managed appropriately. If a child presents with an auricular haematoma, consider NAI.

Retained earrings/butterflies

This is commonest in young girls who have recently had their ears pierced and have small stud earrings. In some cases, the earring/butterfly is partially visible and can be easily removed. If the earring/butterfly is completely embedded, removal can be more difficult.

Management

- Inject the lobe with a small amount of lidocaine.
- Grab the visible earring/butterfly with forceps, and remove.
- A small 'nick' in the posterior surface of the lobe may be required to ease removal in embedded earring/butterflies.
- Despite the lobe being red and swollen, antibiotics are rarely needed.

Auricular haematoma

A bruised, swollen pinna is usually caused by direct trauma from a blunt force, e.g. slap/punch, or in contact sports, most commonly rugby. Failure to correctly treat an auricular haematoma can result in the development of a 'cauliflower' ear. A haematoma to the pinna causes blood to collect between the skin and cartilage of the ear. Pressure from the haematoma can compromise the blood supply to the cartilage and destroy it—giving the characteristic cauliflower appearance.

Management

- Large haematomas should be aspirated using an aseptic technique.
- Apply a pressure bandage to prevent further haematoma development.
- Arrange ENT follow-up.

Nose injury

Many adults and children will seek urgent/emergency care, following a nose injury. Falls and assaults are the commonest causes. If a patient attends after an assault, careful documentation is essential to support any report writing for a subsequent legal investigation. Any epistaxis at the time has usually settled prior to seeking assessment.

Examination

- Swelling and bruising of the nose.
- Deformity.
- Is the nose deviated to one side?
- Inspect the nasal septum using a torch.
  - Is there any evidence of a septal haematoma?
- Is the patient able to breathe through each nostril?
- Feel for tenderness on the bridge of the nose.
- Feel for tenderness around the cheek and infraorbital region.
- Signs of base of skull fracture or CSF leak?

Nasal fracture is a clinical diagnosis, and X-rays are not indicated. If there is significant tenderness, bruising, and swelling, then a diagnosis of nasal fracture can be made.

▶▶ Septal haematoma needs immediate ENT referral.

Management

- Refer obvious displaced fractures to an ENT clinic.
- Pain relief.
- Advise the patient not to blow their nose for 24h.
- Advise the patient that 'black eyes' can develop and bruising can track down the face to the jaw line. This is normal.
- Advise the patient to avoid contact sports until the tenderness has settled.
- If there are any problems regarding the cosmetic result or breathing after ~5 days, ENT follow-up is needed.

Major trauma

Major trauma: introduction

Major trauma is the leading cause of death <45y and a significant contributor to the global burden of disease. The complexities of managing trauma in the older adult are becoming increasingly recognized. Trauma care in the UK over the last 2y has been radically developed, leading to a 20% ↓ in mortality. One of the contributing factors to this has been the development of major trauma networks. The networks consist of major trauma centres, trauma units, and out-of-hospital care provision. One of the fundamental changes has been in the out-of-hospital setting where key decisions are made about interventions and which level of facility the patient requires, bypassing trauma units, where indicated, to take patients with significant injuries to major trauma centres.

Management of the patient with multiple injuries

Patients with multiple injuries can pose significant challenges in prioritization and management. Adopting a systematic approach is fundamental to ensure that the life- and limb-threatening injuries are identified and managed first. Do not be distracted by obvious non-life-threatening injuries.

In trauma, the traditional ABCDE approach is augmented by the addition of another factor <C> for Catastrophic haemorrhage. This is in recognition that some deaths are preventable by the control of haemorrhage. The C reminds us to consider the issue of life-threatening haemorrhage, as we begin assessment and resuscitation.

Following a <C> ABCDE approach will structure your assessment and management. This will consist of a 1° and 2° survey. Do not move on to the next principle until you have effectively managed the previous one.

- <C> Catastrophic haemorrhage[1]—are there visible signs or history of significant blood loss at the scene? Is the patient actively bleeding?
- Airway—with C-spine control. Is the patient able to talk? Is the airway patent and clear? Remove debris. Remember C-spine control in major trauma.
- Breathing. Are they breathing? What is the RR? Tachypnoea may indicate hypoxia or hypovolaemia. Are both sides of the chest rising and falling symmetrically (you can only tell this from standing either at the head or foot of the trolley and looking from chest height)? Any abnormality of the chest wall? Is there good air entry on both sides? Is the chest normally resonant? Is there any point tenderness when palpating the chest? Is there any bony crepitus as you palpate the bony structure? Do you feel any surgical emphysema? Is the trachea central in the neck—deviation is a late sign in tension pneumothorax? What is the O_2 saturation reading? NB. Provide high-flow O_2 to all trauma patients. As part of the B assessment, do not forget to include the neck in the examination—using the mnemonic TWELVE will help to structure the approach (➔ see Guides to assessment, pp. 490–6).
- Circulation. Recheck for <C>. Is there a peripheral pulse? Is there a central pulse? Is the abdomen soft and non-tender? What is the BP? Secure wide-bore cannula access, preferably one line in each arm. What is the blood gas result? Raised lactate and base deficit are sensitive markers for hypovolaemic shock. If initial attempts fail, consider central

or IO access. Consider 'blood on the floor (from external blood loss) and four more'. Is there blood in the head, chest, or pelvis or from long bone fractures? Given the response to fluids or blood products—is there any ongoing haemorrhage?

- *Disability.* What is the GCS score (➔ see Neurological assessment: the Glasgow Coma Score, pp. 726–7) or, in children, AVPU ('alert, verbal, painful, unresponsive' (➔ see Management of the injured child, pp. 118–19). Is sensation intact? Any indication of spinal injury?
- *Exposure.* Fully undress the patient to ensure you have not missed any major injury. In penetrating trauma, check 'hidden areas' such as the axilla, buttock creases, or groin. Check the urinary meatus for any signs of bleeding indicating trauma to the genitourinary system. In ♂, check for priapism—a possible indicator of spinal cord injury.

▶ Temperature assessment and management are crucial. Hypothermia is part of the lethal triad (➔ see The lethal triad, p. 490).

Once the 1° survey and initial imaging (FAST scan (➔ see p. 71) and Trauma CT) are completed and resuscitative measures started, a 2°, more detailed survey, including a 'log roll' may be performed. A log roll should not be performed until significant pelvic injury is ruled out. The 2° survey should not be conducted until the patient has been adequately resuscitated.

Reference

1 Hodgetts TJ, Mahoney PF, Russell MQ, and Byers M (2006). ABC to <C>ABC: redefining the military trauma paradigm. *Emerg Med J* **23**, 745–6.

Guides to assessment

When faced with a patient with major trauma, it can be easy to be distracted by different injuries and to feel overwhelmed. It can sometimes be useful to use mnemonics to help remember things to consider when examining a patient. The following mnemonics may help in the assessment of the trauma patient.

TWELVE

The TWELVE mnemonic can be helpful in structuring the assessment of the neck in trauma.

- *T*rachea—is it central?
- *W*ounds—are there any wounds? With your gloved hands, slide them round the back of the neck. Is there any blood on the gloves from wounds round the back of the neck?
- *E*mphysema—is there any surgical emphysema?
- *L*arynx—is there any evidence of a fracture of the larynx?
- *V*eins—are the neck veins distended/flat?
- *E*very time—you should do this every time as part of your 1° survey!

ATOMFC

The ATOMFC mnemonic can be used to remember life-threatening chest injuries:

- *A*irway compromise;
- *T*ension pneumothorax;
- *O*pen pneumothorax;
- *M*assive haemothorax;
- *F*lail chest;
- *C*ardiac tamponade.

The lethal triad

A combination of three factors have been identified as detrimental in trauma management.

- Hypothermia—hypothermia exacerbates challenges to the clotting cascade. Preventing cooling and promoting active rewarming are advocated.
- Lactate—lactate is a product of anaerobic cellular activity and is evidence of tissue hypoperfusion. The demands for O_2 ↑ in trauma. Measures should be taken to reduced lactate-induced acidosis. High-flow O_2, fluid resuscitation, and haemorrhage control are required.
- Coagulopathy—recognizing and preventing coagulopathy are key in trauma resuscitation. Managing haemorrhage, fluid resuscitation, and an appropriate ratio of blood and clotting blood products, together with administration of tranexamic acid (TXA) for patients with a known or suspected haemorrhage, are fundamental in this process.

Traumatic cardiac arrest

A patient may suffer from a cardiac arrest as a result of major trauma. In some instances, a preceding medical event may cause a cardiac arrest, leading to major trauma, e.g. the driver of the car taken ill and then being involved in an RTC.

In a traumatic cardiac arrest, the key principles are early identification and treatment of reversible causes such as, but not limited to:

• airway obstruction;
• hypoxia;
• hypoventilation;
• tension pneumothorax.

Early recognition of cardiac arrest due to trauma is essential. Look for agonal, absent, or abnormal breathing, or the absence of a central pulse (take no longer than 10s to look for these). If found and a traumatic cause suspected, utilize the traumatic cardiac arrest algorithm (➲ see Fig. 15.1) (Resuscitation Council UK, 2015).

Considering massive haemorrhage

If the patient is showing signs of hypovolaemic shock in trauma, it is important to consider from where they may be bleeding. The phrase 'blood on the floor and four more' is used to prompt thinking about sources of haemorrhage.

Blood on the floor

• Look for signs of external haemorrhage. Can you find the bleeding point? Remember the patient may have a wound on their back that you cannot see. Importantly, consider scalp wounds—they may not look that large, but you can lose a great deal of blood volume from a bleeding scalp wound over a period of time.

Four more

• Chest—any external sign of chest injury? What was the mechanism? Could the chest be injured through a direct blow? Has there been an injury to the great vessels in the chest through a rapid deceleration or crush injury?
• Abdomen—any external signs of abdominal injury? What was the mechanism? Was there a direct blow to the abdomen? What about compression of the abdomen and injury to the small bowel? NB. It is important to remember that some of the organs in the abdomen sit on the border of the chest—a low chest injury on the right may involve damage to the liver and on the left the spleen.
• Pelvis—is there concern about a significant pelvic injury? If so, consider application of a pelvic binder to help compress possible bleeding points and stabilize the pelvis (remember, roll their feet together too, tying them together; this will bring the femurs into a better position for stabilizing the pelvis).
• Long bones—is there a fracture to a long bone(s)? You can lose a considerable amount of blood in the compartment around a long bone. Early traction on a fractured femur will help to reduce muscle spasm, pain, and bleeding. Early splinting of other *long bones will achieve the same.*

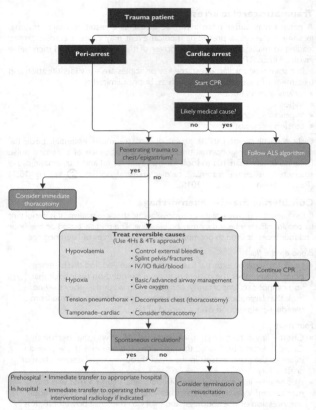

Fig. 15.1 Traumatic cardiac arrest algorithm.
(Reproduced with the kind permission of the Resuscitation Council (UK). 2015 Guidelines.)

Managing major external haemorrhage

If you can see where the bleeding point is, every effort should be made to arrest the bleeding.

Consider the following:
- Compression and elevation.
- *If* possible, apply direct pressure, and elevate the limb.
- Apply pressure for a minimum of 5min.
- Consider the use of a compression-type bandage.

- If the wound is bleeding through, consider adding an additional layer of bandage, and reapply pressure. Removing the first bandage may dislodge any clot that has formed.
- Consider the use of a haemostatic gauze such as Celox™. Gauzes are impregnated haemostatic agents that, when coming into contact with blood, form a gel and assist in the formation of clots. There are a number of products on the market. Haemostatic gauzes are a really useful adjunct to help arrest bleeding in wounds that are not amenable to pressure or elevation.
- Tourniquets—in the case of an arterial bleed, tourniquets placed proximal to the bleeding area can be effective in stopping bleeding. They are used as a temporizing measure—definitive management should be established <2h. Once in hospital, a pneumatic tourniquet should be used to preserve tissue viability and ensure a more controllable pressure is applied to the limb.

Massive haemorrhage

Haemorrhagic shock accounts for 50% of deaths in the first 24h after injury.[2] In the event of a patient presenting to the ED with major haemorrhage (trauma/ruptured AAA/upper GI bleeds/significant PV bleed), prompt action can prevent significant morbidity and mortality.

Massive transfusion is arbitrarily defined as the replacement of a patient's total blood volume in <24h, or as the acute administration of more than half the patient's estimated blood volume per hour. Every ED should have a major haemorrhage protocol in place, and this should include clinical, laboratory, and logistic responses. Familiarize yourself with your department's protocol.

Defining a leader and allocating specific roles will improve team performance.

Logistics

Activation of a major haemorrhage protocol should be instigated by the team leader as soon as the need is recognized (this may be from prehospital alerts).

- Identify an individual to take control of communication.
- Inform blood bank, switchboard, and portering, as per hospital guideline.
- A dedicated 'runner', often a porter or health-care support worker, should convey blood samples, blood, and blood components between the laboratory and clinical area. They should be in radio contact with the resuscitation room at all times. They MUST know where to go.
- A third member will normally be allocated to securing venous access on initial arrival of the patient.

Clinical response

- Gain immediate control of obvious bleeding (direct pressure, tourniquet application, haemostatic dressings).
- Address the priorities (A, B, C).
- Give high-flow O_2 via a face mask.

- Secure adequate venous access (minimum two large-bore IV cannulae/ central access, if appropriate).
- Take baseline bloods, including FBC, U&E, lactate, coagulation screen, and VBG or ABG.
- Send bloods for immediate cross-matching.
- Monitor vital signs, including pulse, BP, SaO_2, and RR.
- Fluid resuscitation should be with warmed blood and blood components.
- Actively warm the patient and all transfused fluids.
- Give early IV TXA 1g over 10min. This acts to inhibit clot breakdown.[3]
- If blood loss is predicted to be from significant/ongoing bleeding, prepare a rapid transfusion device, if available, prior to patient arrival, if possible.
- Consider/prepare for rapid access to appropriate imaging (FAST, ultrasound, radiography, and CT if patient stable, or immediate surgery if unstable).
- Alert the theatre team/interventional radiology about a possible urgent patient transfer and the need for cell salvage autotransfusion devices (these take time to set up).

Transfusion guidelines

In a patient *who is bleeding* and has evidence of a coagulopathy (or is likely to develop a coagulopathy), it is sensible to give blood components *before* coagulation deteriorates and worsens the bleeding.[4]

Current guidelines suggest:
- In traumatized patients with haemorrhagic shock: replace losses with blood. If delays in obtaining blood exist, use a crystalloid fluid for initial volume replacement. Give blood to maintain a palpable radial pulse. The blood type transfused depends on urgency of the situation (➜ see pp. 666–7). The response to blood transfusion should be carefully monitored—an unresponsive patient needs urgent haemorrhage control.
- Further doses of factors to assist with clotting should only be given if bleeding continues and should be guided by the PT and aPTT.
- Platelets are rarely needed in a resus situation, unless the platelet count is below 75×10^9/L, or in multiple or CNS trauma below 100×10^9/L.
- If required, an adult-dose unit of platelets should raise the platelet count by about 50×10^9/L.
- If bleeding continues, monitor the platelet count, as further transfusion may be needed to maintain the target count.
- Finally, cryoprecipitate may be indicated when there is bleeding with a fibrinogen concentration below 1g/L.
- Again familiarize yourself with the different blood products, the volumes they come in, and how they are administered.
- Give FFP (30min to defrost) in an initial dose of 15mL/kg, which is four or five donor units of FFP.

➜ See Fig. 15.2 for an algorithm for the management of major haemorrhage.

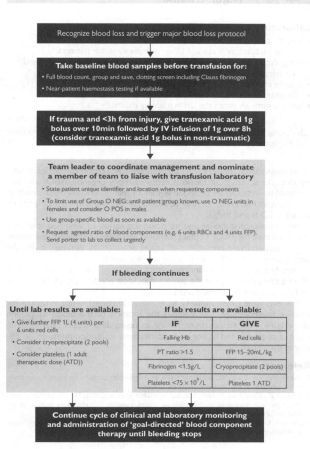

Recognize blood loss and trigger major blood loss protocol

Take baseline blood samples before transfusion for:
• Full blood count, group and save, clotting screen including Clauss fibrinogen
• Near-patient haemostasis testing if available

If trauma and <3h from injury, give tranexamic acid 1g bolus over 10min followed by IV infusion of 1g over 8h (consider tranexamic acid 1g bolus in non-traumatic)

Team leader to coordinate management and nominate a member of team to liaise with transfusion laboratory
• State patient unique identifier and location when requesting components
• To limit use of Group O NEG: until patient group known, use O NEG units in females and consider O POS in males
• Use group-specific blood as soon as available
• Request agreed ratio of blood components (e.g. 6 units RBCs and 4 units FFP). Send porter to lab to collect urgently

If bleeding continues

Until lab results are available:
• Give further FFP 1L (4 units) per 6 units red cells
• Consider cryoprecipitate (2 pools)
• Consider platelets (1 adult therapeutic dose (ATD))

If lab results are available:

IF	GIVE
Falling Hb	Red cells
PT ratio >1.5	FFP 15–20mL/kg
Fibrinogen <1.5g/L	Cryoprecipitate (2 pools)
Platelets <75 × 10⁹/L	Platelets 1 ATD

Continue cycle of clinical and laboratory monitoring and administration of 'goal-directed' blood component therapy until bleeding stops

Fig. 15.2 Algorithm for the management of major haemorrhage.
(Adapted from the BCSH Practical Guideline for the Management of Those With, or At Risk of Major Haemorrhage (2014).)

Laboratory considerations

What to send to the labs?

- A total of 10mL of a clotted blood sample for adult patients.
- If significant blood loss with the potential for major transfusion, send two samples.
- Ensure correct labelling (at the bedside).
- Ascertain from the team leader the blood products required.
- Ensure samples reach the lab in a timely manner.

⚠ Poorly labelled and lost samples will lead to significant delays in receiving requested products and may result in adverse outcomes.

A full cross-match should always be requested. Full blood compatibility testing can take up to 1h. If blood is required more urgently, ABO- and Rh-compatible units can be provided within 15 min. In uncontrolled bleeding, uncross-matched group O Rh −ve blood can be issued immediately (often from the ED blood fridge).

When contacting the labs, write down the names of who you spoke to, and make sure they have contact numbers and names for your department.

Judicious and safe prescribing of blood products at all time—giving the wrong blood can itself cost life and is a never-event.

Identify the patient on anticoagulants (warfarin); haemorrhage control may be compounded, and the patient should be given vitamin K IV 5–10mg and a prothrombin complex product.

It is everyone's responsibility to know your department's protocol for massive haemorrhage; this includes the location of the blood fridge and blood bank, how to get there, having an up-to-date access card or password, if required, and having up-to-date phone extension numbers on display in the department.

References

2 Westerman RW, Davey KL, and Porter K (2008). Assessing the potential for major trauma transfusion guidelines in the UK. *Emerg Med J* **25**, 134–5.

3 CRASH-2 collaborators, Roberts I, Shakur H, Afolabi A, et al. (2011). The importance of early treatment with tranexamic acid in bleeding trauma patients: an exploratory analysis of the CRASH-2 randomised controlled trial. *Lancet* **377**, 1096–101.

4 Norfolk D (2013). *The Transfusion Handbook*, fifth edition. Available at: ℜ http://www.transfusionguidelines.org/transfusion-handbook.

Traumatic brain injury: nursing assessment and management

Serious head injury may be obvious from the initial examination or history, but the possibility must always be considered where there is altered conscious level or coma, in vulnerable groups, e.g. those with alcohol dependency or the elderly. Injury to the brain encompasses both the 1° injury and any 2° damage that develops during the first few hours or days after injury.

⚠ Be aware of the two main contributing factors to ↑ mortality and morbidity: failure to correct hypoxaemia and hypotension, and delay in appropriate surgical management.[5]

Identify patients who have a serious injury from:
• information given by paramedics;
• the mechanism of injury;
• assessment of vital signs, including GCS and CBG;
• motor responses.

Summon senior clinical help without delay, and proceed with full neurological assessment (**➔** see Neurological assessment, pp. 726–7; Physical examination, pp. 176–7). When assessing patients with traumatic brain injury (TBI), also consider the following:
• Consider an associated C-spine injury, and immobilize the C-spine.
• Give analgesia as prescribed, and monitor its effectiveness.
• Consider IV antibiotics as prescribed if there is an open skull fracture.
• Check the tetanus status.
• Clean and suture any head/facial wound, as necessary. This should not take priority over resuscitation or a CT scan, except when controlling haemorrhage is necessary.
• Prepare the patient, and accompany him/her to the CT scanning room.
• Assist medical staff in examining the patient.
• Escort the patient on any transfer to a neurosurgical unit.
• Provide emotional support and explanations to relatives and carers.

Secondary prevention measures for brain preservation

2° brain injury is the result of a complex process, following a 1° brain injury. It is important to understand preventative measures and recognize signs of deterioration, which may include changes in the GCS score, ↑ agitation, or confusion. The causes may be due to cerebral oedema, intracranial hypertension, hydrocephalus, vasospasm, haematomas, electrolyte imbalance, infection, and/or seizures.

Standard therapy for the management of raised ICP in severe TBI includes intubation and sedation, normocapnic ventilation, nursing the patient with the head raised, and ensuring an MAP >90mmHg. An ICP bolt may be inserted to monitor the ICP and guide the management. Alternatively, serial CT scans may reveal improvements or deterioration in ICP. IV mannitol has been used to ↓ raised ICP after severe TBI, as it creates a temporary osmotic gradient and it ↑ serum osmolarity. However, mannitol is contraindicated in patients with TBI who also have renal failure because of the risk of pulmonary oedema and heart failure. Also, it may pass and accumulate in the brain, causing a reverse osmotic shift or rebound effect, ↑ ICP. Recent evidence suggests that hypertonic sodium solutions (HTS) across a range of concentrations are more effective than mannitol in reducing ICP in patients with TBI and should be considered as first-line therapy for these patients.

Indications for neurosurgical referral

- CT shows a recent intracranial lesion.
- The patient meets criteria for CT, but facilities not available locally.
- Persisting coma after initial resuscitation.
- Confusion that persists >4h.
- Deterioration in conscious level.
- Progressive focal neurological signs.
- Seizure without full recovery.
- Depressed skull fracture.
- Definite or suspected penetrating injury.
- CSF leak or other sign of basal skull fracture.[6]

Checklist to ensure patient stable for transport

- Airway safe or secured by intubation:
  - tracheal tube position confirmed by X-ray.
- Breathing:
  - sedation, analgesia, and muscle relaxant;
  - ventilation established on transport ventilator;
  - adequate gas exchange confirmed by ABG.
- Circulation:
  - HR/BP stable;
  - tissue and organ perfusion adequate;
  - any obvious blood loss controlled;
  - circulating volume restored;
  - Hb adequate;
  - minimum of two routes of venous access;
  - arterial line and central venous access.
- Neurology:
  - seizures controlled; metabolic causes excluded;
  - protective measures in place to prevent, where possible, 2° brain insult.
- Trauma:
  - C-spine protected;
  - pneumothoraces drained;
  - where possible, intrathoracic and intra-abdominal bleed controlled;
  - intra-abdominal injuries investigated and appropriately managed, where possible;
  - long bone/pelvic fractures stabilized.
- Metabolic:
  - blood glucose >3mmol/L;
  - K^+ 3.5–6mmol/L; ionized Ca^{2+} >1mmol/L;
  - acid–base balance acceptable;
  - temperature maintained within normal limits.

- Monitoring:
  - ECG;
  - BP—arterial and non-invasive;
  - O_2 saturation;
  - $EtCO_2$;
  - temperature;
  - pupils.
- Documentation:
  - patient records;
  - CT scans, all X-rays;
  - blood results and blood products, if available;
  - referral letter, observation charts, and all nursing records;
  - inter-transfer observation chart;
  - details of neurosurgical unit, telephone number, accepting consultant name, mobile phone number of receiving specialist registrar.

In addition to this checklist, clear instructions must be given to any family members or carers who wish to follow the patient by car (→ also see Transporting the critically ill, pp. 760–1).

References

5 Neurocritical Care Multidisciplinary Team at The National Hospital for Neurology and Neurosurgery (2015). *Acute management of adults with traumatic brain injury*. University College London Hospitals NHS Foundation Trust, London. Available at: ℘ https://www.uclh.nhs.uk/OurServices/ServiceA-Z/Neuro/ANAE/Documents/Traumatic%20Brain%20Injury%20(TBI)%20referral%20guidance.pdf.

6 National Institute for Health and Care Excellence (2014). *Head injury: assessment and early management*. CG176. National Institute for Health and Care Excellence, London. Available at: ℘ https://www.nice.org.uk/guidance/cg176.

Complications of head injury

Intracranial haematoma

- Deteriorating consciousness after head injury may be due to an intracranial haematoma.
- Accurate observation and monitoring are essential in identifying such developments early, as surgical intervention may be lifesaving.
- ↑ agitation or confusion, increasingly severe headache, or persistent vomiting requires reassessment by a senior clinician.
- ⚠ Patients on anticoagulants or those with bleeding disorders are at ↑ risk of developing an intracranial haematoma after head injury.

Extradural haematoma

Extradural haematoma results from rupture of one of the meningeal arteries that run between the dura and the skull. The commonest cause is a linear fracture of the temporo-parietal bone, with associated injury to the middle meningeal artery.

Injury/laceration of this artery may result in a rapidly expanding haematoma that, if not evacuated, may be fatal. These patients may be difficult to assess, as initial injury will often be relatively minor. More than half of cases occur in persons <20y old. The patient may report a period of unconsciousness, followed by full coherence and subsequent ↓ GCS.

Signs and symptoms will be due to rising ICP. The nurse's role with these patients is accurate neurological assessment and consistent monitoring.

Subdural haematoma

A subdural haematoma is a blood clot that forms beneath the dura mater. This type of venous bleed is usually caused by trauma such as a fall, an assault, or acceleration/deceleration patterns associated with an RTC.

There are two main types of subdural haematoma:

- acute—develops within 24h of the initial trauma and is associated with severe brain insult;
- chronic—develops over several days after the initial trauma and often occurs in the elderly and alcoholics. The patient may present with a fluctuating level of consciousness, and there may be a vague, or sometimes no, history of trauma.

A poor prognosis is likely if the subdural haematoma is bilateral or accumulates rapidly, or if there is a >4h delay in achieving definitive neurosurgical management.

Diffuse axonal injury

This is a severe brain injury, often due to rapid deceleration, and the commonest cause of coma and subsequent disability. Patients with diffuse axonal injury are often in a deep coma immediately after injury, despite an initially normal ICP and a normal CT scan.

Overview of maxillofacial injuries

Maxillofacial injuries can be life-threatening and cause significant morbidity. Some of the patients presenting with these injuries have multisystem trauma due to RTCs, assaults, or, in some cases, sporting injuries. These injuries require expert resuscitation and collaborative management between emergency clinicians and surgical specialists in ENT, trauma surgery, plastic surgery, ophthalmology, and oral and maxillofacial surgery.

Many more patients with less life-threatening facial injuries are managed by ENPs. As there is often a forensic component to these cases, nurses need to be aware that they may be called on in the future to account for their examination and findings in court. It is essential to adopt a thorough and systematic approach to examining these patients and to maintain comprehensive records on which to rely at a later date.

Trauma to the maxillofacial anatomy is complex, as contained within the face are systems that control specialized functions, including sight, hearing, smelling, breathing, eating, and speech. Also, vital structures in the head and neck may be at risk, and the psychological impact of disfigurement can be devastating for the patient and his/her family.

Anatomically, the face is divided into three parts:

- the upper face where fractures involve the frontal bone and sinus;
- the midface which is divided into upper and lower parts. The upper midface is where maxillary Le Fort II and Le Fort III fractures occur and/or where fractures of the nasal bones, naso-ethmoidal or zygomatico-maxillary complex, and the orbital floor occur. Le Fort I fractures are in the lower part of the midface;
- the lower face where fractures are isolated to the mandible.

→ See Maxillary fractures, pp. 507–12, and Figs. 15.3–15.5.

Assessment and resuscitation of the patient with facial injuries

Resuscitation

- Follow the <C> ABCDE approach, bearing in mind that the main complication of maxillary fractures is airway obstruction. This may be caused by haemorrhage, oedema, vomit, or facial instability.
- Call for specialist help without delay.
- Look for, and treat, airway obstruction: jaw thrust, chin lift, and suction. Be mindful of a possible associated neck injury.
- As intubation is often difficult or impossible, prepare for a surgical airway, and assist the anaesthetist.
- Establish IV access with two wide-bore cannulae, and collect blood for FBC, clotting, group and save, and cross-match.
- Give IV analgesia as prescribed, and monitor the effect.
- Commence IV infusion as prescribed, and document the fluid regime.
- Record the GCS score (➜ see pp. 726–7).
- Record baseline vital signs. Attach the patient to monitoring equipment.
- Record ECG.
- Administer antibiotic medication as prescribed.
- Check the patient's tetanus status.
- Stay with the patient during X-rays or accompany to CT.
- Prepare the patient for theatre or transfer, depending on the location, for definitive fracture management.
- Reassure and comfort the patient, and keep the family informed as much as possible and as appropriate.

History taking

As in any trauma situation, address all life-threatening injuries first. A systematic approach to the history and physical examination ensures adequate assessment of a maxillofacial trauma. A history is more likely to be obtained from the family, friends, or paramedics.

In most emergency situations, history taking and initial management occur simultaneously. Enquire about the following:

- mechanism and time of injury; loss of consciousness at the time or since;
- location, type, and quality of pain and sensation;
- any symptoms of visual loss, blurred or double vision, photophobia;
- symptoms of headache, dizziness, tinnitus, nausea;
- any loss of hearing;
- past medical history and any relevant previous injury or ENT condition;
- recent drug or alcohol ingestion;
- known allergies.

Examination

Inspection
- Note any swelling, bruising, lacerations, deformity, flattening, or discoloration of face.
- Inspect open wounds for FBs.
- Look for asymmetry in the face.
- Bleeding from the nose or around the teeth; check the position and alignment of the teeth. Check for avulsed teeth.
- Inspect the tongue. Look for intraoral lacerations, bruising, or swelling.
- Nasal deviation and flattening of the nasal bridge.
- Inspect the nasal septum for a haematoma or CSF rhinorrhoea.
- Eyes for pupil size, shape, and level; corneal surface. Subconjunctival haemorrhage without a posterior border suggests an orbital wall fracture; uneven pupil levels may indicate an orbital floor fracture.
- Note lacerations that may involve the lacrimal duct. Refer appropriately.
- Eye movement: compare bilaterally. Note any restriction of movement.
- Jaw position, malocclusion, side-to-side movement of the jaw, mandible protrusion, opening and closing of the mouth.
- Examine the external ear for lacerations and the auditory canal for injury or CSF leaks, integrity of the tympanic membrane, perforation, or mastoid area bruising (i.e. Battle sign).
- Face movements (scrunch up, and close the eyes).

Palpation
Palpate bilaterally for swelling, depressions, crepitus, and specific tenderness in the:
- frontal bone;
- orbital rim;
- zygomatic arch;
- maxilla;
- nasal bones;
- mandible.

Movements
- Check the temporomandibular joint for any pain or clicking, locking, with movement.
- Check for any anaesthesia or loss of sensation in the face, cheek, side of the nose, and upper lip (infraorbital nerve injury).

Neurological Cranial nerve check if you suspect an associated head injury (➔ see Box 15.1).

Box 15.1 The cranial nerves
- CN I, olfactory. Smell.
- CN II, optic. Vision.
- CN III, oculomotor. Eyeball movement; innervation of superior, medial, and inferior recti, inferior oblique, levator palpebrae, and smooth muscle pupilloconstrictor, and ciliary muscle.
- CN IV, trochlear. Eyeball movement; innervation of superior oblique.
- CN V, trigeminal. Sensation from the face. Innervates muscles of mastication.
- CN VI, abducens. Eyeball movement, innervation of the lateral rectus muscle.
- CN VII, facial nerve. Innervation of muscles of the face. Sense of taste. Innervation of salivary glands.
- CN VIII, vestibulocochlear. Equilibrium and hearing.
- CN IX, glossopharyngeal. Taste, salivation, and swallowing.
- CN X, vagus. Taste, swallowing, palate elevation, and phonics.
- CN XI, spinal accessory. Head rotation and shrugging of shoulders.
- CN XII, hypoglossal. Tongue movement.

Frontal sinus fractures

These are due to a severe blow to the forehead. The anterior and/or posterior table of the frontal sinus may be involved. A fracture to the posterior wall of the frontal sinus may result in a dural tear. The nasofrontal duct may also be involved. The patient will present with swelling, tenderness, and crepitus to the forehead. There may be loss of sensation and other symptoms associated with head injury.

• Get specialist help.
• Commence neurological observations; monitor and record meticulously.
• Give analgesia and antibiotics, as prescribed.
• Prepare the patient for admission.

Advise the patient not to blow their nose, and ensure adequate pain relief. Refer the patient to a faciomaxillary specialist.

Zygomatic fractures

These are the second commonest fractures of the facial bones after nasal bone fractures. Concurrent ophthalmic injuries are common. The zygoma is the main supporting bone between the maxilla and the skull. Although it is strong, its prominent location makes it vulnerable to injury. Fracture is usually due to a blow to the side of the face or 2° to RTCs.

• Look for flattening of the cheek, any palpable defect in the orbital margin, diplopia, and subconjunctival haemorrhage.
• A direct blow to the zygomatic arch can result in an isolated fracture involving the zygomatico-temporal suture, which will cause pain on jaw movement.
• Fracture of the arch of the zygoma may be identified by a palpable defect over the area involved.
• Pain upon palpation and limitation of movement of the mandible may be found upon physical examination.

Advise the patient not to blow their nose, and ensure adequate pain relief. Refer the patient to a faciomaxillary specialist and an ophthalmologist, if indicated.

Orbital floor fractures

A direct blow to the eye can result in an isolated fracture of the orbital floor. Herniation of the orbital contents into the maxillary sinus is possible. The incidence of ocular injury is common but globe rupture is rare. Periorbital oedema may be visible.

- Check and record visual acuity.
- Check extraocular movements (EOMs).
- Check for diplopia (lateral and upward gaze dysfunction may result due to entrapment of the medial and inferior rectus muscles).
- Infraorbital nerve damage can cause paraesthesiae of the cheek and upper gum on the affected side.
- Fracture may not be visible on X-ray but may be assumed on the basis of the 'teardrop sign' (soft tissue mass in the roof of the maxillary sinus).

Advise the patient not to blow their nose, and ensure adequate pain relief. Refer the patient to a faciomaxillary specialist and an ophthalmologist.

Mandibular fractures

Direct trauma to the mandible is the commonest cause of mandibular fracture. Fractures can occur in multiple locations 2° to the U shape of the jaw and the weak condylar neck. Fractures often occur bilaterally at sites other than the site of direct trauma. The 'ring bone rule' is applicable to mandibular fractures—'if you identify a fracture or dislocation in a ring bone, look for another fracture or dislocation.' This phenomenon is also referred to as the pretzel/bagel spectrum.

Signs and symptoms

- Facial deformity, malocclusion of the teeth, or loose or missing teeth. Possible bruising or bleeding to the gums, and abnormal mobility of portions of the mandible or teeth.
- Paraesthesiae to the lower lip suggests injury to the inferior dental nerve where it passes through the ramus of the mandible.

Investigations and management

- Request an orthopantomogram (OPG) and condylar views.
- Give analgesia and antibiotics, as prescribed.
- Check the tetanus status.
- Refer to a faciomaxillary surgeon for definitive management.

Dislocation of the temporomandibular joint

The mandible has some degree of flexibility due to mobility around the temporomandibular joints. Dislocation and/or fracture of the mandible can be due to trauma, but dislocation on its own can also occur quite easily, usually spontaneously during a large yawn. Sometimes, it may happen whilst eating, during a dystonic reaction, or during intubation. It is usually an anterior dislocation, but it can be uni- or bilateral. The patient presents with considerable pain, is unable to close the mouth, and dribbles saliva because of difficulty in swallowing.

Management

- Reassure the patient.
- X-ray is only indicated if there is a history of trauma.
- Reduction is usually easily achieved without sedation or analgesia, provided it has only just happened, the clinician is skilled, and the process is properly explained to the patient.
  - Sitting in front of the patient, place both thumbs (covered by gauze swab) onto the lower molars, and press down and backwards at the same time, lifting the chin with the fingers.
- Confirm relocation with an X-ray, if a first episode.
- Delayed presentation may be more difficult to relocate due to muscle spasm.
- Advise the patient to eat a soft diet for 24h and to avoid opening the mouth wide or yawning.

Alveolar fractures

These fractures involve the teeth and their bony support, and can occur in isolation from a direct low-energy force or can result from extension of the fracture line through the alveolar portion of the maxilla or mandible. Clinical findings include gingival bleeding, mobility of the alveolus, and loose or avulsed teeth.

Maxillary fractures

These are classified as Le Fort I, II, or III (➔ see Figs. 15.3, 15.4, and 15.5).

Le Fort I fracture

Is a horizontal maxillary fracture across the tooth-bearing portion of the maxilla and separates the alveolar process and hard palate from the rest of the maxilla. The fracture extends through the lower third of the septum, and there may be facial oedema and mobility of the hard palate and upper teeth. There may be a haematoma of the soft palate and malocclusion.

Le Fort II fracture

Is a pyramidal fracture starting at the nasal bone and extending through the lacrimal bone, downward through the zygomatico-maxillary suture, producing mobility of the midface. Patients may present with pain, facial oedema, subconjunctival haemorrhage, diplopia, telecanthus, mobility of the maxilla, epistaxis, and possible rhinorrhoea.

Le Fort III fracture

Le Fort III fracture, or craniofacial disjunction, is a separation of all of the facial bones from the cranial base, with simultaneous fracture of the zygoma, maxilla, and nasal bones. The entire midface is fractured from the base of the skull.

Clinical features of Le Fort III fractures include extensive oedema, and bruising with facial elongation and flattening. An anterior open bite may be present due to posterior and inferior displacement of the facial skeleton. Movement of all facial bones is in relation to the cranial base with altered pupillary levels. Epistaxis and pharyngeal bleeding may lead to hypovolaemic shock and compromise the airway. CSF rhinorrhoea may also be found upon physical examination.

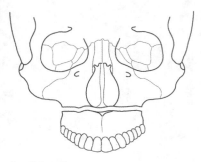

Fig. 15.3 Le Fort I.

(Reproduced with permission from Perry, M. (ed.) (2005). *Head, Neck, and Dental Emergencies*, Fig. 8.31, p. 258. Oxford University Press, Oxford.)

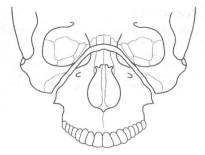

Fig. 15.4 Le Fort II.
(Reproduced with permission from Perry, M. (ed.) (2005). *Head, Neck, and Dental Emergencies*, Fig. 8.32, p. 258. Oxford University Press, Oxford.)

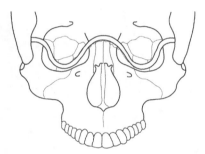

Fig. 15.5 Le Fort III.
(Reproduced with permission from Perry, M. (ed.) (2005). *Head, Neck, and Dental Emergencies*, Fig. 8.33, p. 259. Oxford University Press, Oxford.)

Naso-ethmoidal fractures

These extend from the nose to the ethmoid bones and can result in damage to the medial canthus, lacrimal apparatus, or nasofrontal duct. They also can result in a dural tear at the cribriform plate.

These fractures are characterized by a widened and flattened nasal bridge, epistaxis, rhinorrhoea, periorbital bruising, and subconjunctival haemorrhage. There may also be supraorbital and supratrochlear nerve paraesthesiae.

Chest trauma

In addition to patients presenting with respiratory problems arising from medical causes, many patients will present to an ED each year following a chest injury. The majority of these patients will have suffered from minor chest wall trauma from contact sports, assaults, or falls. However, a small number will have sustained significant chest wall trauma, with underlying damage to the lungs, heart, great vessels, and/or abdominal organs.

Mechanism of injury

Minor mechanisms tend to be falling over (often landing on an arm bent across the chest wall) or receiving a punch or an elbow to the chest wall during sports or an assault. However, just because a mechanism appears minor, a significant underlying lung injury cannot be reliably excluded. More significant mechanisms involve considerable blunt mechanical forces applied to the chest, e.g. falls from heights, RTCs, and pedestrian RTCs. Penetrating chest wall trauma can also cause significant injury, even though the surface wound may appear insignificant.

Nursing assessment

- History of injury. A clearly documented mechanism of injury is a crucial part of assessing the patient's risk of having underlying pulmonary or other organ damage. Generally speaking, the more force involved, the more the risk of underlying damage. However, in the elderly population, a relatively minor mechanism can result in significant chest injuries.
- PMH.
- Patients who smoke or those with pre-existing respiratory problems are more likely to develop respiratory problems from even the most minor of mechanisms.

Signs and symptoms

Assessing for the following signs/symptoms can identify patients who require further assessment or intervention:
- pain—ascertain the site and nature;
- breathlessness—is the patient tachypnoeic or do they find it difficult to breathe due to pain?
- hypovolaemic shock—in significant chest injury, 1500mL of blood can be sequestered in the thoracic cavity;
- respiratory distress—hypoxia and the resultant agitation can indicate a significant underlying injury.

Inspection

Signs of surface trauma to the anterior and/or posterior chest wall can include bruising, lacerations, abrasions (these may have characteristic markings, e.g. from a seat belt). An impaled object is an obvious sign of penetrating chest wall trauma. Look for asymmetrical chest wall movement and/or paradoxical movements; these are significant and can indicate a pneumothorax or flail segment.

Auscultation

Breath sounds should be equal and clear bilaterally. Any abnormality (reduction or absence) will usually require further evaluation with a CXR, except where there is a strong suspicion of a tension pneumothorax; this should be treated immediately with needle decompression (➔ see Needle thoracocentesis, p. 724).

Palpation

The clavicles, ribs, and sternum should be palpated. Crepitus may indicate an underlying fracture. Surgical emphysema detected clinically or on a CXR indicates an 'air leak' somewhere in the pulmonary tree. Pain on palpation is often present and can sometimes be pinpointed to a specific rib/s. However, pain on laughing, coughing, movement, changing position when in bed, or deep inspiration may be present without any chest wall tenderness.

Percussion

Percussion of part of the chest wall may be dull, which indicates fluid. In an acute chest injury, this dullness is likely to be blood. Hyper-resonance on percussion indicates air in the pleural cavity and may indicate a pneumothorax.

Nursing interventions

All patients should have a full set of vital signs recorded, regardless of how minor the mechanism:
- pulse and temperature;
- RR, BP, and O_2 saturations;
- pain score;
- GCS/AVPU.

Further interventions include the following:
- analgesia;
- CXR (➔ see Box 15.2) is indicated if the assessing clinician cannot confidently exclude pneumothorax/underlying pulmonary injury from the history and examination;
- ABG if SpO_2 <93% on air or for all known/suspected significant injuries;
- ECG if there has been blunt anterior chest wall trauma;
- FBC, U&E, and group and save/cross-match if significant injury suspected.

Box 15.2 CXR in chest trauma
- A CXR is a standard X-ray in a multiply injured patient.
- 50% of isolated rib fractures do not show up on a standard CXR.
- In patients with minor chest injuries, a CXR is usually not required.
- CXRs are indicated in patients where the clinician suspects an underlying injury to the lungs or mediastinum from either the history or clinical examination.
- If a tension pneumothorax is suspected, treat it first. Do a CXR afterwards.

Minor chest wall injuries

Patients with a relatively minor mechanism of injury, no overt signs of respiratory distress/difficulty, and normal observations are usually discharged from the ED. The diagnosis is clinical, and the rationale for not X-raying this group of patients may need to be explained (→ see Box 15.2).

Discharge planning

Patients will require analgesia appropriate to their pain score, advice about deep breathing exercises (to prevent the 2° development of a chest infection), and the knowledge that their symptoms may persist for up to 4wk. Patients should also be advised to seek further medical advice if any additional symptoms develop.

Multiple rib and sternal fractures

Multiple rib fractures

Patients with multiple rib fractures (two or more ribs) are diagnosed clinically and often have them confirmed by CXR.

Previously fit, healthy patients with no pre-existing respiratory problems or other injuries can often be discharged home (➔ see Chest trauma, pp. 514–16). Give patients clear written and verbal advice about when to return to the ED. A review several days later is often useful to ensure that no 2° problems, such as a small haemothorax/effusion, have developed.

- The elderly or those with an underlying lung disease may need a short period of hospital admission or intermediate care to ensure adequate pain management and the monitoring of any complications such as chest infection.
- Admission may also be indicated in some patients with multiple rib fractures if an underlying pulmonary contusion is suspected or severe pain requires well-controlled analgesia and/or an intercostal nerve block.

Sternal fracture

Fractures to the sternum are usually caused in RTCs from blunt trauma to the anterior chest wall from either the seat belt or steering wheel. A sternal fracture is acutely painful, and an underlying cardiac or great vessel injury must be ruled out prior to discharge.

Specifically, patients require the following:

- ECG to exclude arrhythmias, MI, or contusion which may be evidenced by ST segment changes;
- an echocardiogram may be undertaken in the resuscitation room in symptomatic patients;
- cardiac troponins—these can identify myocardial damage;
- a sternal X-ray usually shows a transverse fracture (± CXR if associated injuries are suspected).

Admission
Patients should be admitted if there are any signs of cardiac contusion.

Discharge
Patients should only be discharged if they have an isolated sternal fracture with no other injuries and no pre-existing cardiorespiratory problems. Discharged patients require analgesia and advice (➔ see Discharge planning under Minor chest wall injuries, p. 516).

Traumatic pneumothorax

Mechanisms ranging from relatively minor, e.g. elbow to the chest whilst playing rugby, to major trauma can cause a traumatic pneumothorax. Treatment for all but the smallest pneumothoraces is with a chest drain (➔ see Chest drains, pp. 684–6).

Tension pneumothorax

A tension pneumothorax can result from chest trauma or as a consequence of an underlying lung disease (➲ see Fig. 15.6). Although rare, its early detection and prompt treatment are critical to the survival of the patient. Patients with tension pneumothorax rapidly deteriorate, and it is a well-recognized cause of PEA cardiac arrest.

A tension pneumothorax is a pneumothorax that ↑ in size with every breath. A tear in the lung tissue creates direct communication with the pleural space, and the flap of injured tissue acts like a one-way valve. On inspiration, the flap of tissue is forced open, and inspired air passes through it into the pleural space. On expiration, the flap closes, and the air that has passed into the pleural space is trapped. Consequently, with every breath, more air passes through the flap, and the pneumothorax is under 'tension'. It continues to ↑ in size until the lung on the affected side has completely collapsed. The pneumothorax continues to expand, putting pressure on the mediastinum, causing it to shift towards the uninjured side. Pressure on the mediastinum causes compression of the heart and great vessels, which leads to impaired cardiac output, hypotension, and cardiovascular collapse. The larger the tension pneumothorax, the more extreme the patient's symptoms and the greater the chance of cardiac arrest.

Signs and symptoms

- Profound tachypnoea; gasping for breath.
- Tachycardia.
- Acute respiratory distress.
- Altered conscious level: agitated, confused, uncooperative.
- Cyanosis.
- ↓ or absent breath sounds on the affected side.
- Hyper-resonance on the affected side.
- Hypotension.
- Surface trauma to the chest.
- Bony crepitus may be present in injury.
- ↓ chest wall movement on the affected side.
- Engorged neck veins due to impaired cardiac emptying (although this may be absent in a hypovolaemic patient).
- Tracheal deviation, as the mediastinum shifts towards the uninjured side.
  - ⚠ This is a very late sign.

Nursing assessment

▶▶ It is critical that patients in acute respiratory distress are assessed immediately and managed in an appropriate resuscitation area:

- pulse;
- RR;
- BP;
- SpO_2;
- temperature;
- cardiac monitoring;
- AVPU/GCS.

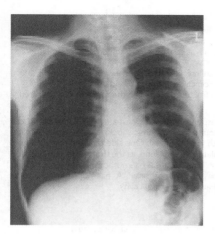

Fig. 15.6 A tension pneumothorax.

(Reproduced with permission from Warrell, D.A., *et al*. (2003). *Oxford Textbook of Medicine*, 4th edn, vol. 2, p. 1520. Oxford University Press, Oxford.)

Nursing interventions
- High-flow O_2.
- Continuous monitoring.
- Preparation for needle decompression.
- Preparation for chest drain insertion.

Management

Immediate needle decompression (➔ see Needle thoracocentesis, p. 724), followed by chest drain insertion (➔ see Chest drains, pp. 684–6).

Haemothorax

A haemothorax is almost always a consequence of blunt or penetrating trauma, although occasionally it can arise from the erosion of a pulmonary vessel by a tumour.

- In penetrating trauma, an intercostal, pulmonary, or great vessel is lacerated, and the thoracic cavity fills with blood.
- In blunt chest trauma, a fractured rib can be the cause of the lacerated vessel.

As well as the obvious respiratory compromise a thorax full of blood can cause, there may be profound hypovolaemic shock, and therefore two life-threatening situations with which to deal. One side of the thorax can hold 30–40% of the total circulating volume, and, as the thorax fills, compression on the mediastinum and shift can occur. A haemothorax causing hypovolae-mic shock is termed a 'massive haemothorax'. A 'haemopneumothorax' is a collection of blood and air in the pleural cavity.

Signs and symptoms

- Tachypnoea.
- Altered conscious level: agitated, confused, uncooperative.
- Cyanosis.
- Respiratory distress.
- Pleuritic chest pain.
- Tachycardia.
- Surface trauma to the chest wall or signs of a penetrating wound.
- Bony crepitus may be present in injury.
- Narrowed pulse pressure (➜ see Box 15.3) as a consequence of shock.
- ↓ or absent breath sounds on the affected side.
- Dullness to percussion on the affected side.
- Hypotension.
- ↓ chest wall movement on the affected side.
- Flattened neck veins, if shocked.
- Tracheal deviation, as the mediastinum shifts towards the uninjured side. This is only present if the haemothorax is massive.

Investigations

- CXR—shows diffuse hyperdensity on the affected side. A fluid level may be visible on an erect CXR.
- ABG—check lactate and base deficit.
- Blood for FBC, U&E, and urgent cross-match.
- Consider O-negative/positive blood in massive haemothorax.

Nursing assessment

▶▶ It is critical that patients in respiratory distress are assessed immediately and managed in an appropriate resuscitation area:

- pulse;
- RR;
- early recognition of changes in lactate and base deficit;
- BP, noting if the pulse pressure (➜ see Box 15.3) is narrowing;
- SpO$_2$;

Box 15.3 Pulse pressure

Pulse pressure is the difference between the systolic and diastolic pressure. Trends in pulse pressure are most easily detected when serial measurements are documented. Changes in pulse pressure reflect physiological changes in the cardiovascular system. Systolic BP reflects the CO; therefore, if the systolic BP falls, the CO is lower. Diastolic BP reflects the systemic vascular resistance (SVR); therefore, as the pressure that the blood exerts within the vessels falls, so does the diastolic BP.

A narrow pulse pressure occurs in the early stages of shock, as peripheral vasoconstriction causes pressure in the vessels to ↑, causing a rise in the diastolic BP. A small elevation in systolic BP may arise as a consequence of this, as 'squeeze' in the vessels ↑ the cardiac preload and therefore the CO.

- temperature;
- cardiac monitoring;
- AVPU/GCS;
- pain score.

Nursing interventions

- High-flow O_2.
- Continuous monitoring.
- Analgesia.
- IV access, two large-bore lines in the antecubital fossa, with IV fluid bolus if signs of hypovolaemic shock.
- Prompt regarding repeat ABG.
- Ensure blood has been sent for cross-match.
- Provide continuous support and reassurance, as the insertion of a drain can be very frightening for the patient and stressful for the relatives.
- Assist with chest drain insertion (➲ see Chest drains, pp. 684–6).

Management

A large-bore intercostal drain should be inserted ≥32FG (➲ see Box 15.4). A large-bore drain helps to ensure that blood clots do not block the tube.

Box 15.4 Monitoring intercostal drainage

This drain requires close monitoring. If the drain collects 1000mL of blood following insertion or subsequently drains 200mL/h, an urgent cardiothoracic opinion is required, and the patient may need urgent transfer for an open thoracotomy.

Flail chest

A flail chest arises when two or more ribs are fractured in two or more places. A segment of rib(s) is now no longer attached and the integrity of the chest wall is compromised (➜ see Fig. 15.7). Following blunt trauma a flail segment affects the patient's ability to adequately ventilate as the chest wall is no longer intact. There may also be an underlying pneumothorax, haemothorax, or pulmonary contusion. Significant alterations in oxygenation are more likely to be caused by underlying pulmonary contusions than the disruption to the mechanics of ventilation. Significant forces need to be applied to the chest wall to create a flail segment, e.g. high speed RTC or a fall from a height. However, with advancing age, osteoporosis, or bony metastases a simple fall can cause multiple fractures and a flail segment.

Signs and symptoms

- Tachypnoea.
- Tachycardia.
- Respiratory distress.
- Agitation.
- Pleuritic chest pain, usually severe.
- Surface trauma to the chest wall: bruising, swelling, bony crepitus.
- Cyanosis.
- ↓ or absent breath sounds on the affected side.
- ↓ chest wall movement on the affected side.
- Paradoxical chest wall movement—the flail segment moves in the opposite direction to the rest of the chest wall with respiration (➜ see Fig. 15.8). This is not always apparent clinically, as the intercostal muscles can splint the segment during the initial phase following injury.

Nursing assessment

- Pulse.
- RR.
- BP.
- SpO_2.
- ABG.
- Temperature.
- Cardiac monitoring.
- AVPU/GCS.
- Pain score.

Nursing interventions

- High-flow O_2.
- Continuous vital sign monitoring.
- IV access.
- Analgesia.
- Assist with chest drain insertion, if indicated (➜ see Chest drains, pp. 684–6).
- Assist with intercostal nerve block, if required.
- Assist with intubation (➜ see Endotracheal intubation, pp. 650–1) and ventilation, if required (➜ see Bag–valve–mask ventilation, p. 660).

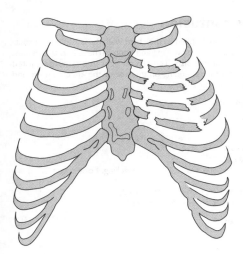

Fig. 15.7 Flail chest.

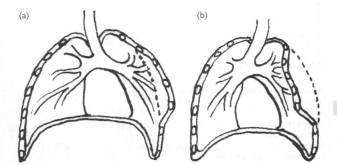

Fig. 15.8 Flail chest on (a) inspiration and (b) expiration.

Management

Most patients can be managed with adequate pain control, which may require a thoracic epidural or an intercostal nerve block. These patients are usually transferred to a high dependency area to enable their respiratory status to be closely monitored. A small number of patients will require intubation and ventilation. This is usually reserved for those who have persisting respiratory inadequacy or 2° complications despite the above management.

Pulmonary contusion

When significant forces are applied to the chest wall, these can be transmitted to the lung tissue and cause swelling and haemorrhage into the tissues. Pulmonary contusions vary in size. The clinical signs and symptoms listed range from mild to severe, depending on the size of the affected area, and usually develop over the first 24h.

Signs and symptoms

- Tachypnoea.
- Tachycardia.
- Agitation.
- Respiratory distress.
- Pleuritic chest pain.
- Surface trauma to the chest wall: bruising, swelling, bony crepitus.
- Cyanosis.
- ↓ or absent breath sounds on the affected side.
- ↓ chest wall movement on the affected side.

Nursing assessment

- Pulse.
- RR.
- BP.
- SpO_2.
- ABG.
- Temperature.
- Cardiac monitoring.
- AVPU/GCS.
- Pain score.

Nursing interventions

- High-flow O_2.
- Continuous vital sign monitoring.
- IV access.
- Analgesia.
- Assist with chest drain insertion, if indicated (➔ see Chest drains, pp. 684–6).
- Assist with intubation (➔ see Endotracheal intubation, pp. 650–1) and ventilation (➔ see Bag–valve–mask ventilation, p. 660), if required.
- Mechanical ventilation.

Open chest injury

Open chest injuries develop as a result of penetrating trauma to the chest wall. An impaling object may still be present—do not attempt to remove this. In the case of gun crime, an entrance ± exit wound may be visible on the chest or abdominal wall or the overflanks. As well as damage to the thoracic content, the abdominal and retroperitoneal organs may also be damaged. Open chest injuries can cause haemothorax, haemopneumothorax, pneumothorax, diaphragmatic rupture, open haemopneumothorax, pulmonary contusion, and rib fracture. Signs and symptoms of respiratory difficulty ± hypovolaemic shock depend on the site and size of the injury and the involvement of other organs.

Nursing assessment

- Pulse.
- RR.
- SpO$_2$.
- ABG.
- BP, noting if the pulse pressure (➲ see Box 15.4) is narrowing.
- Temperature.
- Cardiac monitoring.
- AVPU/GCS.
- Pain score.

▶▶ Observe the patient closely for the development of a tension pneumothorax.

Nursing interventions

- High-flow O$_2$.
- Continuous vital sign monitoring.
- IV access, ensuring blood has been sent for cross-match.
- Analgesia.
- Temporary dressing.
- Assisting with chest drain insertion, if indicated (➲ see Chest drains, pp. 684–6).
- Assist with intubation (➲ see Endotracheal intubation, pp. 650–1) and ventilation (➲ see Bag–valve–mask ventilation, p. 660), if required.
- Mechanical ventilation.
- Prepare for urgent thoracotomy.

Cardiac tamponade

Haemorrhage into the pericardial sac may cause compromise to cardiac function. Accumulation of fluid in the pericardial sac results in reduced ventricular filling and subsequent haemodynamic compromise. It can be caused by penetrating or blunt trauma. If bleeding is ongoing, tamponade may result. Tamponade, causing constriction on movement of atria and ventricles, may lead to cardiac arrest.

Clinical suspicion and signs

- History of injury to chest—penetrating or blunt.
  - ↑ shortness of breath;
  - ↑ distress;
  - ↓ arterial pressure;
  - ↓ venous return.
- Collapse.
- Distended neck veins.

Beck's triad is often referred to as a method of recognizing cardiac tamponade; this can be remembered as 3Ds:
- Distant (or muffled) heart sounds (rare);
- Distended jugular veins;
- Decreased arterial pressure.

⚠ In penetrating trauma, such as stabbing, a formal 'stab check' should be carried out. This includes a close inspection of the anterior and posterior chest, abdomen, and back. There is likely to be limited information about the implement used, length, and direction of travel.

Resuscitative thoracotomy

This may be required for life-threatening emergencies, in particular penetrating chest trauma, causing cardiac tamponade. There is ↑ use of resuscitative thoracotomy in blunt trauma to access and occlude the descending aorta for haemorrhage control. Each Trust should have a protocol for the management of traumatic cardiac arrest, with clear indications for initiating a resuscitative thoracotomy.

Nursing interventions

- Have an understanding of resuscitative thoracotomy and techniques employed, i.e. the Clamshell approach.[7]
- Be familiar with the hospital guidelines for the procedure.
- Be familiar with the equipment required (two large scalpels, two pairs of trauma shears, a Gigli saw, two large Spencer Wells forceps, large sutures ± a Foley catheter—a full theatre thoracotomy set is not required).
- Assist in the procedure, as required.
- Ensure that the team are aware of, and understand, the plan.
- Brief and support relatives.

Reference

7 Wise D, Davies G, Coats T, Lockey D, Hyde A, and Good A (2005). Emergency thoracotomy: "how to do it". *Emerg Med J* **22**, 22–4.

Abdominal trauma

Abdominal injury is the third leading cause of death in trauma. Blunt trauma to the abdomen from either compressive (assault or crush injury) or deceleration forces (high-speed RTC) are the commonest mechanisms injuring abdominal organs. The kidneys are relatively mobile structures and are prone to injury from deceleration forces, which can cause tears in the renal arteries. The ↑ use of guns and knives has resulted in a rise in the number of patients who present with penetrating injuries to the abdomen. All multiply injured patients should have their abdomen evaluated to assess for organ injuries as part of a trauma assessment (➔ see The handover of care, p. 17).

Patients can present with an isolated abdominal injury where the mechanism is clear, e.g. elbow to the abdomen during a rugby tackle. More complex and difficult to diagnose are patients with multiple injuries who may or may not have a significant intra-abdominal problem.

- Life-threatening injuries can occur without any signs of trauma to the abdomen.
- Where bleeding is confined to the retroperitoneal space, examination of the anterior abdomen may be entirely normal.
- Abdominal injuries should be suspected and assessed for in any patient with trauma between the fourth rib and the hips. This will ensure that patients with lower chest injuries have their abdomen appropriately assessed, as the liver and spleen could be injured.
- Assessment of the flanks is also crucial to detect any retroperitoneal injury.
- Penetrating injuries to the chest have the potential to damage both thoracic and abdominal organs.

Vascular abdominal organs

The liver and spleen are solid, extremely vascular organs enclosed in a fibrous capsule. Injuries range from haematomas to lacerations to burst-type injuries. Blood loss can be significant.

Fluid-/gas-filled abdominal organs

The stomach and the small and large bowel are vulnerable to perforation from penetrating injuries. Rupture of the stomach or intestines can also occur from blunt forces. A transient rise in intraluminal pressure causes perforation. Leakage of abdominal contents into the peritoneal cavity causes peritonitis, which develops over a number of hours.

Signs and symptoms of intra-abdominal injury

Signs and symptoms highly suggestive of intra-abdominal pathology are hypovolaemic shock, pain, blood loss, and absent or diminished bowel sounds. However, signs of injury are often subtle and can even be absent initially. The abdomen can sequester large amounts of blood without any obvious distension, and all symptoms can be absent if there is a retro-peritoneal haematoma, competing pain from another injury, drugs/alcohol, reduced level of consciousness, or spinal cord injury. Physical findings are not always accurate. ~ 20% of patients with a significant abdominal injury only have trivial signs.

These are common signs and symptoms of intra-abdominal injury:
- surface trauma to the lower chest, abdomen, or flanks, e.g. bruising, seat belt markings, wounds, impaled objects;
- even the smallest of wounds can cause intra-abdominal injury and perforation of organs. They should not be dismissed until thoroughly explored;
- pain and the pattern: guarding, rebound tenderness, and rigidity all suggest peritonism;
- referred pain (➜ see Table 10.1);
- hypovolaemic shock;
- dullness on percussion may indicate fluid within the abdomen;
- hyper-resonance on percussion may indicate air within the peritoneum;
- haematuria can indicate renal, urethral, or bladder injuries;
- scrotal bruising can indicate urethral trauma.

Nursing assessment
- Vital signs.
- Pain assessment and score.
- Urinalysis.
- ABG or VBG—particular attention to lactate and base deficit.
- FBC, U&E, amylase/lipase, LFTs, group and save, cross-match.

Nursing interventions
- O_2.
- IV access.
- Fluid resuscitation

⚠ Aggressive fluid resuscitation in an unstable patient with a penetrating injury can worsen their prognosis. A systolic BP of 90mmHg in a conscious adult patient is acceptable prior to emergent transfer to theatre.

- Analgesia.
- NG tube.
- Urinary catheter.
- IV antibiotics.
- Secure impaled objects. These should only be removed in theatre.
- Cover wounds.
- Prepare for FAST scan or CT.
- Prepare patients urgently for theatre when signs of peritonitis and/or hypovolaemic shock are present.

Further investigations
- USS (FAST scan) is increasingly performed at the bedside in the resuscitation room. It is non-invasive and repeatable. However, it is operator-dependent and may miss some bowel and pancreatic injuries.
- CT scan with contrast is often used and has high accuracy. However, it usually takes time to organize and perform. Therefore, the patient has to be relatively stable or, if unstable, a full trauma resuscitation team should accompany the patient.

Spinal fractures

The spinal cord is vulnerable and may be injured as a consequence of the fracture sustained or may be at risk of additional injury if not carefully handled following trauma. Nurses caring for any patient who has sustained trauma should act to immobilize the C-spine where the history, signs, or symptoms suggest possible spinal injury. It should also be borne in mind that people with degenerative conditions, such as osteoporosis, neoplasm, or other underlying conditions that affect bone, can sustain fractures with minimal trauma or even through normal activity. The commonest spinal injuries occur in the C-spine and at the thoracolumbar junction.

Most patients with a C-spine injury are young, with ~80% of patients aged 18–25y. ♂ are four times more likely to sustain this injury than ♀. These patients are most likely to be brought to the ED by ambulance but may self-present.

Patients with vertebral fractures 2° to trauma should be evaluated and treated in a systematic way. Initial priorities are twofold: attention should be focused toward the patient's airway, breathing, and circulation (ABC), whilst simultaneously adhering to C-spine precautions. In the multiply injured patient, diagnosis of spinal cord injury is challenging and may be made once all imaging and other interventions are complete. Findings on physical examination in cervical and thoracic spinal cord injury may include the following (however, they may present later in the patient's clinical course):

- spinal shock—loss of motor and sensory tone below the lesion, resulting in:
  - *flaccidity*;
  - *arreflexia*;
  - *loss of anal sphincter tone*;
  - *faecal incontinence*;
  - *priapism*;
  - *loss of bulbocavernosus reflex*.
- neurogenic shock—loss of sympathetic response to bleeding, resulting in:
  - *hypotension*;
  - *paradoxical bradycardia*;
  - *flushed, dry, and warm peripheral skin*;
  - autonomic dysfunction;
  - paralytic ileus;
  - urinary retention;
  - poikilothermia—where the patient takes on the ambient temperature.

Specific nursing points to remember with spinal injury

- Immobilize the C-spine by placing one hand on either side of the patient's head and maintaining alignment with the rest of the body.
- Give the patient 100% O_2, and perform simple airway opening manoeuvres if the airway is not open, whilst maintaining in-line immobilization of the C-spine. Apply a hard collar, with head blocks and tape. Attach the patient to an O_2 saturation monitor.

- Observe the breathing pattern, bearing in mind that cord ischaemia/ oedema can compromise breathing by paralysing the nerves that supply the diaphragm and intercostal muscles. Observe for diaphragmatic breathing (jerky, abnormal movements between the chest and abdomen) and the use of accessory muscles of respiration.
- Insert two wide-bore cannulae, and commence IV fluids, as prescribed, and collect blood samples, as needed.
- Record an ECG. Initiate ongoing monitoring of BP, being mindful that hypotension may indicate hypovolaemia or neurogenic shock. Potential sites of bleeding should be investigated in the presence of hypotension.
- A full neurological examination will be performed as part of the expanded 1° or 2° survey. Assist the clinician in examining the pelvic and perineal areas, and extremities. Consider the need for a urinary catheter.
- A rectal examination is indicated, especially if the patient has weakness in the extremities. A full explanation should be given before this is carried out. Assist in log rolling the patient to examine the spine and rectum. Remove the spinal board if it has not already been removed.
- Reassure the patient constantly, and ensure privacy and dignity. Keep the relatives informed.
- Keep the patient warm.

Incomplete cord injury patterns

These will generally be diagnosed once the examination and diagnostic imaging (including MRI) are completed.

Anterior spinal cord syndrome This is usually a result of compression of the artery that runs along the front of the spinal cord. These patients usually have complete loss of strength below the level of injury. Sensory loss is incomplete. Generally, sensitivity to pain and temperature is lost, whilst sensitivity to vibration and proprioception is preserved.

Posterior cord syndrome Injury to the posterior cord. Preservation of motor function, sense of pain and light touch, with loss of proprioception below the level of the lesion.

Brown-Séquard syndrome This is incomplete spinal cord injury caused by hemisection of the cord. This results in loss of motor function and proprioception on the side of the lesion, and loss of sense of pain and temperature on the opposite side.

Central cord syndrome This is an incomplete spinal cord injury, resulting in greater neurological involvement in the upper extremities than in the lower extremities.

Pelvic fractures

Pelvic fractures are orthopaedic *and* vascular emergencies. Pelvic injuries can lead to severe uncontrollable haemorrhage and death. When the pelvic ring is disrupted through injury, damage to the internal and external iliac arteries can result in exsanguination. Compound fractures of the pelvis have a mortality of up to 50%. Associated bladder and urethral injury is not uncommon.

For guidance about management of pelvic injuries, ➔ see Fig. 15.9.

Symptoms

A patient with a pelvic ring fracture may have severe pelvic pain.

Signs

- Abnormal vital signs; signs of severe shock.
- Pelvic asymmetry.
- Differences in leg length and external rotation of a leg, without an associated limb fracture.
- Flank, perianal, or scrotal swelling and bruising.
- Look for any injury to the groins, perineum, and genitalia. A swollen testicle may suggest testicular rupture, requiring surgical decompression. Examine the penis for blood at the meatus, suggestive of urethral damage.
- Check the femoral pulses on both sides. Absent pulses may indicate vascular damage. Get help, as surgery may be necessary to preserve the limb of the affected side.
- Examine the vulva, and inspect the vagina and urethral meatus for blood.
  - Where no evidence of urethral injury, insert a urinary catheter.
  - If urethral injury is likely, suprapubic catheterization may be necessary for bladder decompression. This applies to ♂ and ♀.
- A rectal examination should be performed to test sphincter tone. A reduction in tone is suggestive of a sacral fracture.
- Any blood from the rectum may be indicative of a rectal tear. This will require surgery.

Specific interventions

- Initial management focuses on fluid replacement, haemorrhage control, stabilization of fractures, and pain management.
- In the haemodynamically unstable patient, activate the major haemorrhage protocol.
- Give opiate analgesia, as prescribed, and monitor the effect.
- Use a pelvic splinting device.
- Fluid replacement should be guided by the patient's haemodynamic state. The patient's haemodynamic condition and response to fluids should be continuously monitored during this period.
- Give prophylactic antibiotics, as prescribed, for wounds, as there is a risk of infection from faecal flora.
- Patients with obvious pelvic fractures should *not* be log rolled. Enough people should be enlisted to perform a straight lift.

- Keep the patient NBM, and prepare, as appropriate, for theatre or interventional radiology.

Sacral fractures are often associated with other pelvic fractures as a result of major trauma. Transverse fractures result from directly applied forces to the sacrum. Vertical fractures occur as part of complex pelvic fractures. Stress fractures are usually vertical and near the sacroiliac joint.

MRI or bone scan are useful to detect stress fractures. Sacral fractures can be quite subtle and are easily missed.

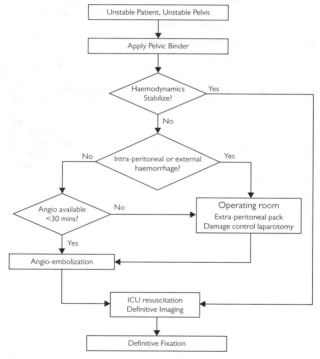

Fig. 15.9 Pelvic injury management.

(Reproduced from Brohi 'Management of Exsanguinating Pelvis Injuries' (2008), ☜ www.trauma.org with permission of Karim Brohi.)

Femoral fractures

❶ Any injured limb should be assessed for the presence of the 'five Ps' that might indicate neurovascular compromise:
- pain;
- pallor;
- pulselessness;
- paraesthesiae;
- paralysis.

Fractures of the femur fall into three anatomical categories: proximal, mid-shaft, and distal. Check for signs of hypovolaemia, as blood loss from a shaft of femur fracture can be 1000–1500mL.

Management priorities

Two main management priorities exist in the ED: preventing 2° damage and pain control. Preventing 2° damage includes managing blood loss by initiating IV fluid replacement. Reduction in blood loss and significant pain reduction can be achieved by correct application of an appropriate traction splint such as a Thomas splint. These stabilize the fracture until definitive repair can take place.

In doing this, the extent of the trauma to surrounding soft tissue is minimized. Pain is reduced, because bone ends are immobilized. Distal and proximal pulses, capillary refill, and sensation should be rechecked after splint application. If the fracture is open, broad-spectrum antibiotics should be given, and the patient's tetanus status checked. The wound should be covered with a wet dressing.

Knee dislocation and tibial plateau fractures

Knee dislocation

Knee dislocations are rare. Most are due to high-energy injuries such as RTCs or industrial accidents. They are an orthopaedic emergency, as there is a high incidence of neurovascular damage associated with this injury. Multiple ligament injuries are required for knee dislocation. Usually both cruciates and one or both collateral ligaments are injured. Injury to the popliteal artery or nerve is common.

- Check and record pulses and sensation. Look also for associated bony injury of the femur and lower limb.
- Reduction will require analgesia and sedation. Get specialist help.
- Post-reduction, immobilize in a full long-leg back slab, and continue to check and record circulation.
- Prepare the patient for admission.

Tibial plateau fractures

The principal bones involved in tibial plateau fractures are the femur and tibia. Fractures of the tibial plateau commonly occur in association with other injuries resulting from a fall or an RTC. Isolated fractures of the tibia are not fatal but may be associated with injuries to neighbouring structures such as the popliteal artery, ligaments, peroneal nerve, soft tissues, and menisci.

Signs and symptoms

- Patients usually present with pain over the fracture site and inability to weight-bear.
- Swelling can vary, and there is often a haemarthrosis.

Treatment

- Fractures of the tibial plateau may require elevation and open reduction and internal fixation with bone grafting as the preferred management.
- Conservative treatment in POP is less preferable because of the risks of long immobilization, especially in older patients. Ensure adequate analgesia before immobilizing the limb in a long-leg POP back slab, and refer to the orthopaedic team.

Tibial and fibular shaft fractures

Tibial fractures

A direct blow to the tibia is the commonest cause of fracture, as the tibia has little muscle protection. Significant injury may also be caused by falls or jumps from a height and, in recent years, gunshot wounds to the lower leg. Spiral fractures to the tibia or fibula may occur during violent twisting injuries from sport.

Undisplaced stress fractures can occur, particularly in adults involved in sports, and may not always be evident on X-ray. Persistent symptoms suggestive of stress fracture should be followed up in fracture clinic.

Diagnosis of a tibial fracture is relatively easy. Inability to weight-bear on the affected leg and a visible malformation of the leg are often presenting features.

Pain is usually severe, but this can vary. Any wound proximal to the fracture site should be regarded as a potential open injury. A tibial fracture should be considered among the differential diagnoses after trauma, especially in a patient with an altered mental status who cannot provide a reliable history. A tibial shaft fracture will be treated according to the type of fracture and alignment of the bone.

Treatment

- POP is appropriate for tibial shaft fractures that are minimally displaced or undisplaced and are well aligned. The cast must extend from above the knee to below the ankle (a long-leg cast). These fractures tend to heal well, and casting avoids the potential complications of surgery such as infection. Patients with casts must be monitored for the development of compartment syndrome and to ensure satisfactory healing of the tibia and to ensure the bony alignment is maintained.
- Open reduction and internal fixation are required when fractures are unstable. Factors that contribute to instability are the type of fracture, location of fracture, and degree of comminution—also associated fibular fractures.

▶▶ Open fractures are orthopaedic emergencies, and a specialist should be consulted immediately.

- Rarely, such fractures can be treated conservatively.
- Most patients need to be prepared for theatre for debridement and irrigation within 6h of injury. Longer intervals have been shown to ↑ the rate of infection.
- On occasions, especially in multiple trauma, the definitive fracture treatment may be delayed. If surgery must be delayed, leg appearance and compartmental pressure must be monitored carefully.
- The risk of compartment syndrome is high. ∴ Admission for 24h observation and limb elevation should be considered in very swollen proximal tibial fractures.

Fibular fractures

- These occur in combination with tibial fractures or as a result of direct trauma to the lateral aspect of the calf. Distal fibular/malleolar fractures occur with excessive rotational forces (➲ see Ankle injuries, pp. 320–1)
- Isolated fibular fractures are not common. The patient may present with pain over the fracture site. Because the fibula is not a weight-bearing bone, the patient may be walking with discomfort. Swelling is usually minimal.
- The common peroneal nerve may be damaged in proximal fibular injuries, so it is important to examine specifically for weakness of ankle dorsiflexion and ↓ sensation of the lateral aspect of the forefoot.

Depending on the degree of pain, isolated fractures are treated by either plaster cast or compression bandage.

Maisonneuve fracture

Is a fracture of the proximal fibula, in addition to a fractured medial malleolus (or injured deltoid ligament). Patients present with proximal fibular pain, in addition to medial ankle pain. This is an unstable ankle injury.

Open fractures

An open fracture (compound fracture) is a broken bone that penetrates the skin and is open to the air. Open fractures are usually caused by high-energy injuries such as RTCs, falls, or sports injuries. High-energy fractures can be life- and limb-threatening. Mangled or severe open fractures need timely emergency management as soon as life-threatening injuries have been dealt with.

▶▶ Open fractures are orthopaedic emergencies requiring immediate specialist intervention because of high risk of infection and potential associated neurovascular damage. Surgical intervention is usually required to adequately assess the injury, clean the area, and stabilize the fracture. Even with prompt surgical intervention, these injuries are often slow to heal and may result in some level of disability for the patient. Early IV antibiotics are a priority for specific management of severe open lower limb injuries (see BOAST 4 guidelines, available at: ✎ https://www.boa.ac.uk/wp-content/uploads/2014/12/BOAST-4.pdf).

Nursing interventions

- Ensure ABCs are managed effectively before dealing with the open fracture.
- Assess pain. Administer opiate analgesia and an anti-emetic, as prescribed.
- Immobilize the wound as much as possible.
- Record baseline observations to include temperature, HR, BP, and CBG. Report any abnormalities.
- Record pedal pulses half-hourly on the affected limb.
- Apply dressing to the wound to protect against further contamination. Leave fracture blisters (if any) intact, as, once broken, they are likely to become more contaminated.

- Establish the tetanus immunization status of the patient, and consider the need for tetanus Ig—open fractures are classed as high-risk for tetanus.
- Establish IV access, and collect blood for FBC, U&E, group and save, as the patient will need surgical intervention.
- Administer IV antibiotics, as prescribed.
- Record the presence/absence of distal pulses before covering the wound, and continue to monitor.
- Remove any obvious foreign bodies before applying a sterile soaked dressing.
- Reassure and support the patient and family, as these are very frightening injuries.
- Prepare the patient for theatre.

Gunshot wounds

Gunshot wounds are unfortunately an ↑ presentation in the ED. In the UK, the police must be notified if a patient presents with a gunshot wound. It helps to have some understanding of the nature of ballistics in caring for patients with gunshot injuries. Ballistics refers to the study of projectile motion and is divided into three categories: internal, external, and terminal ballistics. Wound ballistics is a subset of terminal ballistics and is the most important aspect of ballistics for clinicians to understand.

A bullet wound is different to a knife wound. When a projectile strikes, it dissipates energy. The energy of a body is $e = mv$ where e is energy, m is mass, and v is velocity. Thus, kinetic energy KE is proportional to mass and to the square of its velocity, so injury is more dependent on velocity than mass.

Bullet injuries are most serious in friable solid organs, such as the liver, where damage may be caused by temporary cavitation away from the actual bullet track. Bone and SC fat are more resilient to bullet injury. Bones slow down the course of the bullet.

Assessment of gunshot wounds

History may be obtained from the paramedic crew, the police, or the patient, if conscious, or relatives/friends. In these situations, it is important to ensure the safety of staff, so allow only immediate next of kin into the resuscitation room. Try to establish what kind of weapon was used, and check that the weapon is not still with the patient.

Nursing interventions

- Make an assessment of the general state of the patient. Remember that a young person compensates for blood loss, and even tachycardia may be a fairly late feature, whilst hypotension suggests very marked blood loss.
- Give high-flow O_2, and monitor saturation.
- Establish IV access as soon as possible with two wide-bore cannulae for fluid replacement, and collect blood for FBC, U&E. Cross-match for an initial 6 units, or activate the major haemorrhage protocol.
  - In hypovolaemic shock from penetrating trauma/injuries, fluid replacement should be carefully titrated to achieve a lower than normal systolic BP. In the prehospital care setting, boluses of 250mL of fluid can be titrated against the presence or absence of a radial pulse. Evidence suggests that over-administration of crystalloids in the prehospital setting may be harmful. Once in the hospital, the emphasis must be on early operative intervention to control the source of haemorrhage.
- Apply pressure to any obvious bleeding points. Open or sucking chest wounds must be covered immediately.
- Record baseline observations, and maintain frequent monitoring of vital signs; blood gases.
- Attach to ECG monitoring.
- Request CXR.

- Be prepared. Have a chest drain ready and equipment for emergency thoracotomy if there is any deterioration or cardiac arrest.
- Do not consider 1° closure of a wound before full exploration and debridement, as bullets cause considerable tissue damage.
- Consider tetanus prophylaxis.
- Give IV antibiotics, as prescribed.
- Give prescribed analgesia, as needed.
- Assist in full medical examination.
- Prepare the patient for theatre/ICU.

Points to consider

Chest injuries

May involve the heart, lung pleura, great vessels, mediastinum, diaphragm, and abdominal contents. The most frequent injury is a haemopneumothorax from damage to the lung and chest wall. This requires a chest drain. Injury to the mediastinum may cause a cardiac tamponade.

Abdominal injuries

Most deep penetrating wounds of the abdomen need an exploratory laparotomy.

Limb injuries

Nerves, tendons, and vessels may be damaged. Examine the limb in a good light, and check for pulses, but remember that finding a pulse does not exclude vascular injury. Record sensation/skin temperature/sweating. Apply direct pressure to bleeding points.

Blast injuries

Blast injuries are devastating and can be caused by domestic, industrial, or bomb explosion injuries. They are categorized as 1°, 2°, tertiary, and quaternary.

- 1° blast injuries affect those closest to the explosion and are caused by the impact of a blast wave on the body surface. The lungs, GI tract, middle ear, and other gas-filled structures are most vulnerable. Types of injury ensuing from a 1° blast are tympanic membrane rupture, blast lung or pulmonary barotraumas, abdominal perforation and haemorrhage, eye injuries, and concussion without any apparent head injury.
- 2° blast injuries are caused by flying debris and bomb fragments. These include penetrating or blunt injuries and shrapnel injuries. Penetrating eye injuries can be occult.
- Tertiary blast injuries are caused by people being thrown by a blast. Injuries can be very severe and can include serious head injuries, amputations, and fractures.
- Quaternary blast injuries include all explosion-related injuries, illness, or disease not attributable to 1°, 2°, or tertiary mechanisms. Also include exacerbation of existing conditions, e.g. angina. Injuries include partial- and full-thickness burns, inhalation injuries, crush injuries, and open or closed brain injuries.

Nursing interventions

Management of such seriously injured patients is a team effort; ensure life-threatening injuries are prioritized. However, these patients need very intensive support and understanding, and must have assigned a nurse to ensure continuity of care.

Proceed with nursing assessment as usual, but give special consideration to the following points.

- Respiratory injuries. Consider blast lung in patients who are wheezing or who have a hypoxic result in blood gas analysis. Blast lung is the commonest fatal blast injury and presents as a triad of apnoea, bradycardia, and hypotension. These symptoms may or may not be evident at initial presentation. Pulmonary contusion or acute lung injury may evolve over the initial 48h from injury, so these patients need meticulous observation. Protective ventilation strategies may be needed if this injury is suspected. Be aware that wheezing may also be due to inhalation of fumes/dust/gases or pulmonary oedema.
- Renal injury. Urinalysis should be routine at initial assessment to identify any renal trauma. Haematuria may be indicative of rhabdomyolysis, suggesting compartment syndrome. This may occur as a result of swelling and ↑ pressure in muscle compartments (2° to the blast injury).
- Abdominal injuries. Consider delayed perforation and intestinal mural contusions. Unexplained hypovolaemia may indicate severe intra-abdominal injury.

- Ruptured tympanic membrane. All victims of a blast should be examined by an ENT specialist.
- Ophthalmology. All victims of a blast should be assessed by a specialist.
- Head injury. Patients can suffer from concussion without having sustained an apparent head injury.

▶ Frequent recording of vital signs is paramount. It is equally essential that staff show compassion and support for these very traumatized patients.

Traumatic amputation

Traumatic amputation is the accidental severing of some, or all, of a body part. A complete amputation refers to the total severing of the limb. In a partial amputation, some of the tissue remains attached.

Trauma is the leading cause of amputation. The majority of patients are <30y old and ♂. RTCs, especially those involving motorbikes, and the use of heavy gardening equipment and power tools are attributable causes. Industrial and agricultural workers traditionally have been more vulnerable to such trauma. More recently, traumatic amputations have been caused by explosions.

Haemorrhage is variable, depending on the site and nature of injury. On arrival in the ED, decisions will be made about the viability of the severed part and the potential of successful reattachment. Various limb salvage scoring systems are used to aid surgeons in making these difficult decisions. These are:
- mangled extremity severity score (MESS);
- predictive salvage index (PSI);
- limb salvage index (LSI).

Nursing interventions
- The injured limb should be gently cleaned with a sterile solution and covered with a moist sterile dressing.
- Loose tissue should be supported in its normal position, whilst waiting for theatre.
- Establish the tetanus status of the patient, and consider the need for tetanus Ig.
- An amputated body part should be wrapped in a sterile towel, sealed in a plastic bag, and kept cool till definitive care.
- Analgesia.
- Elevation of the affected limb, if possible.
- Offer reassurance for the patient and family.

Trauma in pregnancy

Pregnant patients are more vulnerable to trauma than non-pregnant patients, especially during the second and third trimesters, because of the ↑ size and change in the position of the uterus. Trauma may be caused by common mechanisms such as falls, RTCs, or assaults. However, emergency nurses need to be vigilant and aware of the evidence that suggests that pregnant women are more prone to domestic violence. Injuries that are inconsistent with the history should be regarded with suspicion and reported to the midwife caring for the patient.

- Whilst there are two lives to be considered, give priority to resuscitating and stabilizing the mother, as this offers the best chance for both.
- In assessing the patient, it is essential to bear in mind the physiological changes in pregnancy (➋ see The pregnant patient, pp. 146–7).
- ▶▶ Obtain specialist obstetric and paediatric help at the outset.
- The type of injury will determine treatment, but, in the first instance, follow a systematic <C> ABCDE approach in assessing the patient.
- Determine the stage of pregnancy (➋ see Fig. 5.2).
- Establish and maintain an airway. Remember, due to delayed gastric emptying in later pregnancy, there is ↑ risk of regurgitation and vomiting; therefore, have suction available. Early anaesthetic help may be required.
- Give 100% O_2. Remember ↑ O_2 consumption and ↑ Vt in pregnancy.
- Establish venous access, and collect blood for FBC, U&E, clotting, and cross-match. Send to the lab as a matter of urgency.
- Ongoing assessment of haemodynamic status is essential. Pregnant women have a physiological ↑ in circulating volume; therefore, they can lose a significant amount of blood before appearing truly 'shocked'.
- Consider early crystalloid fluids or blood products, as prescribed, if haemorrhage is suspected.
- Relieve pressure on the inferior vena cava by raising the mother's right hip with a (Cardiff) wedge or pillow, or manually displace the uterus.
- Once a C-spine injury has been excluded, nurse the patient in the left lateral position to prevent compression of the inferior vena cava.
- Establish the presence of a fetal heart and the rate (use a Pinard stethoscope or Doppler probe).
  - Consider continuous monitoring if the fetal HR is abnormal.
- Palpate the fundal height, and mark the skin. A higher than expected fundus may indicate intra-abdominal bleeding. Feel for fetal movements, and document.
- Observe for any PV bleeding or rupture of membranes. Collect any evidence of blood loss such as towels/clothing/clots.
- Insert a urinary catheter, and record the fluid intake/output.

- Insert an NG tube to minimize vomiting or aspiration. Consider an orogastric tube in head trauma.
- Administer pain relief, as prescribed.
- Consider anti-D Ig if the patient is Rh-negative.
- Consider tetanus prophylaxis if appropriate (pregnancy is not a contraindication).
- Assist with investigations and diagnostic procedures indicated by the injury.
- Prepare the patient for possible surgery or an emergency Caesarean section.
- Stay with the patient throughout, offering consistent support and realistic assurances.
- Keep the partner and family informed of proceedings.
- Keep meticulous records of all interventions.

Endocrine and metabolic emergencies

Overview

Many patients presenting to the ED may have disordered metabolism due to an underlying endocrine disease. These patients are often critically ill and require rapid assessment and intervention to prevent further complications, coma, and death. Emergency care staff need to have an understanding of how these diseases present and their initial management. As the incidence of type 2 diabetes continues to rise, ED staff need to have a good understanding of the complexity of this disease process and how it impacts on health and well-being.

Hypoglycaemia

▶ Do not ever forget glucose!

Pathophysiology

The normal glucose range is 3.5–5.5mmol/L. Hypoglycaemia can therefore be defined as a blood sugar <3.5mmol/L, although many areas identify that values <3.0mmol/L represent clinical significance.

Hypoglycaemia develops when there is an imbalance between the rate of glucose uptake by tissues, in contrast with hepatic glucose output and/ or glucose intake.

- Patients taking insulin are most at risk, especially in relation to a misjudged dose, insufficient or delayed food intake, exertion that was not accounted for, or infection.
- Oral hypoglycaemics, such as sulfonylureas (e.g. gliclazide), can also lead to hypoglycaemia, whereas metformin does not have this effect.
- Alcohol is also responsible for hypoglycaemia, as alcohol inhibits hepatic gluconeogenesis, whilst patients who are malnourished or have liver disease have ↓ glycogen reserves.
- In addition, although gluconeogenesis occurs mainly in the liver (via substrates such as glycerol and lactate), the renal cortex also has a 2° role in this process. Hence, hypoglycaemia can be a feature of profound renal failure.
- Other causes include insulinomas in the pancreas, Addison's disease, pituitary insufficiency, and self-harm/poisoning via insulin or oral hypoglycaemics.
- Hypoglycaemia can also rapidly develop in children in the face of overwhelming physical insult, e.g. sepsis. This leads to a depletion of glucose stores (especially in infants). Thus, it is essential that blood sugars are monitored and corrected in such situations.

Clinical features

Early signs of hypoglycaemia relate to the sympathetic nervous system response and may include sweating, pallor, and tachycardia. Most diabetics are able to identify these early signs and take remedial action. It is particularly noteworthy, however, that β-blockers will inhibit this sympathetic response and thereby blunt these early warning signs. This is one reason why β-blockers should be generally avoided in diabetic patients. β-blockers can inhibit gluconeogenesis, which can lead to hypoglycaemia.

Signs and symptoms of hypoglycaemia become particularly notable at <2.5mmol/L. As glucose levels fall, the neurological impairment becomes more apparent. This reflects that 50% of the body's available glucose is consumed by the brain. Patients can therefore present with a ↓ level of consciousness, seizures, aggression, confusion, and even isolated hemiparesis. Recurrent hypoglycaemic episodes are associated with ↑ morbidity and mortality 2° to microvascular damage and brain injury.

Assessment/diagnosis

In relation to the 1° survey, blood sugar monitoring is a vital component of the disability assessment. Diagnosis is based upon presenting signs and symptoms in association with a blood sugar <3.5mmol/L, initially tested using a blood glucose monitoring meter.

To verify the result, a formal venous blood glucose sample should also be sent to the laboratory. However, treatment should not be delayed, whilst awaiting this formal result.

If the cause for the hypoglycaemia is uncertain, a metabolic screen may be required before treatment is commenced.

Management

The mode of treatment will depend upon the severity of the patient's signs and symptoms and their compliance. Patients presenting with early signs of hypoglycaemia can be treated with fast-acting oral carbohydrate (10–20g glucose), e.g. a sugary drink with two teaspoons of sugar (= 10g) or dextrose sweets. This can be followed by slow-release carbohydrate such as a sandwich, banana, or milk.

Patients presenting with more profound hypoglycaemia can be treated in a number of ways.

- Glucose gel is especially useful in the prehospital environment and can be rapidly absorbed from the buccal mucosa.
- Glucagon 1mg SC, IM, IV. This is again very useful prehospital or when venous access is problematic. Glucagon is unlikely to be effective in hypoglycaemia associated with liver failure or chronic alcoholism, as, in these instances, there will be limited hepatic glycogen stores for the glucagon to affect. If there is no significant improvement in a patient's condition 10min after administration of glucagon, consider IV glucose.
- Glucose IV infusion. Glucose 10% is used in such situations—either given as 50mL aliquots or as one 250mL infusion. This reduces the risk of extravasation and subsequent thrombophlebitis. The 50mL aliquots, in particular, are associated with less rebound hyperglycaemia. The paediatric dose is 5mL/kg of 10% glucose.

With appropriate treatment, most patients show significant signs of improvement within 10–20min and can be discharged home if blood sugar readings remain stable and there are no complications. If neurological signs and symptoms do not improve, despite normalization of blood sugars, coexistent pathology should be sought, e.g. stroke or cerebral oedema 2° to hypoglycaemia. Patients presenting with an insulin overdose may need prolonged glucose infusion, and potassium (K$^+$) levels will need to be closely monitored due to associated hypokalaemia.

Diabetic ketoacidosis

Pathophysiology

DKA is almost always associated with type 1 diabetes and is only very rarely a feature of type 2 diabetes. Apart from the first presentation of type 1 diabetes, DKA is usually precipitated by ↑ physiological stress, especially infection (e.g. urinary and chest infections), but also MI, stroke, and trauma. This stress ↑ circulating levels of glucagon, catecholamines, and glucocorticoids, which all ↑ blood glucose levels. In tandem with this physiological stress, there is insufficient insulin to both homeostatically 'brake' these hormonal processes or to 'drive' glucose into cells. This is especially true if insulin has been either omitted or insufficiently augmented at times of illness. The consequences are as follows.

- Rising blood sugars lead to a hyperosmolar state. This provokes a diuretic response and ultimately leads to hypovolaemia and electrolyte derangement. Although there is an overall total body K^+ deficit 2° to the diuresis, the plasma K^+ is actually raised in a third of cases and usually normal in the rest. This reflects extracellular shifts in K^+.
- ↑ levels of glucagon (normally inhibited by insulin) lead to ↑ lipolysis and ↑ production of free fatty acids, from which ketone bodies are derived. This ketone rise results in an acidosis.

Consider metabolic acidosis in any patient who is hyperventilating.

Clinical features

- Hyperventilation (Kussmaul respiration).
- Polydipsia.
- Polyuria.
- Hypotension.
- Tachycardia.
- Acetone breath is virtually pathognomonic of DKA.
- Nausea/vomiting.
- Abdominal pain (often missed in adolescents).
- Altered consciousness.

Diagnosis

Diagnosis is made on the basis of ↑ blood glucose, metabolic acidaemia, and the presence of ketones in the urine. The following tests therefore need to be obtained:

- bedside and laboratory glucose (blood glucose >11);
- urine dipstick checking for ketones >2+, glucose, and signs of infection;
- ABG or VBG (HCO_3^- <15mmol/L, pH <7.3).

Other investigations should include the following:

- CXR (as chest infection may be present).
- ECG (looking for signs of ACS or hypo-/hyperkalaemia).
- U&E, FBC, CRP, LFTs, and/or blood cultures.

Patients with infection in the context of DKA may be apyrexial.

Nursing interventions

- Ensure airway patency, and administer high-flow O_2.
- Fluid replacement. Refer to local protocols. Fluid is generally 0.9% sodium chloride. In adults, the first litre is usually given over 60min, and the second litre over 2h.
- When blood glucose is <15mmol/L following insulin therapy, switch from 0.9% sodium chloride to 5% glucose. This reduces the risk of hypoglycaemia and an over-rapid correction of osmolality and cerebral oedema.
- Beware excessive rehydration. Coexisting cardiac pathology may lead to pulmonary oedema, whilst cerebral oedema 2° to rapid fluid shifts (most commonly affecting children and young adults) is associated with high mortality.
- Insulin (= 0.1 unit/kg/h of Actrapid® or Humulin S®) should be commenced (sliding-scale insulin is no longer recommended). Refer to local policies.
- Electrolyte replacement. Fluid and insulin therapy can lead to rapid intracellular movement of K^+. If the plasma K^+ value is <5.5mmol/L, K^+ needs to be added to the replacement fluids.
- Seek and treat any underlying cause, e.g. infection, MI.
- Consider: NG tube if persistent vomiting; urinary catheter (especially if the patient is oliguric or anuric); CVP monitoring in the critically ill patient.
- ⚠ Ensure thromboembolic prophylaxis (patients with DKA have a hypercoagulable state).
- Patients who are profoundly acidaemic/critically ill will need an ICU/HDU opinion.

Hyperosmolar non-ketotic hyperglycaemia

Pathophysiology

Hyperosmolar non-ketotic hyperglycaemia is associated with type 2 diabetes. It has a gradual onset of days, and even weeks, and is associated with a significant mortality rate of ~10%. As with DKA, the main precipitating factor is concurrent illness (especially infection). Glucagon, catecholamines, and glucocorticoids lead to a significant rise in blood glucose levels and a resultant profound homeostatic imbalance 2° to marked hyperosmolality. Although there may be a small rise in ketones, patients with hyperosmolar non-ketotic hyperglycaemia are, by definition, not ketoacidotic.

Clinical features

- Hypovolaemic (2° to hyperosmolar diuresis).
- Hypotensive.
- Tachycardic.
- ↓ level of consciousness, especially in the elderly.
- Electrolyte imbalance.
- Signs and symptoms of thromboembolic disease (such as stroke, MI, PE, DVT) 2° to an underlying hypercoagulable state. This is a major cause of mortality.

Diagnosis

Diagnosis is made on the following basis:
- ↑ bedside and laboratory glucose (often >30mmol/L);
- ↑ urine and blood osmolality;
- there may be a coexistent lactic acidaemia 2° to hypoperfusion, but ketones are absent or minimally present.

Nursing interventions

- Ensure airway patency, and administer high-flow O_2.
- Full set of vital signs, including ECG.
- Establish IV access. Collect blood for FBC, U&E, clotting, glucose, CRP, cultures if pyrexial.
- Commence IV fluid resuscitation cautiously.
- Rapid dilution of the blood and a rapid drop in osmolality ↑ the risk of rebound cerebral oedema.
- If not shocked, fluid replacement needs to be gradual. A rate of 200mL/h of 0.9% sodium chloride is often appropriate.
- If plasma Na^+ is very high, use 0.45% sodium chloride slowly.
- Urinalysis, and monitor urine output.
- A general guide is that a half dose of the insulin usually required for DKA should initially be infused, e.g. 3 units/h of Actrapid®, rather than 6 units/h.
- Give LMWH, as prescribed, to minimize risks associated with hypercoagulable blood.

Acid–base disorders

Normal blood pH is 7.35–7.45, and a number of homeostatic mechanisms ensure that this narrow normal range is maintained. For example, respiratory and renal adjustments alter the plasma levels of CO_2 and HCO_3, respectively, and thereby ensure an optimal pH. Variations away from these normal values can have a deleterious effect upon cellular and organ function. For example, cardiac function deteriorates in the face of profound acidaemia.

Terminology

- Acidaemia relates to a plasma pH <7.35 (hydrogen ion (H^+) >45nmol/L). This is 2° to an acidotic process (respiratory, metabolic, or mixed) that leads to a rise in H^+ concentrations. Such acidotic processes, however, do not always lead to an acidaemia, as respiratory or metabolic compensation can occur.
- Alkalaemia relates to a plasma pH >7.45 (H^+ <35nmol/L). This is 2° to an alkalotic process (respiratory, metabolic, or mixed) that leads to a fall in H^+ concentrations. Again, such alkalotic processes do not always lead to an alkalaemia, as metabolic or respiratory compensation can occur.

Respiratory and metabolic acidaemia

Respiratory acidaemia

CO_2 combines with water to form carbonic acid, and hence ↑ arterial CO_2 tension ($PaCO_2$) leads to a more acid environment and a ↓ pH. For example, patients with acute ventilatory failure develop ↑ $PaCO_2$ (>6.0kPa) 2° to insufficient alveolar gas exchange, and hence a respiratory acidaemia ensues. Renal compensation, via the ↑ renal retention and secretion of HCO_2 and ↑ renal excretion of H^+, takes time.

Normal values
- pH = 7.35–7.45.
- H^+ = 35–45nmol/L.
- $PaCO_2$ = 4.5–6.0kPa.
- HCO_3 = 22–26mmol/L.
- Base excess = −2 to +2mmol/L.

However, it is often notable that patients with chronic hypercapnia have a coexisting raised HCO_2 to maintain homeostasis. Short-term management of respiratory acidaemia relates to treating the underlying cause, e.g. bilevel positive airway pressure (BiPAP) for ventilatory failure 2° to an exacerbation of COPD.

Metabolic acidaemia

A metabolic acidaemia is characterized by a pH <7.35 and HCO_3 <22mmol/L (base excess <−2), and is caused by a gain of acid and/or a loss of base. A number of processes can lead to these results:
- ↑ acid intake, e.g. poisoning with salicylates (aspirin) or ethylene glycol (antifreeze);
- ↑ acid production, e.g. lactic acid 2° to hypoperfusion and ↑ ketones in DKA;
- ↓ acid excretion, e.g. in acute renal failure;
- ↑ base excretion, e.g. diarrhoea and fistulae.

A falling HCO_3 level therefore most commonly reflects the ↑ utilization of HCO_3 in its attempts to neutralize excess acid.

Respiratory compensation may fully or partially counteract a metabolic acidosis. The respiratory centre in the brainstem detects ↑ H^+ and provokes ↑ alveolar ventilation to lower the $PaCO_2$ (e.g. Kussmaul respiration in DKA). This drop in $PaCO_2$ leads to ↓ production of carbonic acid and therefore ↑ pH.

Hypokalaemia

Hypokalaemia (serum K^+ <3.5mmol/L) may occur due to ↓ dietary intake, or ↑ GI and renal losses (e.g. diarrhoea and vomiting, DKA, diuretic use).

Clinical signs

- Skeletal muscle weakness.
- Constipation.
- Paralytic ileus.
- Hypotension and arrhythmias (e.g. SVT and VT).
- ECG: T wave flattening, ST segment depression, and U waves.

Nursing interventions/management

Based on treating the underlying cause of the hypokalaemia:

- full set of vital signs and ECG; commence continuous cardiac monitoring;
- mild cases can be treated with oral supplements;
- IV replacement may be necessary—20mmol/h;
- an accelerated regimen has been proposed by the Resuscitation Council (UK)[1] (e.g. 20mmol over 10min) for life-threatening arrhythmias. Central access is preferable in such circumstances, and full ECG monitoring is required, as well as expert help.

Reference

1 Resuscitation Council UK (2010). *Advanced life support*, sixth edition. Resuscitation Council, London.

Hyperkalaemia

Hyperkalaemia (serum K^+ >5.5mmol/L) may occur due to renal failure, cell injury (e.g. rhabdomyolysis and burns), and endocrine diseases such as hypoadrenalism and DKA. Hyperkalaemia can ensue due to the body's attempt to correct an ion imbalance. Thus, one should always consider acidosis as a 1° cause before attempting to treat the hyperkalaemia.

Features

- Muscle weakness.
- Abdominal cramps.
- Paraesthesiae.
- Hypotension and arrhythmias (e.g. heart block, VT).
- ECG may show changes such as peaked, tented T waves, prolonged PR intervals, and widened QRS complexes.

Nursing interventions/management

- Full set of vital signs, and commence continuous cardiac monitoring.
- In severe cases (K^+ >6.5mmol/L and ECG changes), administer 10mL of 10% calcium gluconate IV over 5min, as prescribed, to give immediate cardioprotection.
- Administer by salbutamol 5mg nebulizer (may be repeated). This shifts K^+ into cells.
- Correction of metabolic acidaemia with 50mL of 8.4% sodium bicarbonate IV over 5min.
- Ten units of soluble insulin in 50mL of 50% glucose IV over ~15–30min shifts K^+ into cells.
- Polystyrene sulfonate resins (e.g. Calcium Resonium®) can also be either rectally or orally administered to promote GI excretion.
- Diuretics (e.g. furosemide) can be administered to ↑ renal excretion of K^+.
- The underlying cause should be sought and treated, e.g hydrocortisone for an Addisonian crisis; dialysis for renal failure.

Hyponatraemia

Hyponatraemia (serum Na^+ <135mmol/L) is often associated with a low osmotic pressure. Caution is therefore required to avoid overly vigorous Na^+ correction, as the rapid intravascular rise in osmotic pressure can lead to rapid fluid shifts from tissues, especially the brain (pontine demyelination). Rates of correction of 0.5mmol/L/h may be appropriate.

Features of hyponatraemia

- Nausea, vomiting.
- Headache.
- Fatigue.
- Seizures and coma.

Causes of hyponatraemia

- Too little Na^+ intake (depletional hyponatraemia).
- Too much water (dilutional hyponatraemia), e.g. $2°$ to fluid overload, syndrome of inappropriate antidiuretic hormone (SIADH), nephrotic syndrome.
  - If symptomatic, diuretics, such as furosemide, can be used, and hypertonic saline (e.g. 1.8% sodium chloride) can be given in judicious aliquots to replace urinary Na^+ losses.
  - Fluid restriction can be utilized in asymptomatic patients.
- Loss of both Na^+ and water (but $Na^+ >$ water), e.g. diarrhoea and vomiting, overdiuresis.

Management

- If symptomatic, emergency treatment includes the judicious use of hypertonic 1.8% sodium chloride.
- Asymptomatic patients can receive 0.9% sodium chloride to gradually raise Na^+ levels.

Hypernatraemia

Hypernatraemia (serum Na$^+$ >145mmol/L) is often associated with a high osmotic pressure. Caution is therefore required to avoid an overly vigorous reduction in Na$^+$ levels, as the rapid reduction in intravascular osmotic pressure can lead to rapid shifts of fluid into the tissues, especially the brain (cerebral oedema).

Features of hypernatraemia

- Thirst.
- Lethargy.
- Seizures and coma.

Causes of hypernatraemia

- Too much Na$^+$, e.g. excess IV sodium chloride.
- Cushing's and Conn's syndromes.
- Too little water, e.g. diabetes insipidus.

Management

- If hypovolaemic, emergency management consists of fluid resuscitation with either colloid or 5% glucose. Thiazide diuretics can be utilized in conjunction with these fluids to promote renal Na$^+$ excretion.
- Loss of both Na$^+$ and water (but water > Na$^+$), e.g. consider judicious use of 0.9% sodium chloride, or 0.45% sodium chloride in severe cases (both Na$^+$ and water need to be replaced, but water is proportionately more necessary).

Anion gap

When aiming to determine which metabolic process is responsible for a metabolic acidaemia, the calculation of the anion gap can prove valuable.

Anion gap = plasma $(Na^+ + K^+) - (HCO_3^- + Cl^-)$

Normal range = 8–16mmol/L.

To maintain electroneutrality, cations (positive ions such as Na^+ and K^+) and anions (negative ions such as HCO_3^- and Cl^-) need to balance. The differential which therefore exists when calculating the anion gap represents those anions not routinely measured in the laboratory, e.g. phosphates, lactic acid, and ketones. A widening anion gap suggests ↑ numbers of these anions and is especially associated with ↑ acid ingestion or production, or ↓ acid excretion, as represented in the following mnemonic.

A MUDPILE CAT
- Alcohol.
- Methanol.
- Uraemia.
- DKA.
- Paraldehyde.
- Iron/isoniazid.
- Lactic acidosis.
- Ethylene glycol.
- Carbamazepine.
- Aspirin.
- Toluene.

Respiratory and metabolic alkalaemia

Respiratory alkalaemia

A respiratory alkalaemia is characterized by a pH >7.45 and ↓ $PaCO_2$ (<4.5kPa) 2° to hyperventilation (which leads to a corresponding reduction in carbonic acid production). Causes of hyperventilation leading to alkalaemia include:

- anxiety;
- pain;
- drugs such as the early stages of salicylate poisoning;
- hypermetabolic states, e.g. fever;
- hypoxia, e.g. PE or anaemia.

The cause of hyperventilation needs to be sought, and treatment initiated, e.g. rebreathing exhaled CO_2 in cases of anxiety (via a paper bag) or O_2 therapy if hypoxic.

Metabolic compensation for respiratory alkalaemia occurs via the kidneys, as both HCO_3 excretion and H^+ secretion ↑. This process, however, takes time. Hence, it may take a couple of days for full compensation to be achieved.

⚠ Never dismiss hyperventilation as hysterical—you may miss a serious underlying pathology.

Metabolic alkalaemia

A metabolic alkalaemia is characterized by a pH >7.45 and a raised plasma HCO_3 (>26mmol/L, base excess >2mmol/L), and is caused by a loss of H^+ (acid) and/or a gain in HCO_3.

The underlying cause needs to be sought and treated, e.g. fluid and electrolyte replenishment. Respiratory compensation may also be noted. Hypoventilation leads to ↑ $PaCO_2$ and, as a result, ↑ carbonic acid levels. Such compensation, however, is limited by hypoxia, which ultimately restimulates ventilation.

Hypoadrenal crisis

Pathophysiology

1° hypoadrenalism (Addison's disease) is most commonly caused by auto-immune processes that lead to the destruction of the adrenal cortex. These patients therefore require long-term steroid replacement therapy (e.g. hydrocortisone, which has both a glucocorticoid and mineralocorticoid effect). A hypoadrenal ('Addisonian') crisis may therefore ensue if there is either a sudden withdrawal of steroid therapy or if there is an insufficient ↑ of steroid therapy at times of physiological stress (e.g. infection, trauma, MI).

In contrast, patients develop 2° hypoadrenalism when the whole hypothalamus–pituitary–adrenal axis is suppressed, most commonly due to long-term steroid use for non-endocrine disease, e.g. COPD, or to avoid transplant rejection. These patients are also prone to a hypoadrenal crisis if steroid therapy is suddenly curtailed (hence the necessity for weaning such patients off steroid medication).

Clinical features

- Glucocorticoid deficiency can lead to weakness, vomiting, hypoglycaemia, weight loss, abdominal pain, and coma.
- Mineralocorticoid deficiency can lead to dehydration, hyponatraemia, hyperkalaemia, postural hypotension, and hypovolaemic shock.

Diagnosis

These patients are treated on clinical suspicion, as formal diagnosis is based upon plasma cortisol and adrenocorticotrophic hormone (ACTH) levels, and Synacthen® tests.

Nursing interventions/management

- Ensure airway patency and oxygenation. Full set of vital signs and ECG.
- Fluid replacement. If shocked, consider colloid; otherwise utilize 0.9% sodium chloride.
- Give hydrocortisone 100mg IV stat, as prescribed.
- Manage hypoglycaemia and hyperkalaemia.
- Seek and treat any underlying co-morbidity, e.g. infection, MI.

Thyrotoxic crisis

Pathophysiology

This is a rare condition, sometimes known as a thyroid storm. Patients tend to have pre-existing hyperthyroidism, most notably 'Graves' disease' (thyroid-stimulating autoantibodies lead to ↑ levels of triiodothyronine (T_3) and thyroxine (T_4)). The crisis itself is usually precipitated by ↑ physiological stress, including infection, trauma, surgery, and diabetic emergencies. However, cessation of anti-thyroid therapy and thyroxine overdose can also provoke a crisis.

Clinical features

Features include:
- hyperpyrexia;
- tachycardia and arrhythmias (especially AF);
- cardiac failure;
- irritability, agitation, confusion, and coma.

Deterioration can be rapid. Mortality is ~10%.

Diagnosis

The diagnosis is confirmed by standard thyroid function tests (TFTs) (i.e. T_3, T_4, and thyroid-stimulating hormone (TSH)). Treatment, however, should not be delayed, whilst awaiting formal test results. Hence, the clinical history (especially a history of existing hyperthyroidism) and signs/symptoms should initially guide management.

The following investigations can aid diagnosis:
- ECG (for identification of arrhythmias);
- CXR (for identification of heart failure or chest infection);
- U&E, FBC, blood cultures, glucose, and urinalysis.

Nursing interventions/management

These patients may be very agitated and frightened, and need a competent reassuring response.
- Ensure airway patency and oxygenation.
- Full set of vital signs:
  - CBG;
  - ECG, once more settled.
- Commence continuous cardiac monitoring.
- IV access and gradual fluid replacement (initially with 0.9% sodium chloride).
- Maintain strict fluid balance.
- Routine bloods, including TFTs.
- Acute agitation can be treated with titrated IV or oral benzodiazepines.
- Consider antipyretics for hyperpyrexia, but avoid aspirin, as it ↑ circulating thyroxine levels.
- Give corticosteroids (e.g. hydrocortisone 100mg IV), as prescribed. These suppress many of the features of hyperthyroidism.
- Give other medications, as prescribed (potassium iodide and carbimazole are used to inhibit T_4 synthesis).
- Be aware of possible underlying co-morbidity, e.g. infection, DKA.

Myxoedema (hypothyroid) coma

Pathophysiology

This is a rare condition, associated with profound hypothyroidism. Precipitating factors include infection, surgery, MI, stroke, and cold weather. The elderly are predominantly affected, especially in the context of pre-existing hypothyroidism.

Clinical features

The usual clinical features associated with hypothyroidism are profoundly exacerbated. These include:

- hypoventilation;
- bradycardia and cardiac failure;
- confusion and coma;
- metabolic and respiratory acidaemia;
- hypothermia.

Diagnosis

TFTs lead to a definitive diagnosis, but management should initially be based upon clinical suspicion 2° to history and examination.

Nursing interventions

- ICU involvement may be necessary from the outset.
- Ensure airway patency and oxygenation.
- Full set of vital signs, CBG, ECG.
- Ensure continuous cardiac monitoring.
- Establish IV access, and collect routine bloods, including TFTs, CRP, and blood cultures if pyrexial.
- Observe for hypotension, cardiac failure, bradycardia, and seizures.
- Use a warming blanket to gradually rewarm the patient.
- Give low-dose T_4 replacement, as prescribed.
- Give corticosteroids (e.g. hydrocortisone 100mg IV), as prescribed. These may be necessary, as coexisting hypoadrenal crisis may be masked by myxoedema.
- Ensure the patient has one-to-one continuous nursing, as these patients are highly dependent and very unwell.

Heat illness

Pathophysiology

The hypothalamus regulates the temperature to ensure homeostasis, utilizing mechanisms, such as sweating and vasodilatation, to achieve temperature control. At times, however, these homeostatic processes are inadequate to ensure thermoregulation, especially when ambient temperatures and humidity rise, prolonged activity is undertaken (e.g. intense physical exertion), and fluid and electrolyte intake does not match losses. Children and the elderly are particularly at risk of heat illness, but other risk factors include coexistent alcohol use, cardiac disease, and recreational drugs such as ecstasy and cocaine. More recently, marathon runners have been brought to the ED suffering from heat illness.

- Heat cramps and heat exhaustion signify mild to moderate heat illness (temperature <40.5°C). Cramps occur 2° to electrolyte deficiencies following hypotonic fluid replacement, whilst exhaustion occurs 2° to both water and electrolyte losses. Both forms of presentation are eminently treatable.
- Heat stroke, however, signifies severe heat illness (core temperature >40.5°C). The physiological response to the ↑ body temperature is completely overwhelmed, and, as a result, there is a derangement in fluid and electrolyte balance, as well as multiorgan damage, e.g. cerebral oedema, renal failure, and coagulopathies. The overall mortality rate approaches 10% but is higher in the elderly population.

Clinical features of heat cramp/exhaustion

- Core temperature <40.5°C.
- Muscle cramps.
- Fatigue.
- Headache.
- Nausea and vomiting.
- Collapse (often 2° to postural hypotension).

Clinical features of heat stroke

- Core temperature >40.5°C.
- Circulation: hypotension, tachycardia, arrhythmias, and signs of DIC such as petechial and purpuric rashes.
- Neurological: confusion, seizures, and coma.
- Metabolic: acidaemia, hypoglycaemia, and signs of jaundice.
- Renal: features of rhabdomyolysis, such as haematuria and myoglobinuria, may be present.

Diagnosis

Diagnosis is based upon the accurate measurement of temperature (e.g. rectal), in conjunction with underlying signs and symptoms.

⚠ If the patient's clinical condition is more severe than would be expected for a given temperature, remember that cooling may have occurred in transit to the ED. Failure to take this into account may lead to a significant under-appreciation of the multiorgan damage that has already ensued, with a corresponding delay in initiating emergency treatment.

Nursing interventions/management

Heat cramp/exhaustion

Simple cooling techniques (e.g. removing clothing, cooling ambient temperature), in conjunction with oral rehydration/electrolyte solutions, are usually sufficient. IV fluid replacement may be required if signs/symptoms are more significant.

Heat stroke

- Ensure airway patency, and administer high-flow O_2. Seek ICU assistance, as appropriate:
  - full set of vital signs;
  - CBG;
  - ECG.
- IV fluids (e.g. 0.9% sodium chloride) should be commenced, but judicious fluid replacement is required to avoid precipitating cerebral/pulmonary oedema. Invasive monitoring may be required to assist with clinical decision-making.
- Urinary catheter, and strict fluid balance initiated.
- Collect blood for FBC, U&E, coagulation, CK, and glucose.
- Request CXR.
- Seizures should be managed with benzodiazepines first-line.
- Cooling. All clothing should be removed, and a cooling rate of 0.1°C/min should be aimed for. This is best achieved with evaporative cooling, e.g. cool water is sprayed onto the patient, and fans are utilized to blow air over the patient. In addition, ice packs over areas, such as the groin, axillae, and neck, can directly cool circulating blood, but caution is required to avoid direct thermal injury to the skin. In the face of refractory hyperthermia, more aggressive management may be required such as gastric, peritoneal, pleural, and/or bladder lavage with cold water or cardiopulmonary bypass if available.
- Antipyretics, such as paracetamol, are not indicated, as the pathophysiological processes of fever and heat illness differ.
- Adjuncts to the resuscitation process should include a urinary catheter, so that an accurate fluid balance can be determined.

Frostbite

Pathophysiology

Frostbite occurs when tissue temperatures fall below 0°C. This leads to extracellular ice crystal formation which directly results in cell membrane damage, but also leads to an ↑ in osmotic pressure. This can ultimately lead to cell dehydration and death. In tandem, peripheral vasoconstriction ↓ blood flow and encourages the development of microthrombi—this leads to tissue ischaemia, and ultimately tissue necrosis. As with any ischaemia, a penumbral region surrounds the necrotic core, and this can be potentially salvageable. Treatment is therefore directed at limiting further damage to this area and restoring perfusion.

Clinical features

- Symptoms usually relate to the severity of the exposure. Paraesthesiae and anaesthesia are the commonest presenting features,
- Initial sensory deficits, such as in light touch and pain, are replaced by complete sensory loss, as ischaemia and neuropraxia progress.
- Distal extremities are most at risk, including toes, fingers, ears, nose, and penis. Tissues may initially appear mottled or white.
- Rewarming is associated with the development of reperfusion erythema, even in the most severe cases, as well as the development of an aching, throbbing pain that may last for a significant period (even months).
- Rewarming may also lead to blister and oedema formation. Their presence is often a better prognostic indicator in severe cases than their absence.
- In the most severe cases, black necrotic tissue develops, reflecting irreversible ischaemic damage.

Diagnosis

There is often a poor correlation between the initial presentation and the eventual outcome. For this reason, the extent of the cold injury is often based upon retrospective analysis:

- superficial frostbite = no eventual tissue loss;
- deep frostbite = tissue loss.

In the initial management phase, however, diagnosis is based upon a sound assessment of the patient. This includes a thorough history, especially the time of exposure, and a thorough clinical examination, including an assessment of sensation, colour, function, and the development of erythema and blisters on rewarming.

More long-term diagnostic and prognostic perspectives can be gained from comparison X-rays, angiography, and MRI. In severe cases, the final assessment and demarcation of viable from non-viable tissue can take up to 3 months to determine. For this reason, there is often a corresponding delay prior to any surgical intervention.

Intervention/management

- If rewarming can be successfully undertaken prehospital, then it should be attempted.
- Immersion of the injured body part in water at 40–42°C leads to rapid rewarming, which has been shown to be more efficacious than gradual rewarming.
- Friction massage should be avoided, as it worsens tissue damage.

Emergency department

- Treat concurrent hypothermia if present.
- Immerse the affected body part in water maintained at 40–42°C until distal erythema is noted (may take up to 30min).
- Subsequently, dry the injured area, and elevate, where possible, to limit post-thaw oedema.
- Any open wounds should be dressed appropriately.
- The vast majority of patients will require hospital admission. Therefore, refer to the appropriate specialty (perhaps orthopaedics or specialist plastics/burns unit, where available).
- Ongoing monitoring will be required to determine the extent of the injury and for the management of complications, e.g. compartment syndrome and infections.

Hypothermia

Pathophysiology

The term hypothermia relates to a core body temperature <35°C. The following classification is often used in practice:

- mild hypothermia—temperature 32–35°C;
- moderate hypothermia—temperature 30–32°C;
- severe hypothermia—temperature <30°C.

Hypothermia most commonly occurs 2° to environmental exposure to cold conditions (such as poorly heated housing in winter, exposure to wet and windy conditions when undertaking outdoor pursuits, or cold water immersion). Added risk factors include immobility (e.g. following injury, ↓ level of consciousness 2° to alcohol or drug use, and comorbidity in the elderly) and thermoregulatory/metabolic impairment (e.g. infants, the elderly, and those with hypothyroidism). The elderly are at further risk in the presence of cognitive impairment, such as dementia, leading to ↓ cold awareness.

As the body cools, both brain and cardiovascular function begins to fail—essentially the body begins to 'shut down'. Paradoxically, this can provide some protection to both the brain and other vital organs in the face of profound hypothermic insult. The ultimate sequelae, however, are complete cardiovascular collapse and death, often 2° to arrhythmias.

Clinical features

- Hypotension and arrhythmias.
- Sinus bradycardia is followed by AF, VF, and asystole sequentially.
- Respiratory depression.
- Lethargy, confusion, and coma.

Diagnosis

A low reading rectal thermometer is required to confirm diagnosis. In cases of profound hypothermia, signs of life should be sought for up to a minute before declaring cardiac arrest, e.g. via palpation of the carotid artery in conjunction with ECG trace and signs of breathing. The pulse may be very slow, irregular, and small in volume.

Management

Patients with cardiac output

Patients with profound hypothermia should be handled carefully, as undue movement can precipitate arrhythmias and cardiac arrest.

- A. Ensure airway patency and ICU involvement, as required.
- B. Warmed, humidified O_2 should be utilized, where available.
- C. Ensure ECG monitoring and IV access. Warmed fluids should be given if the patient is hypotensive, but caution is required to avoid precipitating pulmonary oedema.
- D. Hypoglycaemia should be sought for and corrected, where necessary.
- E. Wet clothing should be removed, and the skin dried.

- Passive rewarming is appropriate for mild/moderate hypothermia and includes a warm clinical environment, blankets, bonnets for the head, and the use of warm air delivery systems, such as the Bair Hugger™, where available.
- As a general rule, patients who have cooled slowly need to be warmed slowly, especially if elderly. In such cases, 0.5°C/h is probably appropriate and helps to limit the development of cerebral/pulmonary oedema.
- Active rewarming is required in cases of severe hypothermia or cardiac arrest. Warmed fluids (40–45°C) can be instilled into the bladder, stomach, and peritoneal and pleural cavities. The fluid is left *in situ* for 10–20min, and then replaced to ensure that warming is optimized.
- Cardiopulmonary bypass, however, is the mode of choice, where available, and can lead to very rapid rewarming.
- Adjuncts should include blood investigations, ABG, CXR, and NG tube and urinary catheter, as required.
- An ECG should be obtained, both to seek arrhythmias and also to determine whether J waves are seen at the junction of the QRS complex and ST segment. These waves may appear at temperatures <32°C.

Patients in cardiac arrest

Once cardiac arrest has been diagnosed in a hypothermic patient, the following factors should be considered, in conjunction with the standard approach to resuscitation.

- Warmed, humidified O_2 and active rewarming techniques should be used.
- IV drugs should be withheld until the temperature is >30°C, and subsequently time intervals between doses should be doubled until the temperature is >35°C, in order to reflect slower drug metabolism associated with hypothermia, and hence the ↑ potential for toxic drug dosages.
- VF/pulseless VT should be treated initially with defibrillation. If three shocks have not been effective, and the temperature is <30°C, further attempts should be withheld until the temperature is >30°C.
- Prolonged resuscitation may be necessary. Death should not be confirmed until either the patient has been rewarmed (e.g. >32°C) or attempts to raise the core body temperature have failed.
- If resuscitation has been successful, aim to maintain the patient's temperature at 32–34°C.

Drowning

Pathophysiology

Drowning incidents involve respiratory impairment 2° to submersion or immersion in a liquid. This liquid, normally water, prevents the victim from breathing air. ∴ The ultimate sequela of drowning incidents is death 2° to suffocation. Almost half of deaths involve children <4y old.

Specific patterns of drowning have been noted.

- 'Wet drowning'. Fluid is aspirated into the lungs, leading to pulmonary damage such as alveolar–capillary membrane dysfunction and surfactant loss. Survivors often develop ARDS 2° to such damage, which has been termed 'secondary drowning'.
- 'Dry drowning'. Post-mortem studies have revealed that ~10–20% of drowning deaths are 2° to intense laryngospasm following a small amount of water entering the larynx. Minimal lung aspiration is therefore found.

Hypothermia may occur concurrently with a drowning incident, and this may offer some protection to vital organs, especially if the hypothermia develops rapidly, e.g. submersion in water <5°C. In addition, young children can gain neurological protection after prolonged immersion (even >60min) 2° to the diving reflex, especially in combination with hypothermia. Cold water and hypoxia lead to a reflex bradycardia and peripheral vasoconstriction, with subsequent redistribution of blood to the brain and heart.

There is no evidence that drowning in either fresh or salt water alters initial presentation or management. However, there is evidence that prolonged immersion in water leads to a 'hydrostatic squeeze' on the body. On removal from water, this pressure is alleviated, intravascular pressures drop, and hypotension and cardiovascular collapse ensue. Removing such patients from the water in a horizontal position, rather than a vertical position, helps to lessen such cardiovascular consequences.

Clinical features

Patients involved in drowning incidents may present with a wide range of signs and symptoms, which may range between cardiac arrest, hypoxic coma, or a normal clinical examination.

Patients presenting with a significant history of a drowning incident should be closely monitored for signs of developing ARDS, e.g. dyspnoea, hypoxia, or pulmonary oedema.

Nursing interventions/management

In the presence of cardiorespiratory arrest, full ALS should be implemented. Consider also concurrent neck injury and hypothermia.

For patients who are spontaneously breathing and with a cardiac output, the following management should be considered.

- A. C-spine injury. Immobilization should be considered, and the patient treated accordingly and the airway maintained. Suction may be required to remove fluid and debris from the upper airway.
- B. High-flow O_2 should be utilized. CPAP may be required if ARDS develops.

- C. IV fluids should be administered if the patient is hypotensive, but caution is required to avoid fluid overload.
- D. Hypoglycaemia should be considered and treated, if necessary.
- E. Wet clothing should be removed, and a core temperature obtained. Rewarm, as indicated.
- Adjuncts include blood investigations, CXR, and ECG.
- An NG tube will assist with gastric decompression if water has been swallowed.
- Antibiotics may be required if the water was contaminated with sewage or other waste.
- Consider also the tetanus status if there are cuts or abrasions to the skin.

Outcome depends upon a number of factors. Patients with a brief submersion/immersion time and who receive prompt medical assistance have the best prognosis. Patients who are asymptomatic in the ED should be closely observed for at least 6h prior to discharge, and only then discharged if ABGs and clinical examination remain normal.

Diving emergencies

Barotrauma

Barotrauma relates to injury to air-containing body systems following changes in atmospheric pressure or, in the case of diving, water pressure.

On descent, the water pressure ↑, and hence air is compressed or 'squeezed'. As a result, the middle ear, in particular, is prone to trauma from these compressive forces, especially if the Eustachian tube is congested, thereby limiting pressure equalization. As a consequence, the tympanic membrane can perforate, with resultant conductive hearing loss and/or the development of a nystagmus and vertigo if cold water reaches into the middle ear itself. In such instances, prophylactic antibiotics are often indicated to avoid otitis media. Similarly, pressure changes in the inner ear can lead to vestibular damage and resultant tinnitus, vertigo, and hearing loss.

Barosinusitis

Leads to pain over ethmoid, frontal, and/or maxillary sinuses. This is commoner in those with polyps, mucosal thickening, or other history of sinus problems.

Facial barotraumas with resultant facial bruising, swelling, and subconjunctival haemorrhage can result if the negative pressure in a diver's face mask is not equalized during a dive by occasional nasal exhalation.

Pulmonary barotrauma

This is typically a complication of ascent, as the volume of air in the lungs will expand as the diver comes to the surface. Exhalation on ascent will usually overcome this issue, but rapid ascent with breath-holding (e.g. in an emergency) or air trapping 2° to asthma or other lung pathology can result in trauma. Pulmonary barotraumas can thus result in the following conditions.

Arterial gas embolism

Complications include cardiac ischaemia, arrhythmias, and stroke, as oxygenated blood is mechanically obstructed by the air and therefore does not reach the tissues. Arterial gas embolism (AGE) should be suspected in any patient who develops neurological, cardiac, or breathing symptoms on, or shortly following, ascent (typically <10min). Management centres upon hyperbaric treatment.

Pneumomediastinum and subcutaneous emphysema

Air from alveolar rupture travels into the neck, mediastinum, and/or pericardium. Features include:

- hoarse voice;
- retrosternal chest pain;
- crepitus may be felt SC at the neck.

High-flow O_2 is usually sufficient to deal with this clinical situation.

Pneumothorax
Air from alveolar rupture can pass into the pleural cavity. Further air volume expansion on ascent can lead to a tension pneumothorax. Standard treatment is advocated.

Alveolar haemorrhage
Haemoptysis 2° to alveolar rupture may occur independently or in conjunction with the other conditions listed here.

Decompression sickness

Diving at depth leads to an accumulation of dissolved nitrogen in tissues and blood. On ascent, this dissolved nitrogen comes out of solution and begins to form small nitrogen bubbles. In a controlled dive, these bubbles are transported to the lungs and exhaled before significant problems ensue. Decompression sickness (DCS), however, arises when nitrogen comes out of solution faster than it can be excreted, and hence larger bubbles form in the tissues and blood. These can lead to ischaemia and tissue hypoxia.

- Type I DCS affects the musculoskeletal system and skin, and produces classic aching joints associated with 'the bends', especially in the shoulders and elbows. This pain is aggravated by movement.
- Type II DCS involves other organs and tends to be more serious. In such cases, signs and symptoms can be very similar to those of AGE, and it can be very difficult to differentiate between the two pathological processes. Typically, however, DCS develops >10min following ascent. Management is with hyperbaric treatment.

Risk factors for the development of DCS include ↑ duration and depth of dive, rapid ascent, frequent dives without full excretion of nitrogen between dives, obesity, heavy exertion on a dive, and air travel soon after diving. In addition, if one diver develops DCS, it is advisable to fully assess any fellow diver who may have been with them as a 'buddy'.

Hyperbaric treatment

Hyperbaric therapy is the only definitive treatment for both DCS and AGE. Speed is of the essence—recompression within 5min of surfacing for patients with AGE carries a mortality rate of 5%, whereas recompression delayed to 5h or more carries a mortality rate of 10%. Hyperbaric treatment relieves mechanical obstruction by reducing the size of air or nitrogen bubble volume, ↑ nitrogen excretion, and ↑ O_2 delivery to the tissues. The pressure and duration of recompression are calculated using predetermined charts.

Nursing interventions

Whilst waiting for hyperbaric treatment to commence, 100% O_2 should be administered. This speeds the excretion of nitrogen.

- Entonox® should *never* be used.
- Intubated patients need to have the ETT cuff inflated with water, and not air—otherwise the cuff will deflate on recompression.
- Ground transportation is preferable to air transportation for patients requiring hyperbaric treatment, as altitude ↑ gas bubble size.

Altitude-related illness

Those at risk of developing altitude-related illnesses are people who do not normally live at altitude, but who have recently ascended to mountainous areas without gradual acclimatization (especially over 3000m). At high altitude, the atmospheric partial pressure of O_2 is lower. As a result, people arriving at high altitude become hypoxic, with a ↓ partial pressure of O_2 in arterial blood (PaO_2). This causes a hypoxic ventilatory response (HVR). The HVR for any individual can vary, depending upon a number of factors such as genetics, co-morbidity, and even alcohol and caffeine intake. Patients most at risk of developing altitude illness have a poor HVR, resulting in hypoxaemia, and this, in turn, can lead to acute mountain sickness (AMS), high-altitude cerebral oedema (HACO), and high-altitude pulmonary oedema (HAPO).

Acute mountain sickness and high-altitude cerebral oedema

Hypoxaemia can result in ↑ cerebral blood flow and volume and ↑ vascular permeability, leading to the development of cerebral oedema. Patients with AMS may have early signs of rising ICP and present with headache, nausea, vomiting, and fatigue.

- AMS often develops within a few hours, is fairly common, and begins to resolve in most cases within a few days, as acclimatization ensues. Management involves halting any further ascent. More severe cases can be treated with O_2, simple analgesics (not opiates, as these can further depress the HVR), and acetazolamide (which speeds the acclimatization process).
- The most severe form of AMS is HACO, which reflects a significant rise in ICP. Cerebellar ataxia may be an early indicator, followed by seizures, focal deficits, and coma. Management involves immediate descent, where possible, O_2, dexamethasone, diuretics (e.g. mannitol), and hyperbaric therapy.

High-altitude pulmonary oedema

Hypoxaemia can also lead to pulmonary artery hypertension and ↑ vascular permeability in the lungs, with resultant pulmonary oedema. Features include dyspnoea at rest, cough, and haemoptysis in severe cases.

▶▶ Early recognition is vital, as death can rapidly ensue. Management involves immediate descent, where possible, O_2 (with CPAP, if available), diuretics, and hyperbaric therapy in severe cases.

Haematological emergencies

Overview

Patients with haematological disease may be immunocompromised, due to their condition or the treatment prescribed for their condition. These patients are usually treated in outpatient clinics or have chemotherapy as day cases, and are often advised to attend their local ED if they develop new symptoms. Patients may be neutropenic as a result of treatment, and thus be vulnerable to infection. It is not uncommon for patients with haematological disease to present in the ED with life-threatening complications of their disease. In addition to recognizing shock (⊋ see Shock, pp. 278–9), it is also important for the nurse to understand haemostatic mechanisms.

Haemostasis

This is the process of clot formation in the walls of damaged blood vessels to prevent blood loss, whilst, at the same time, maintaining blood in a fluid state within the vascular system. Blood disorders occur when there is an imbalance in haemostasis.

- If blood becomes too thin, it loses the ability to form the blood clots that stop bleeding.
- If blood becomes too thick, the risk of blood clots developing within the blood vessels ↑, creating a potentially life-threatening condition such as DIC.

Abnormalities of haemostasis

People with bleeding disorders bleed easily and may lose excessive amounts of blood as a result of injuries, surgery, or dental surgery. Severe bleeding disorders may even cause spontaneous bleeding without any injury. Injury to a blood vessel initiates a series of events that result in the formation of a clot (haemostasis). The ability of the blood to clot is a vital part of the body's natural defence. This process of forming a clot is referred to as coagulation. Further chemical interactions are required to dissolve the blood clot, as the body heals.

A shift in haemostasis can result in coagulation that is either too slow or too fast. Blood disorders result from imbalances in haemostasis. Haemostatic disorders can be acquired or inherited. Acquired disorders are by far the commonest, particularly thrombocytopenia. Bleeding is to be expected where there has been blunt or penetrating trauma, but a clotting disorder should be considered if bleeding is excessive and not responding to conventional pressure, or if it is evident from uninjured sites.

Von Willebrand's disease

- Von Willebrand's disease is the commonest bleeding disorder.
- It affects up to 1% of the population and occurs in both sexes.
- Symptoms of Von Willebrand's disease are usually mild, and many people may not even be aware that they have a clotting deficiency.
  - People with Von Willebrand's disease bruise easily and may suffer from frequent nosebleeds.
  - Women with Von Willebrand's disease may have heavy periods.
- Treatment is usually with factor VIII concentrate.
- Factor VIII is often given prior to operative procedures, tooth extraction, etc., in order to prevent excess haemorrhage.
- TXA has also been used to ensure haemostasis and should be given if haemorrhage is not controlled.

Haemophilia

Haemophilia, which is perhaps the best known of the bleeding disorders, is a genetic disease caused by mutations of genes on the X chromosome.
- Because the mutated gene is recessive, the majority of haemophiliacs are ♂.
- Patients with haemophilia A may present with haematuria or bleeding into large joints.
- Intracranial bleeding is a major cause of death in this patient group.

Disseminated intravascular coagulation

DIC is a syndrome of widespread intravascular coagulation. It may be a serious complication of septicaemia (➲ see Shock, pp. 278–9), extensive tissue injury, or other diseases, in which fibrin is deposited in the vascular system and many small and medium-sized vessels are thrombosed. The ↑ consumption of platelets causes bleeding to occur at the same time. The overall picture is one of widespread tissue ischaemia due to clot formation, and bleeding due to consumption of clotting factors and platelets.

Causes of disseminated intravascular coagulation

These include the following:

- infection (especially Gram-negative infection);
- vascular causes (e.g. aortic aneurysm);
- trauma, especially burns and head injuries;
- obstetric causes (e.g. placental abruption, severe pre-eclampsia, intrauterine death);
- malignancy (e.g. carcinoma of the prostate, ovary, lung, or pancreas);
- other causes (e.g. drug reactions, incompatible blood transfusions);
- massive blood transfusion (➲ see Blood transfusion, pp. 666–7).

Signs of disseminated intravascular coagulation

The signs of DIC are complex.

- Clotting problems include:
  - VTE;
  - skin necrosis or gangrene;
  - coma due to cerebral infarction;
  - multiorgan failure.
- Bleeding problems include:
  - spontaneous bruising;
  - bleeding from venepuncture sites;
  - bleeding from the GI system;
  - post-operative bleeding.

Nursing assessment and interventions for patients with bleeding disorders

- Initial assessment of the patient should be guided by the principles of ABC, remembering that any traumatic bleeding into the neck or pharynx may rapidly compromise breathing.
- Obtain a brief medical history, whilst you are assessing the patient. Consider:
  - allergies;
  - medication (both prescribed and over-the-counter);
  - herbal remedies and supplements.
- Undress the patient, and record their temperature, remembering that hypothermia aggravates any bleeding disorder, whereas a raised temperature may indicate sepsis.
- Obtain a pain score.
- Record RR and O_2 saturation, and give high-flow O_2.
- Record and monitor BP and pulse. Tachycardia and hypotension are indicative of shock.
- Attach the patient to a cardiac monitor if they are complaining of chest pain. Obtain a 12-lead ECG.
- Record blood sugar levels.
- Record neurological vital signs, and consider intracranial haemorrhage in any patient with a headache or an altered level of consciousness.
- Obtain a urine sample, and test for haematuria.
- IV access needs to be established, but this should be done by a clinician skilled in this procedure, in order to avoid further bleeding.
- Central line insertion should only be considered *in extremis*, as uncontrollable haemorrhage may occur.
- The use of IM injections should be avoided.
- TXA may be the drug of choice if haemorrhage is not controlled.
- Blood samples should be collected for FBC, group and save, and cross-matching.
- Before giving any drug, check whether it may aggravate the condition or interfere with any other medication the patient is taking.
- Ensure the patient's comfort and privacy, and give emotional support to their family.

▶▶ If the patient is known to have a bleeding disorder and presents with haemorrhage or a history of trauma, summon senior help.

Sickle-cell disease

Sickle-cell disease occurs in people of Afro-Caribbean, Middle Eastern, and, in some cases, Mediterranean origin. It is an inherited disorder of Hb synthesis. The resulting abnormality produces a normocytic haemolytic anaemia with multiple diversely shaped RBCs that are susceptible to morphological transformation into a sickle shape. The sickle cells cause thrombosis and obstruction in small vessels, leading to ischaemia and necrosis of distal tissue, which results in severe pain. Patients with sickle-cell anaemia have chronic anaemia (Hb concentration in the range of 8–10g/dL) and are particularly prone to infection.

Sickle-cell crisis may occur for no apparent reason or as a result of infection or dehydration. The crisis may involve thrombosis, haemolysis, marrow aplasia, or acute splenic or liver sequestration. Cerebral sickling may present with strange behaviour, confusion, or fits. Because of these different processes, patients may complain of severe pain anywhere in the body, with some symptoms resembling acute medical or surgical emergencies. They may also present with jaundice or priapism.

- Joint pain—osteomyelitis and septic arthritis occur more frequently in sickle-cell disease.
- Acute chest syndrome presents as chest pain, hypoxia, tachypnoea, and wheezing. This may be severe and is a leading cause of death in patients with sickle-cell disease.
- Acute splenic sequestration—large numbers of RBCs aggregate in the spleen, causing an enlarged spleen, hypovolaemia, and thrombocytopenia. The patient may present in a state of shock. This presentation is commoner in young children.

Nursing assessment and interventions specific to sickle-cell disease

Follow the general assessment approach described in ➲ Nursing assessment and interventions for patients with bleeding disorders, p. 585, bearing in mind that the priorities for these patients are as follows.

- Pain relief—as pain is always severe, it needs to be managed with titrated opiate analgesia.
- O_2.
- IV access if the patient is dehydrated and not drinking.
- IV fluids.
- FBC, coagulation studies, U&E, and CRP.
- Give medication, as prescribed.
- Transfusion should be commenced promptly if the patient has severe acute chest syndrome with hypoxia, has had a CVA, or has priapism.

▶ It is vital to be understanding and to provide emotional support for patients with sickle-cell disease, who are usually young and disadvantaged because of their condition. It is especially important not to dismiss their pain, which can be unremitting and severe.

Overdose and poisoning

Overview

Acute and chronic poisoning by drugs, chemicals, traditional remedies, plants, and bites of animals (e.g. snakes, insects) is a common presentation in the ED. Poisoning may be accidental or intentional. Accidental poisoning is commoner in children, whereas intentional poisoning is commoner in adolescents and young adults. Poisoning can also affect all the members of a household, workplace, or community, due to multiple exposures from a common source. This may occur through ingestion from a contaminated food or water supply, or through inhalation of toxic gases or sprays.

Poisoning in children

Accidental poisoning is the term used when a child becomes exposed to a poison as a result of natural exploratory behaviour or of imitating adults without knowing the possible consequences. This type of poisoning occurs from the ages of around 6 months to 5y, with a peak between 18 months and 2y. Frequently, this type of ingestion is of minimal toxicity, but the incident causes great concern to the parents.

The other types of poisoning that may occur in small children are iatrogenic and non-accidental.

- Therapeutic poisoning occurs in particular in premature infants and neonates, in whom a small error in dose can cause life-threatening toxicity (especially with drugs such as chloramphenicol, theophylline, and digoxin).
- Non-accidental (i.e. intentional) poisoning may range from a carer's attempt to sedate a child in order to quieten them, to Munchausen's syndrome by proxy.

Poisoning in teenagers and adults

- In teenage children, deliberate self-harm (DSH) and substance misuse are the commonest causes of poisoning.
- In early adulthood, DSH in the form of parasuicidal gestures is common.
- All through adult life, poisoning can occur in industrial settings.
- Serious suicidal attempts become commoner, and are more likely to be successful, in men over 45y of age. There may be underlying factors such as mental or physical illness, alcohol or substance misuse, unemployment, and relationship problems.

History taking

Obtaining a history may be difficult, especially if the patient is drowsy. Note that the information obtained from the patient may be unreliable, so a history from their family or friends may be more accurate.

The diagnosis of poisoning is most often apparent from the history and circumstances, but the nurse may need to consider poisoning if the patient presents with unexplained symptoms, collapse, or coma without any apparent cause. Intentional poisoning of a child or an adult by another person may present with a misleading history and clinical findings that do not fit with a medical illness. The patient who insists that they have been poisoned must be listened to carefully in order to consider whether their suspicions are justified and whether the symptoms are consistent with poisoning. A minority of these individuals may indeed have been poisoned. Others may be suffering from a paranoid delusion of poisoning—in these cases, the alleged source of the poisoning is vague, and the symptoms are ill-defined.

It is common practice to measure salicylate and paracetamol levels when it is known or suspected that these drugs have been ingested. This is especially important in the case of paracetamol, as there may be no symptoms, even in a potentially fatal overdose.

When taking the history, the nurse needs to ask the following questions.

- What drugs or chemicals have been taken? This should include the time and the amount, and whether they were ingested, injected, or inhaled.
- Has the patient vomited since taking the poison?
- What other medications are they taking?
- Does the patient have any known allergies?
- Does the patient have any other medical conditions?
- Is there any previous history of depression, mental illness, or attempted suicide?

Nursing assessment and interventions

The overall aim of the nursing assessment is to identify the cause, maintain the safety of the patient in terms of airway, breathing, and circulation, and minimize the risk of further absorption, whilst providing both physical and emotional supportive measures to the patient who may be very distressed. Further information about drugs ingested can be obtained from TOXBASE® (℅ http://www.toxbase.org). Emergency nurses should be aware of the various antidotes that are kept in their departments.

General assessment and interventions

Airway

- Establish and protect the airway.
- Airway adjuncts or intubation may be necessary.
- Suck out any secretions, and remove dentures if they are causing an obstruction.
- If the patient's gag reflex is reduced or absent, they will require intubation.
  - ▶▶ Call the anaesthetist.
- Once the airway has been secured, high-flow O_2 should be administered.
- Record O_2 saturations. Assess respiratory rate and effectiveness.
  - Respiration may be slowed by opiates, barbiturates, or tricyclic antidepressants.
  - Wheezing may be evident after inhalation of chlorine gas.

Circulation

- Establish venous access using a wide-bore cannula, and collect blood samples for FBC, group and save, U&E, coagulation studies, toxicology screening, and also prescribed medication screening.
- Observe the skin for cyanosis or fresh needle marks.
- Observe any burns or swelling around the nose, mouth, and throat.
- Inspect the nose for FBs, singed nasal hair, or drug remnants.
- Serum glucose levels should be established on arrival in the ED, and corrected if abnormal.
- Attach the patient to a monitor.
- Commence meticulous recordings of BP, HR, RR, and O_2 saturations.
- Record a 12-lead ECG.
  - Tricyclic antidepressants can cause tachycardia, tachyarrhythmias, and hypotension.
  - Cocaine can also cause tachyarrhythmias and even MI.
  - Bradycardia may be caused by organophosphate insecticides or β-blocker medication.
- If the patient is hypotensive, give IV fluids as prescribed.

Neurological monitoring

- Record the GCS score, and make sure that the patient's neurological status is frequently reassessed. Meticulous monitoring and frequent reassessment are crucial in order to detect any further deterioration in the level of consciousness.
  - ▶ Remember that changes in the GCS score may be more significant than the overall score.

- Observe pupil size and reaction.
  - Pinpoint pupils may be caused by narcotics.
  - Dilated pupils may be caused by cocaine, amphetamines, atropine, or tricyclic antidepressants.
- Seizures may be caused by withdrawal from drugs or alcohol, but may also be due to poisoning from overdose. Seizures are dangerous, because they cause hypoxia and acidosis and can lead to cardiac arrest. Drugs that may cause seizures in overdose include mefenamic acid, theophylline, and tricyclic antidepressants.

Specific interventions

- Hypothermia can occur in response to any drug that causes coma, especially barbiturates and phenothiazines. Check the patient's rectal temperature using a low-reading thermometer. Use a warming blanket and warm IV fluids to restore the patient's temperature.
- Hyperthermia may be caused by amphetamines, cocaine, Ecstasy, monoamine oxidase inhibitors (MAOIs), and theophylline. Convulsions or seizures are common.
  - ▶▶ Summon help (➲ see Heat illness, pp. 570–1).
- If the eyes and/or skin have been contaminated by corrosive agents or pesticides, the eyes must be attended to first and washed out continuously with water for 10–15min. The skin should be washed with soap and water, paying particular attention to the thinner areas of the skin (axillae, groins, and face).
- Ingestion of corrosive agents, acids, or alkalis should be treated by immediately giving the patient a few cups of water to drink in order to dilute the substance and so prevent damage to the tissues. However, after 10 or 20min, this action may well be too late and the patient may be unable to swallow.
- The National Poisons Information Service (✆ http://www.toxbase.org) provides detailed information about signs and symptoms, toxication, and management.

Gastric lavage
(➲ See Gastric lavage, pp. 704–6.)

The stomach should only be emptied by gastric lavage on the advice of the poisons unit. If the ingestion occurred <1h previously, activated charcoal may be given as a suspension in water. This is specially prepared charcoal with a large surface area that gives it a high adsorbent capacity. It adsorbs most drugs and poisons in a ratio of about one part poison to ten parts charcoal. The dose is 25–50g for an adult, and 1g/kg body weight for a child. Exceptions include iron, lithium, alcohol, methanol, ethylene glycol, corrosive agents, acids, and alkalis, for which oral antidotes or medication need to be given.

Whole bowel lavage
This is another method of decontaminating the intestine. It involves giving isotonic fluid, using solutions that are normally used to prepare the bowel for X-ray procedures. The adult dose ranges from 500mL/h to 2L/h, given until the effluent is clear. It can be used to clear the gut of sustained-release preparations, iron, lithium, heavy metals, and illicit drug packets.

Ipecacuanha

This has been widely used in the past, but there is no evidence to suggest that it reduces drug absorption. It is now contraindicated, as it may lead to prolonged vomiting, drowsiness, and aspiration pneumonia.

Psychosocial care

Serious overdoses require medical admission. Less serious overdoses are usually managed in the observation ward of the ED. Admitting these patients allows some time for more pastoral care and assessment by the psychiatric team. Every deliberate self-poisoning should be assessed in an objective and sympathetic way to ensure that every effort is being made to help these patients, with the aim of preventing further occurrence.

Poisoning from therapeutic drugs

Paracetamol

Paracetamol is the most readily available analgesic worldwide. It is safe in therapeutic use, but an overdose of >300mg/kg can cause liver failure and sometimes also kidney failure. It is important to note that, during the first few hours, the patient remains conscious, and there may be few or no symptoms, apart from malaise, nausea, and vomiting. More advanced signs, such as jaundice and elevated LFTs, may take 2–3 days to appear. Some patients are at ↑ risk of liver damage such as those taking enzyme-inducing agents (e.g. phenytoin, rifampicin, heavy alcohol users) and those who are malnourished or who have been fasting recently.

The updated treatment nomogram for paracetamol overdose is as follows.

- All patients with a timed plasma paracetamol level on or above a single treatment line joining points of 100mg/L at 4h and 15mg/L at 15h after ingestion should receive acetylcysteine (Parvolex® or generics), based on the new treatment nomogram, regardless of risk factors for hepatotoxicity.
- If there is doubt about the timing of paracetamol ingestion, including cases where ingestion occurred over a period of 1h or more (staggered overdose), acetylcysteine should always be given without delay (the nomogram should not be used).
- Administer the initial dose of acetylcysteine as an infusion over 60min to minimize the risk of common dose-related adverse reactions.
- Hypersensitivity is no longer a contraindication to treatment with acetylcysteine.

Salicylates

Common features of toxicity from aspirin and other salicylates include vomiting, dehydration, tinnitus, deafness, sweating, warm extremities, and hyperventilation. Severe poisoning is likely to cause coma, convulsions, pulmonary oedema, and cardiovascular collapse. If any of these occur, the outcome is likely to be fatal. However, the patient is likely to remain conscious and alert for many hours, even after a large overdose. Repeated measurements of drug levels are needed, as drug concentrations can rise for many hours after ingestion of a large dose.

Tricyclic antidepressants

- Symptoms of overdose include tachycardia, dilated pupils, cardiac arrhythmias and widened QRS complex, hypotension, hot dry skin, and dry mouth.
- Cardiac monitoring should be continued for at least 6h after ingestion.
- Convulsions, respiratory depression, and coma can occur.
- If the patient presents within 1h of ingesting a potentially toxic amount, give activated charcoal.

Selective serotonin reuptake inhibitors

These may cause few or no symptoms, even after large overdoses. However, many patients experience GI upset and drowsiness, whilst some develop tachycardia, muscle stiffness, and hypertension. Convulsions may occur. If the patient presents within 1h of ingesting a potentially toxic amount, give activated charcoal.

Benzodiazepines

These are relatively safe when taken in overdose, although they can cause life-threatening problems, particularly in older people and patients with severe chronic obstructive airways disease.

- Symptoms of overdose range from drowsiness, ataxia, and nystagmus to hypotension, respiratory depression, and coma, particularly if benzodiazepines are taken with alcohol or other CNS depressants.
- The effects of benzodiazepines can be reversed with flumazenil, but it is safer to protect the airway and allow the patient to recover.

Iron tablets

- Early symptoms of iron overdose include nausea, vomiting, abdominal pain, and diarrhoea. The patient's vomit and stools may be grey or black.
- Haematemesis and rectal bleeding may occur. In severe cases, coma and shock may occur.
- Most patients, especially children, will require measurement of serum iron levels, possibly gastric lavage, and desferrioxamine treatment, even if their symptoms have resolved within a few hours.
- AXR may show the location of the tablets.

Cardiac glycosides

Chronic therapeutic toxicity may occur with drugs (e.g. digitoxin, digitalis), or plant material from foxglove (*Digitalis purpurea* or *Digitalis lanata*) or oleander (*Nerium oleander* or *Thevetia peruviana*) may be used in self-poisoning.

- Nausea, vomiting, cardiac arrhythmias, hypotension, and death may result.
- The patient should be given activated charcoal if they are able to swallow, with subsequent close observation of ABCs.
- A plasma K^+ concentration of >5.3mmol/L is an indication of severe poisoning.
- If available (and they should be ordered at once), digoxin-specific (Fab) antibodies should have sufficient cross-reactivity to bind with all of the cardiac glycosides.

Drug misuse

Alcohol

Alcoholic drinks cause the typical signs of intoxication (slurred speech, ataxia, confusion, and aggression). Larger amounts can cause vomiting, coma, and hypoventilation, with the risk of aspiration of vomit. If the patient is unconscious on arrival, assess and manage as described for the comatose patient (➔ see pp. 176–7). This subject is discussed in more detail in the section on alcohol misuse (➔ see Alcohol misuse, pp. 602–4).

Opioids

- Features of opioid poisoning include progressive depression of the CNS, leading to drowsiness, coma, respiratory depression, and ultimately respiratory arrest.
- The patient will usually have pinpoint pupils and a slowed RR.
- There may also be hypotension and tachycardia.

Initial management depends on the patient's level of consciousness.
- If the patient is conscious and presents within 1h of ingesting a potentially toxic amount of an opiate, give activated charcoal.
- If respiration appears to be inadequate, call the anaesthetist.
- In respiratory depression or impaired consciousness, consider prescribing naloxone 0.8–2.0mg IV, and repeating the dose every 2–3min up to a maximum of 10mg (this can be given by IM or SC injection if the IV route is not feasible). Give naloxone as prescribed.

The duration of action of some opioids (e.g. dihydrocodeine, dextropropoxyphene, and methadone) can exceed that of an IV or IM dose of naloxone, and deterioration may occur later, despite initial reversal. Repeated doses or an infusion of naloxone may be required. Naloxone may not reverse the effects of buprenorphine, so improvement may be delayed. Such patients require very close monitoring and frequent reassessment.

Illicit drugs

Illicit drugs are an ↑ problem in every society. Many different substances can be misused, from glue or petrol sniffing to cannabis to 'hard' drugs. The popularity of a particular substance varies with age and social scene.

Heroin

This is responsible for the most serious problems, and poisoning can be caused by an excessive dose in a naive user, as well as by a 'regular' dose in a person who has lost their tolerance. It is important to remember that 10mg of heroin IV could be fatal for a non-user, but the average user who presents to an addiction centre for help is taking 750mg daily. Tolerance starts to be lost within a couple of days of abstinence, and toxicity can then be caused by the user's normal dose. Management of toxicity is described under ➔ Opioids above. In addition to toxicity, abscesses and infectious illnesses are also associated with heroin use.

Cocaine

This causes massive surges in BP due to widespread constriction of blood vessels, and chest pain is the commonest complication requiring medical attention. It usually resolves within a few hours without causing any apparent long-term damage. Every patient with symptoms following cocaine use should be given IV diazepam in relatively large doses, and those with chest pain should be given aspirin, as for any patient with acute cardiac chest pain. Hallucinations, aggression, convulsions, and CVAs may also follow cocaine use. Long-term users can develop accelerated atheroma.

Hallucinogens

LSD (lysergic acid dimethylamide), some types of mushrooms, and some plant material can lead to a sought-after hallucinatory experience, in which visual images are distorted and pleasant. However, the experience may also be disturbing or frightening, and physical restraint may be necessary. If possible, try to 'talk down' the patient on a one-to-one basis in a quiet, dimly lit setting. If this fails, IV diazepam is the most effective drug for calming the patient.

Ecstasy (MDMA)

This is now popular for use as a 'dance drug'. Some people may develop hyperthermic collapse due to dancing for too long without replacing fluid, and the urgent treatment is IV fluid, which should bring down the pulse rate and enable normal temperature regulation. Rarely, some people drink too much fluid and become confused or develop convulsions, because this drug causes a surge in levels of antidiuretic hormone. Most patients will recover naturally, so long as no more fluid is given.

Rohypnol® ('date-rape' drug)

Rohypnol® (flunitrazepam) is a sedative that causes muscle relaxation, confusion, memory loss, dizziness, and impaired coordination.

Poisoning from other substances

Lead

- In children, lead poisoning most commonly results from pica (pica is the persistent eating or ingestion of substances such as dirt or paint that have no nutritional value), due to ingestion of lead paint from old buildings. Surma (a coloured eye cosmetic made from lead sulphide) is another cause.
- In adults, lead poisoning may result from contaminated water supplies or occupational causes (e.g. painting, manufacturing).
- Children usually present with anaemia and failure to thrive.
- Adults present with abdominal pain, constipation, muscle weakness (wrist or foot drop), and, in the most severe cases, encephalopathy with convulsions.
- The diagnosis may be suspected on finding punctate basophilia on a blood film, and confirmed by measuring blood lead concentrations.

Caustic chemicals

Ingestion of caustic chemicals may cause severe burns and oedema of the mouth, pharynx, upper airway, and upper GI tract.
- If the patient is conscious and able to swallow, give water or milk (three cupfuls) immediately to dilute the acid or alkali.
- Do *not* give neutralizing chemicals, as the heat released can cause further injury.
- If vomiting occurs, the oesophagus may be damaged.

Carbon monoxide

CO is produced when carbon-containing fuels burn in air, and more is produced when insufficient O_2 reaches the fire, leading to poisoning. Motor exhaust fumes are an important cause of CO poisoning.
- Immediate features of exposure include headache, weakness, tachypnoea, dizziness, nausea, and agitation (➲ see Carbon monoxide poisoning, p. 606).
- Vomiting, impaired consciousness, respiratory failure, MI, and cerebral oedema may occur in severe cases.
- If several people experience symptoms, such as headache and vomiting, it is important to consider CO poisoning as a possible cause.
- Give O_2 at a high concentration, whilst assessing the patient. If the patient is vomiting, use nasal cannulae.

Organophosphates and carbamates

Organophosphorus and carbamate insecticides are used to control insects in domestic, garden, and agricultural settings. They can cause serious poisoning, which may be fatal, through inhalation, skin contact, or ingestion. The amount that causes toxicity varies from one chemical to another. Some products contain petroleum distillate, which can cause pulmonary oedema if aspirated.

- The onset of symptoms may be delayed for up to 12h.
- Symptoms include confusion, exhaustion, nausea, vomiting, diarrhoea, wheezing, sweating, salivation, and fasciculation of the muscles.
- The patient may have miosis, bradycardia, incontinence, and seizures.
- Pulmonary oedema and loss of consciousness are serious signs.
- After clearing the airway of secretions, the most important treatment is to give atropine in large doses (2mg at a time) until the mouth is dry.
- Diazepam can be given to relieve anxiety and control seizures.

Prognosis and long-term care

The long-term outlook following acute poisoning is generally good. The great majority of poisonings cause no permanent damage. The main limitation is when the poisoning has been due to DSH, and the patient may be suffering from depression or schizophrenia, sometimes with alcoholism as another complicating factor. In these cases, there is a risk of further episodes of self-poisoning or of suicide by another method, and long-term antidepressant or antipsychotic medication may be indicated.

If a patient has been poisoned in the course of their occupation, one needs to decide whether the exposure has been intentional, whether carelessness has been involved, and whether safety practices are inadequate or absent. The practitioner can then advise the patient and their employers appropriately.

Poisoning due to substance misuse carries risks associated with both the substance and the mode of use (e.g. IV injection, which may lead to serious bacterial or viral infections). Long-term contact with an addiction centre or agency may help to minimize the dangers and improve the prognosis.

In a small number of poisonings, there may be long-term morbidity. CO and organophosphates (➥ see Poisoning from other substances, pp. 598–9) are important examples. Lead poisoning in children may lead to developmental delay and permanent mental impairment, whereas, in adults, eventual full recovery is the rule, even after severe poisoning.

Food poisoning

Food poisoning is caused by the ingestion of foods that contain bacteria or toxins. *Salmonella* is a bacterium that is usually found in poultry, eggs, unprocessed milk, and in meat and water. It may also be carried by pets (e.g. turtles, birds).

The *Salmonella* bacterium affects the stomach and intestines, and, in more serious cases, it may affect the blood. It can infect all age groups and both sexes. However, children, the elderly, and people who already have medical problems are likely to be more adversely affected.

Symptoms

Symptoms include the following:
- diarrhoea or constipation, possibly with blood in the faeces;
- abdominal pain;
- nausea and vomiting;
- fever, headache, and exhaustion.

In the case of less serious infections, there are fewer symptoms (usually only diarrhoea two or three times a day for a couple of days). Most mild types of *Salmonella* infection will resolve on their own in a few days without requiring any intervention other than rest and plenty of fluid.

Severe infection may cause excessive diarrhoea, stomach cramps, and general malaise. In such cases, stool samples should be sent for investigation, as treatment with antibiotics may be indicated.

Alcohol misuse

Alcohol misuse is a worrying problem for EDs. About 14 million people are treated in EDs in the UK every year. It is estimated that a significant number of these have consumed alcohol before attending the ED, and this figure rises after midnight. The number of alcohol-related deaths in the UK has more than doubled, from 4144 in 1991 to 8758 in 2006.[1] In addition, the UK has the third highest rates for binge drinking in Europe.[2]

Emergency presentations associated with, or caused by, alcohol may be physiological, psychological, social, or all three. ED nurses should bear in mind that alcoholics are more vulnerable to heart attacks, strokes, and injury, and they should therefore maintain a high level of suspicion during assessment. Accurate assessment of patients and helping those whose conditions are complicated by alcohol are challenging, but essential aspects of practice.

Binge drinking

The NHS definition of binge drinking is the consumption of large amounts of alcohol in a short space of time, or drinking in order to get drunk or to feel the effects of alcohol. The amount of alcohol a person needs to drink in a session in order to be classed as bingeing is less clearly defined, but the marker used by the Office for National Statistics and the NHS is drinking more than double the daily unit guidelines for alcohol in a single session. This will cause the blood alcohol concentration (BAC) to rise very quickly, resulting in severe intoxication. Binge drinking and underage drinking (which is becoming increasingly common) are hazardous for the person concerned and consumes disproportionate resources in the ED.

History taking and assessment

- Taking an alcohol history should be standard, wherever possible.
- Never label a patient as 'drunk', as such labels are not only judgemental, but can also obscure a serious pathology and delay urgent intervention.
- Patients who are perceived as being under the influence of alcohol and who are being disruptive should not be removed by the police before they have been medically examined.
- Basic vital signs and a CBG level should be obtained at the very minimum.

A sound understanding of the pathophysiological impact of alcoholism is essential for ED nurses and should be a powerful impetus to intervene in the case of hazardous or binge drinkers by referring them to appropriate services. It is significant and of concern that hazardous drinkers continue to miss the opportunity for effective interventions, often because of their behaviour, but also because of staff inaction in this area.

Acute intoxication

Acute alcohol intoxication occurs after the ingestion of a large amount of alcohol. Inexperienced drinkers, or those sensitive to alcohol, may become acutely intoxicated and suffer from serious consequences after ingesting smaller amounts of alcohol.

Signs of acute intoxication

These include:

- slurred speech;
- nystagmus;
- incoherence/confusion;
- facial flushing;
- unsteady gait.

Careful assessment is essential, as these signs may mask or coexist with other pathology (e.g. head injury). These patients are vulnerable and need close observation.

Alcohol withdrawal

Alcohol withdrawal fits are grand mal seizures that occur hours or days after the last alcoholic drink. These patients are often well known to the ED. Nevertheless, it is essential to check the patient's CBG levels and exclude a head injury as another possible cause of fitting. Fitting is controlled by IV or PR diazepam.

Alcoholic ketoacidosis

This is a metabolic complication of alcohol use and starvation, characterized by hyperketonaemia and anion gap metabolic acidosis, without significant hyperglycaemia. It may present in chronic alcohol misusers, following sudden cessation of, or reduction in, alcohol consumption. It is often confused with DKA.

Wernicke's encephalopathy

This is a neurological disease caused by thiamine deficiency. It has two components—Wernicke's encephalopathy and Korsakoff's psychosis. Wernicke's encephalopathy is a potentially reversible, but severe, condition, whereas Korsakoff's psychosis is a chronic and debilitating condition. Wernicke's encephalopathy presents as acute confusion, nystagmus, ophthalmoplegia, ataxia, and polyneuropathy. The signs of Wernicke's encephalopathy may be misinterpreted as a head injury. This patient group, who can be abusive and obstructive, often walk out without treatment. As Wernicke's encephalopathy is a treatable and reversible condition, it is imperative that clinical staff act in the patient's best interest and encourage them to stay for treatment. Treatment is with parenteral thiamine (Pabrinex®) IV over 30min. The patient should be given oral thiamine and multivitamins on discharge.

Korsakoff's psychosis

Some alcoholic patients with Wernicke's encephalopathy may also develop Korsakoff's psychosis. This is a chronic, irreversible condition characterized by severe memory loss. These patients may confabulate or lie in response to their acute confusion and memory loss. The patient may also have an abnormality of the gait due to polyneuropathy. Visual disturbance with eyelid drooping and abnormal eye movements may also be evident.

Delirium tremens

This is a severe manifestation of alcohol withdrawal, which is characterized by hallucinations, delusions, disorientation, and confusion. This is a most distressing condition, in which the patient is vulnerable to arrhythmias, which may be the result of infection, acidosis, electrolyte imbalance, or cardiomyopathy. Initial treatment consists of IV diazepam to control fitting.

Alcoholic cirrhosis

This is the most advanced form of alcohol-induced liver disease. It also affects other organs (e.g. brain, kidneys). Signs and symptoms reflect this involvement but also include portal hypertension, splenomegaly, ascites, renal failure, confusion, and even liver cancer (➔ see Alcoholic liver disease, pp. 366–7).

References

1 Office for National Statistics (2015). *Alcohol-related deaths in the United Kingdom, registered in 2013*. Office for National Statistics, London. Available at: ℘ http://www.ons.gov.uk/ons/dcp171778_394878.pdf.

2 Anderson P and Baumberg B (2006). *Alcohol in Europe: a public health perspective. A Report to the European Commission*. Institute of Alcohol Studies, London.

Nursing interventions for patients with alcohol-related problems

Apart from the standard physical assessment, the nursing role in relation to patients with alcohol-related problems is to deliver care in a non-judgemental way. Nurses are in an optimum position to use the 'teachable moment' in the ED when patients are more receptive to advice. It is imperative that nurses as health promoters use each opportunity as it presents to highlight hazardous drinking and counsel patients. Nurses may be reluctant to intervene with abusive or violent patients, but some patients may be receptive to intervention. A number of screening tools are currently used for assessing hazardous drinking and dependency. These include the Paddington Alcohol Test (PAT) and the CAGE screening tool.

Useful organizations

Drinkline—National Alcohol Helpline. Tel: 0800 917 8282.

Alcoholics Anonymous Great Britain. PO Box 1, 10 Toft Green, York YO1 7NJ. Helpline: 0845 769 7555. ℘ http://www.alcoholics-anonymous.org.uk.

Al-Anon Family Groups UK and EIRE. 61 Great Dover Street, London SE1 4YF. Tel: 020 7403 0888. ℘ http://www.al-anonuk.org.uk.

British Liver Trust. 2 Southampton Road, Ringwood BH24 1HY. Tel: 0800 652 7330. ℘ http://www. britishlivertrust.org.uk.

Alcohol Research UK. ℘ http://alcoholresearchuk.org/.

Further reading

Henry JA and Wiseman H (eds) (1997). *Management of poisoning: a handbook for healthcare workers*. World Health Organization, Geneva.

Carbon monoxide poisoning

Pathophysiology

CO is produced by the incomplete combustion of carbon-containing materials and may therefore be emitted from car exhausts, blocked central heating vents, and house fires. CO has a very strong affinity for Hb and therefore preferentially binds with this to form carboxyhaemoglobin (COHb). As a result, the O_2-carrying capacity of the blood is ↓, as is the release of O_2 from blood to tissues. In severe cases, this can lead to tissue hypoxia and cell death.

Clinical features

Initial features include:
- headache;
- nausea and vomiting;
- dizziness and signs of confusion.

Severe CO poisoning leads to coma, seizures, hypotension, and metabolic acidaemia, all of which can result in cardiac arrest and death. The classic cherry red skin colour is most likely to be seen post-mortem, rather than in live patients (except in the immediate peri-arrest period).

Diagnosis

This is based on clinical suspicion, history, examination, and COHb levels measured on ABG. COHb in non-poisoned healthy patients is usually <5% but may be up to 8% in smokers. A value >10% certainly suggests CO poisoning.

▶▶ Pulse oximetry values will be meaningless, as the COHb levels will contribute to the percentage reading.

Nursing interventions and management

- Ensure removal of the patient from the CO source.
- Ensure the airway is patent, and administer high-flow O_2 (100%).
- The half-life of CO is ~5h on breathing air, 1h on 100% O_2, and 40min with hyperbaric therapy. If hyperbaric therapy is not locally available, its value is debatable, as COHb levels may already be significantly ↓ with high-flow 100% O_2 by the time a transfer is arranged. Those most likely to benefit from hyperbaric treatment include patients with a history of unconsciousness, a COHb level of >20%, pregnancy (due to fetal Hb levels), and cardiac complications such as MI and arrhythmias.
- Managing the critically ill patient in a hyperbaric chamber presents its own problems and may not, in fact, be practicable.

Patients who present with CO poisoning will feel confused and unwell, and need support and reassurance.

Further reading

Henry JA and Wiseman H (eds) (1997). *Management of poisoning: a handbook for healthcare workers.* World Health Organization, Geneva.

Mental health emergencies

Overview

Patients suffering from mental illness may turn to the ED in times of crisis or when their behaviour is of concern to their family or other health-care professionals. However, it is increasingly recognized that EDs often fall short in the care that they offer this vulnerable group. The management of such patients often causes anxiety among emergency nurses, as they may be unsure of how to assess and manage patients who are withdrawn or disturbed. Many EDs now have a dedicated psychiatric liaison service, but ED nurses will still have a major part to play in their care, especially at triage or in generally looking after the patient. Patients presenting with mental health problems often have complex needs, and ED nurses need much greater understanding to be skilled and competent in assessing and caring for them.

Assessing the patient with mental health problems

The initial assessment of the patient is of vital importance for ascertaining the severity of the patient's condition and determining the risk of harm to self or others.

- When assessing a patient who is presenting with a mental health problem, the nurse should ensure that there is another member of staff present if there are concerns about the patient's behaviour.
- Triage areas should have alarms and be designed so that an easy escape route is available.
- The nurse should greet the patient in a calm and welcoming manner, in an attempt to put them at ease. They should maintain eye contact throughout.
- Skilful questioning by the triage nurse is important in order to obtain relevant and pertinent information about the patient's condition.
  - ▶ Do not be afraid to ask probing questions about the patient's current mental state (e.g. 'How is your mood today?' or 'What was your intention when you harmed yourself?').
- Visual assessment of the patient is also important and can assist greatly in determining the severity of the patient's condition. The nurse should observe the following.
  - The patient's appearance. Look for any signs of self-neglect (e.g. poor hygiene).
  - Posture. Is the patient adopting a poor posture or displaying abnormal movements such as rocking or twitching? If so, note whether the patient is maintaining eye contact.
  - Speech. Is it difficult to engage the patient in conversation, or is their speech quick and hurried (pressurized speech)? Noting the content of speech is also important to identify any delusions or hallucinations.
- Another aspect of the initial assessment may involve speaking to the patient's family and friends to find out about previous or current psychiatric care.

Many emergency nurses are unsure of how to assess the risk of further self-harm or suicide attempts. As already mentioned, questioning is an important part of the initial assessment, and staff should not be afraid to ask questions (e.g. relating to the self-harm act and the intentions of this).

Emergency nurses need to understand that very agitated patients cannot tolerate waiting and so are at high risk of absconding. In order to minimize this risk, they should be assessed as soon as possible, but it is also essential to have a written description of the patient that can be given to the police in the event of the patient absconding.

Deliberate self-harm

DSH is an increasingly common presentation in the ED. It can involve self-inflicted injury such as cuts, burns, or scratches, or the ingestion of poisons or overdose (➔ see Poisoning from therapeutic drugs, pp. 594–5).

Although the incidence of DSH and suicide is apparently ↑ due to various social and psychological issues, many of those who engage in DSH may have a treatable mental disorder or substance abuse/dependence at the time of presentation to the ED.

Identifying the risk of further self-harm is an important component of the assessment. The triage nurse must ensure that their concerns are not only clearly documented, but also communicated to the team, so that all relevant staff are aware of the patient's vulnerability. The use of a scoring system, such as the Modified SAD PERSONS score, may be helpful (➔ see Table 19.1).

- All DSH patients need to be in an area where they can be safely observed.
- Some patients may need to be persuaded to stay for psychiatric assessment. If the patient is unwilling to stay but has obvious mental illness or reduced capacity, urgent mental health assessment is indicated, and appropriate measures should be taken to prevent the patient from leaving.[1]

Treatment

- Many of the superficial injuries that are inflicted can be easily treated with simple first aid and wound care, but some of the deeper lacerations and stab wounds (e.g. wounds to the face or those involving underlying structures such as nerves or tendons) need to be fully assessed and may require a specialist opinion.
- If objects have been swallowed or inserted (into the anus or vagina), the patient may also need referral to the appropriate specialty.
- Self-poisoning may be treated by administering activated charcoal, which reduces absorption of the substance. However, treatment will be dependent on the substance and route of ingestion, and advice should first be sought from the local poisons information centre (⌖ http://www.toxbase.org) (➔ see Poisoning from other substances, pp. 598–9).
- Attempted asphyxiation is traumatic for all those involved. Attempted hangings can cause injury due to cerebral hypoxia as a result of asphyxiation or, less commonly, spinal cord injury, although the latter requires a strong noose and a high drop height.
  - On arrival, the patient should undergo the usual ATLS procedures and may require respiratory assistance.
  - C-spine fractures should be considered, and the patient should be C-spine-immobilized until a fracture has been ruled out (➔ see Spinal fractures, pp. 532–3).
  - Injury to the neck can cause soft tissue swelling and airway obstruction, so close observation of the patient's RR, colour, and O_2 saturation is required.

General principles
- Unless the patient is unconscious or has a low GCS score, treatment should take place in a private and secure part of the ED in an area free of any potential means of further self-harm (e.g. sharps bins, O_2 tubing).
- As far as possible, the patient should not be left alone and should be in an area where maximum observation is possible.
- Wounds and self-poisoning should be treated by the emergency physician or ENP, and a basic mental health assessment should be performed to determine the risk of further self-harm and the patient's desired outcome from self-harming.
- Security staff may be required to assist clinicians.
- The patient should then be reviewed by a mental health professional who will conduct a full mental health assessment and recommend admission or follow-up care.

Table 19.1 Modified SAD PERSONS score: guide for referral and admission

	Score
Sex ♂	1
Age <19y or >45y	1
Depression/hopelessness	2
Previous suicide attempts or psychiatric care	1
Excessive alcohol or drug use	1
Rational thinking loss (psychotic or organic illness)	2
Separated, widowed, or divorced	1
Organized or serious attempt	2
No social support	1
Stated future intent (determined to repeat or ambivalent)	2
Interpretation of total score:	
<6: may be safe to wait for psychiatric assessment in majors.	
6–8: urgent psychiatric assessment is needed.	
>8: constant vigilance is necessary, whilst awaiting urgent assessment.	

Reference

1 National Institute for Health and Care Excellence (2004). *Self-harm in over 8s: short-term management and prevention of recurrence*. CG16. National Institute for Health and Care Excellence, London. Available at: ℜ http://www.nice.org.uk/guidance/cg16.

Obsessive–compulsive disorder

Obsessive–compulsive disorder (OCD) is characterized by the presence of obsessions, compulsions, or both.

- *Obsessions* are defined as unwanted intrusive thoughts, urges, or images that repeatedly enter a person's mind. Often they are perceived by the person to be excessive or unreasonable. Some common obsessions are contamination, fear of harm, obsession with order and symmetry, or the urge to hoard useless possessions.
- *Compulsions* are repetitive behaviours or mental acts that the individual feels driven to perform.
  - A compulsion can often be seen by others (e.g. checking that a door is locked or that a tap has been turned off). This is commonly referred to as 'ritual'.
  - A compulsion may also be a more covert or mental act that is not obvious to others (e.g. repeating a certain phrase in the mind). This is often known as 'rumination'.

Patients are unlikely to present to EDs exclusively with OCD, but this may be related to other conditions such as depression, acute anxiety, eating disorder, drug and alcohol addiction, and schizophrenia. Nurses should therefore bear in mind that OCD may be a symptom of a more serious underlying mental health problem.

Patients with such ideas need to be cared for in a quiet environment that is free from excessive stimuli. Nurses should adopt a calm and understanding approach when dealing with patients with such symptoms.

The most important fact for emergency nurses to remember is that these obsessions and compulsions are real to the patient.

Post-traumatic stress disorder

After any traumatic event, it is usual to experience a range of symptoms, including anxiety, depression, dramatic recollections of the event, and a heightened sense of awareness and arousal. Most individuals find that these symptoms will lessen after a period of a few weeks.

However, some patients find that the symptoms persist over a longer period of time. It is important that emergency nurses realize that some patients who present to EDs may go on to experience symptoms of post-traumatic stress disorder, particularly those who are victims of sexual assaults, road traffic accidents, or episodes of violence.

Anxiety and panic attacks

Patients who experience acute episodes of anxiety or panic are common presentations in the ED. A panic attack can be described as an episode of extreme fear and is usually combined with a multitude of symptoms that have a rapid onset and can occur spontaneously or be associated with certain stimuli (e.g. crowded places).

- Common symptoms associated with anxiety are tachycardia and palpitations, chest pain, shortness of breath and hyperventilation, dizziness and fainting, shaking, and numbness of the limbs.
- These symptoms may be associated with other conditions such as cardiac and respiratory conditions, drug misuse, thyroid dysfunction, and diabetic conditions.
- Basic investigations should be performed to rule out a physical cause (e.g. CBG, routine set of blood tests, and basic observations).
- Performing simple observations is often therapeutic and reassuring to these patients, who commonly feel that there is something seriously wrong with them. The basic treatment in the ED, whilst excluding a medical cause, should be supportive and reassuring.
  - Try to care for the patient in a calm environment.
  - In severe cases, benzodiazepines may be helpful for relieving acute anxiety and fear.
- Referral to the psychiatric liaison service may be of benefit for managing the condition in the longer term.
- Organic causes of the symptoms must be ruled out before the diagnosis of a panic attack is made. This is a high-risk area for missing an acute physiological problem.

Phobias and phobic disorders

A phobia is an unreasonable fear of a certain situation or the presence of a certain object. This causes ↑ anxiety in the patient, often to a high level. These disorders can be divided into three categories.

- *Agoraphobia* is an unreasonable fear of specific places or events, and is commonly described as a fear of open spaces. It can also include a fear of crowds, fear of being left outside, and fear of travelling, especially alone.
- *Social phobia.* The patient suffers from ↑ anxiety in social situations and may find that they are unable to speak or interact in even the smallest social gatherings.
- *Specific phobias.* Anxiety is ↑ in specific situations such as the response to a certain object (animate or inanimate), place, or procedure. Examples of causes of specific phobias include spiders, cars, hospitals, X-rays, and needles.

The symptoms and treatment will be similar to those for acute anxiety, although the patient may require longer-term help to rationalize and conquer their fear.

Acute psychosis

This is one of the main psychiatric conditions that emergency nurses will encounter.

- Acute psychosis can be a result of certain psychiatric conditions such as schizophrenia, bipolar disorder, or depression.
- It can also be caused by recreational drugs (e.g. crack cocaine).
- It may present in some physical illnesses (e.g. HIV and AIDS, alcohol withdrawal), and even in elderly patients with sepsis or altered renal function.

Evaluation of the symptoms of psychosis in the ED should focus on excluding underlying organic causes of the symptoms and includes recording of vital signs, ECG, CXR, and blood and urine analysis.

Features of psychosis

Hallucinations

Hallucinations are false sensory perceptions that occur whilst a person is awake and conscious.

Common types of hallucination include the following.

- Auditory—hearing voices when no one has spoken. The patient often blames the auditory hallucinations for telling them to self-harm, to harm others, or to carry out acts that they would not normally perform.
- Visual—seeing objects or beings that are not present.
- Tactile—feeling a crawling sensation on the skin.
- Olfactory—related to taste or smell (these are less common).

Whether hallucinations have psychiatric or physical causes, it is important to remember that the patient may become agitated and frightened by them, and should not be left unattended.

Delusions

Delusions are beliefs that are clearly false. They are irrational and defy normal reasoning, but remain firmly held in the mind, even when overwhelming evidence is presented to refute them.

Delusions are a common feature of several psychiatric conditions, including schizophrenia and bipolar disorder. They can also feature in illnesses that have an organic or physical cause such as dementia.

Delusions fall into five categories.

- Persecutory—the patient experiences feelings of paranoia and has an unshakeable belief that a person or persons are plotting against them or attempting to harm them.
- Grandiose—these delusions focus on an overinflated sense of self-worth. The patient may believe that they have a unique mission in life or are of extreme importance.
- Jealousy—these delusions usually focus on the fidelity of the patient's partner, especially the belief that their partner has been unfaithful.

- Erotomanic—these delusions focus on the patient's belief that another person—often someone famous or important—is in love with them.
- Somatic—these delusions involve the patient's belief that they are suffering from a serious medical problem.

Management

Irrespective of the reason for a patient presenting to the ED with psychotic symptoms, they will be upset and frightened, and they may exhibit aggressive or violent behaviour. Emergency nurses must be competent and able to deal with these patients and to ensure their own safety and that of the patient.

- Many NHS trusts offer training in the management of violence and aggression. This includes the teaching of de-escalation techniques, which can be extremely useful in these situations.
- Patients should, where possible, be cared for in an environment that is calm and has minimal external stimuli.
- Where possible, the same individuals should care for the patient, as this is important for developing a relationship of trust with the patient.

Sedation and restraint of patients

Sedation

This is frequently a contentious issue in EDs, as it is often difficult to balance the need for sedation against the need for a patient to be able to undertake a full psychiatric assessment.

Restraint

This is another area that emergency nurses find difficult.

- Only those who have received training in restraint techniques should undertake this task, as wrongly applied restraint can lead to injury of the patient and the staff members involved.
- Some NHS trusts offer training in control and restraint techniques, and often combine this with de-escalation techniques that may reduce the need for restraint. All emergency nurses should undertake such training.
- Patients do not have to be under arrest or section to be restrained. Common law allows restraint if a person is assessed by trained staff to be a risk to themselves or others.
- Restraint should use a level of force that is reasonable and appropriate, and for the minimum amount of time necessary.
- One member of staff should lead the team and also be responsible for the patient's head and neck and for observing the airway, etc.[2]
- Rapid tranquillization or restraint should only take place when all other efforts to calm the patient have failed and it is obvious that harm will come to the patient or others if such action is not taken.

It is important for ED staff to recognize the signs of impending disturbed or violent behaviour in a patient, as measures can be implemented to diffuse the situation, thus eliminating the need for restraint or medication.

Common features of impending violence in an individual may include restlessness, anger, ↑ RR and BP, and ↑ rate of speech.

Methods of chemical restraint

- Before sedative medication is given to a patient, the nurse must ensure that resuscitation equipment is available nearby for use in the event of any adverse reaction.
- Risks associated with sedation include loss of consciousness, airway obstruction, and cardiac or respiratory problems.
- Use of anaesthetic drugs in restraint is rare and should only be carried out in the resuscitation area in the presence of an anaesthetist.
- NICE has produced guidelines on the rapid tranquillization of violent patients.[2]

Oral tranquillization

This is the preferred option.

- Non-psychotic: 1–2mg lorazepam.
- Psychotic: 1–2mg lorazepam plus an antipsychotic such as haloperidol.

Intramuscular tranquillization

Use IM tranquillization in cases where oral tranquillization has failed or has been refused by the patient.

- Non-psychotic: 1–2mg lorazepam (maximum of 4mg in 24h).
- Psychotic: 1–2mg lorazepam plus 0.5–10mg haloperidol.

Intravenous tranquillization

This is used where immediate tranquillization is essential.

- 2mg lorazepam or 0.5–10mg haloperidol.
- The *BNF* recommends that lorazepam should be diluted with a similar amount of water for injection.

Reference

2 National Institute for Health and Care Excellence (2005). *Violence: short-term management for over 16s in psychiatric and emergency departments*. CG25. National Institute for Health and Care Excellence, London. Available at: ℬ http://www.nice.org.uk/guidance/cg25.

Depression

Patients suffering solely from depression are unlikely to present to the ED. However, depressive symptoms may be part of a wider picture.

- Patients who are severely depressed may present to the ED as a result of self-harm or poisoning (e.g. overdose) or as a result of self-neglect (e.g. not eating or drinking).
- Depression may also be the result of an ↑ in alcohol consumption or drug addiction.
- On occasion, depression may be due to a serious physical illness, such as HIV/AIDS, or any chronic illness.

Depression can be a debilitating condition. People often say 'I am so depressed', and everyone feels sadness from time to time, but this is very different to someone suffering from major or chronic depression who may experience feelings of worthlessness, low self-esteem, and lack of purpose or achievement in their life. They may also experience disturbed sleep and feel constantly tired.

Major depression

- Symptoms of depression include:
  - feelings of gloom and doom;
  - loss of interest in work, home, family, and leisure activities;
  - weight loss or weight gain;
  - changes in sleep pattern (early-morning wakening is common);
  - constant tiredness;
  - suicidal thoughts.
- Recreational drugs, such as cannabis and cocaine, can also cause the symptoms of depression, and depression can be a side effect of some prescription medicines.
- Depression can occur in reaction to an event or situation (e.g. the death of a loved one, loss of employment, financial and personal problems).
- Seasonal affective disorder (SAD) is a reaction to the change from summer to winter, and is usually prevalent in the autumn months when the clocks change and the nights become longer. SAD is characterized by an ↑ in levels of anxiety, overeating, and extreme fatigue.
- Post-natal depression affects some women following childbirth.
- Manic depression as part of bipolar disorder is discussed in the section on bipolar disorder (➲ see Bipolar disorder, p. 621).

Bipolar disorder

Bipolar disorder is an illness that is characterized by two phases—the depressive phase and the manic phase. EDs are more likely to encounter patients with bipolar disorder in the manic phase of the illness.

The symptoms of the depressive phase are described under ⊃ Depression, p. 620. The manic phase is thought to present after 2–4 episodes of the depressive phase. Symptoms may include the following:

• insomnia;
• pressure of speech;
• a feeling of all being well, with many new ideas, delusions, and hallucinations;
• grandiose delusions are prevalent;
• the patient may also change their appearance in this phase (e.g. wearing vividly coloured clothes and make-up).

Treatment of the manic phase in the ED will focus on calming the patient and ensuring a safe environment. In extreme cases, hospital admission is often necessary.

Admission to hospital of the patient with a psychiatric illness

Admission to hospital of patients with mental health conditions is less common now, due to the ↑ availability of care in the community. Many acutely ill patients may be cared for in their own homes by community psychiatric nurses or separate teams who manage the acute episode of the illness (e.g. crisis teams).

Occasionally, admission to an inpatient ward is necessary. Patients presenting with mental illness in the ED may be admitted to hospital informally, where the patient agrees voluntarily to admission, or they may be admitted under a section of the Mental Health Act 1983.

Admission under a section of the Mental Health Act 1983

▶ Note that mental health legislation is different in Scotland.

The Mental Health Act is a long and complicated document that outlines the conditions for application for, and detention of, patients with mental illness. It also sets out the rights of patients detained under the Act and the appeals process if a patient disagrees with detention.

Where a patient is acutely unwell and is considered a danger to him- or herself or another person, the law allows for compulsory admission to a mental health facility. The Mental Health Act has many different parts, but the following main areas will be encountered by ED staff.

Section 2
- This is a compulsory admission either for assessment or for assessment and treatment.
- In the ED, the usual procedure is that the patient is assessed by a mental health practitioner, and, if it is felt that admission may be required and the patient is unwilling, a team of two doctors and a social worker will then assess the patient. If compulsory admission is necessary, an application for admission to hospital under the Mental Health Act is made.
- In the ED, the application for admission is normally made by an 'approved social worker' (i.e. a social worker who is specially trained in mental illness and approved by the borough in which they are working to assess mentally ill patients).
- The patient's nearest relative can also make the application.
- Two doctors, one of who must be approved by the Secretary of State or health authority as being experienced in assessing the mentally ill, must also examine the patient. Both must give a recommendation for admission and treatment, and this must be recorded on the section forms.
- Section 2 can last for up to 28 days.

Section 3
- This is a compulsory admission to undertake treatment.
- The procedure for application and implementation is the same as for Section 2. This section can last for up to 6 months and can be renewed after this.

Section 4
- This is a section for admission in the case of an emergency, and lasts up to 72h to allow full assessment and examination to take place. After this, a further longer section may be applied.
- Section 4 is similar to Sections 2 and 3, but only one doctor need make the medical recommendation.

Section 136 (Place of Safety Order)
- The police apply this section when a person in a public place is acting in a manner which suggests that they may harm themselves or others.
- The police may apply Section 136 to allow removal of the person to hospital for examination.
- Some EDs are not considered to be a place of safety, and, in this case, the place of safety could be the nearest mental health unit.

Management of compulsory admission

Compulsory admission may be very upsetting for the patient and their family, and sensitivity is required when dealing with these cases.

Often admissions from EDs to mental health facilities may involve the patient being transferred to another site.

Where a section has been applied, the patient should be escorted by a nurse and the approved social worker, who will bring the section papers to the admitting facility.

Transport to the admitting hospital must be carefully planned, and the patient should be in a stable condition and safe enough to travel.

Emergencies in older patients

Overview

Elderly patients are frequent attenders in EDs with a wide range of problems of a medical and psychosocial nature. Pathologies associated with ageing make them different to other patients, and these differences must be recognized if their needs are to be met in an individualized and timely way.

Older patients are vulnerable, and decisions about their care should be influenced by quality of life, rather than age. Making such decisions can be difficult in the emergency situation when there is minimal information and little time available, and scarce resources have to be allocated. Clinical assessment of frail older people can be challenging, because they often present with non-specific problems (e.g. falls, immobility, reduced oral intake, delirium) which can make the immediate diagnosis obscure. History taking may be difficult because of sensory impairment, dementia, or delirium. Additional information and collateral history, which is needed but which may not be readily accessible in the emergency setting, and time pressures mean that staff can only focus on what appears to be the immediate problem. Moreover, due to a poor understanding of the functional life changes in older people, well older people are often overlooked, whilst there is a real need for expert knowledge, advocacy, and expediency with regard to those who are sick.

Older patients, although increasingly in a majority, tend to stay longer in the ED, are more likely to be admitted, and have a longer stay in hospital. The use of screening tools can help to predict those who are more likely to experience adverse health status (➲ see Fig. 20.1). Many do not need admission, and early specialist intervention in the ED setting is desirable and may prevent a simple problem from becoming more complex and difficult to manage, with poor outcomes for the patient. It is essential therefore that ED nurses have a sound understanding of, and are able to recognize and respond with alacrity and compassion to, the older patient with urgent care needs. It is also vital and logical to engage the patient and their carers, wherever possible, in history taking and care planning. All clinical staff in emergency and urgent care settings should familiarize themselves with the Silver Book,[1] which is a set of standards and guidelines for patients over the age of 70y accessing urgent and emergency care. Moreover, all staff (including ancillary staff) should have, at the very minimum, a rudimentary training in dementia care.

Reference

1 British Geriatrics Society. *Quality care for older people with urgent and emergency care needs. The Silver Book.* Available at: ℜ http://www.bgs.org.uk/campaigns/silverb/silver_book_complete. pdf.

Dementia

Dementia currently affects over 840 000 people in the UK, and it is estimated that about 25% of all hospital beds are occupied by people with dementia, many of whom do not have a formal diagnosis.

- Dementia is a syndrome with many causes, characterized by a progressive decline in cognitive function, personality, and behaviour.
- Dementia is commoner in the older patient population, but it may occur in a younger patient. Higher mental functions are affected first, in the early phase of the disease.
- As the disease progresses, the patient may become more disorientated and present in an acute confusional state, not knowing where they are or what day of the week, month, or even year it is. They may also not recognize their carers.
- Patients with existing cognitive impairment have a 5-fold higher risk of experiencing episodes of delirium.
- Some mental illnesses, such as depression and psychosis, may also cause symptoms which must be differentiated from both delirium and dementia.

Delirium (acute confusional state)

- Delirium is essentially reversible brain failure, and it is a medical emergency.
- It is a rapidly developing disorder of disturbed attention that fluctuates with time.
- It commonly goes unrecognized and untreated in the acute setting, as it is often confused with dementia.
- Around 20% of older patients in hospital will develop delirium, but it can occur at any age.

Causes

- Infection.
- Pain.
- Dehydration
- Constipation.
- Recent injury or surgery.
- Admission to hospital.
- Prescribed medication.

Although the signs and symptoms of delirium vary from patient to patient, there are several characteristic features that help to make the diagnosis:

- fluctuating conscious level that is typically worse as the day progresses and at night;
- disorientation that is more marked than usual;
- hallucinations and/or psychosis;
- ataxia;
- incontinence;
- dysarthria;
- the patient may be withdrawn and listless, but can also be hyperactive and/or disruptive.

The ED is a frightening and disorientating place for patients who have any level of confusion. It is also very stressful for carers. Therefore, it is imperative that these frail elderly patients are prioritized and transferred to quieter, more appropriate environments as soon as it is clinically safe to do so. Relatives and carers have a key role in the safe and effective management of these patients, so engaging them at the outset is essential to identifying the causes of delirium and initiating treatment.

Frailty

Frailty, which is characterized by physiological deterioration, especially a loss of muscle mass and bone density in the elderly, is not widely recognized or understood, and the risks associated with it (e.g. delirium, subtle deterioration in well-being, and loss of function) are often missed. The five dimensions of frailty are:

- weight loss;
- exhaustion;
- weakness;
- slowness;
- low levels of activity.

Those who fulfil at least three of the criteria are defined as 'frail', whereas those who do not meet any of the five criteria are defined as 'robust'. The commonest signs of frailty are deterioration in activities of daily living (ADLs), mobility, nutritional status, or cognition. There is no gold standard for the measurement of frailty, but the presence of one or more dimensions of frailty should indicate the need for a more detailed and comprehensive geriatric assessment.

Falls

- Falls are a common and serious problem of older people, leading to injuries, functional decline, fear of falling, social isolation, reduced quality of life, and potentially admission to long-term care.
- Patients who attend the ED with a fall are at high risk of future falls and other adverse events.
- Prompt referral to a Falls Prevention Programme may avoid some of these outcomes.

Assessment of falls patients

- Establish whether the fall was mechanical or whether it was preceded by dizziness, chest pain, or other symptoms.
- Screen all of these patients for infection, particularly UTIs, as these are common and may be a contributing factor.
- Assessment of gait and balance should also be considered.
- All older people with a history of recurrent falls or at ↑ risk of falling should be considered for an individualized multifaceted intervention, including evidence-based strength and balance training, home hazard assessment, and intervention.[2]

Reference

2 National Institute for Health and Care Excellence. Guidelines on care of older people. National Institute for Health and Care Excellence, London. Available at: ℘ http://www.nice.org.uk.

Parkinson's disease

Parkinson's disease is a neurodegenerative disorder, in which cells in the part of the brain called the substantia nigra become damaged and die. As cells are damaged, the amount of dopamine that is produced is reduced. A combination of the reduction in the number of cells and a low level of dopamine in the cells in this part of the brain affects neurotransmitters, causing nerve messages to the muscles to become slowed and abnormal. Patients with Parkinson's disease are particularly vulnerable to falls, and so may be regular attenders in the ED.

Signs of Parkinson's disease
- Tremor.
- Stoop and slowness of movement.
- Rigidity/freezing.
- Rigid facial expression.

Symptoms of Parkinson's disease
- Bladder and bowel problems.
- Eye problems.
- Falls and dizziness.
- Freezing of movements.
- Pain.
- Restless legs syndrome.
- Constipation.
- Skin problems.
- Sleep problems.
- Speech and language problems.
- Swallowing problems.

Patients with Parkinson's disease are also more vulnerable to mental health problems, which include:
- anxiety;
- dementia;
- depression;
- hallucinations and delusions;
- memory problems.

It is important to be aware that patients with Parkinson's disease require rapid access to relevant medications such as levodopa. These medications must be kept in the ED and administered without delay.

Safeguarding older people

Context

- Sadly, abuse of older people is common. It is important to consider safeguarding and know how to respond if any type of abuse is suspected.
- The Mental Capacity Act (2005)[3] introduced a new criminal offence of wilfully neglecting a person without capacity.
- All EDs should have access to local policies and procedures for adult safeguarding which will assist the team in identifying and responding to concerns.

Types of elder abuse

- Physical abuse.
- Psychological abuse.
- Financial or material abuse, including theft, fraud, exploitation, and pressure with regard to wills.
- Sexual abuse.
- Neglect.

Reference

3 Department of Constitutional Affairs (2007). *Mental Capacity Act 2005: code of practice*. The Stationery Office, Norwich. Available at: ℬ http://www.gov.uk/government/uploads/system/uploads/attachment_data/file/224660/Mental_Capacity_Act_code_of_practice.pdf.

Depression

Depression is the commonest mental health problem in old age, and factors, such as loneliness, social isolation, and chronic illness, predispose the older patient to higher risk.

The Geriatric Depression Score-5 is a quick and useful tool for screening for depression. Shorter versions are available that might be suitable for brief screening in the ED.[4]

Reference

4 Sheikh JI and Yesavage JA (1986). Geriatric Depression Scale (GDS): recent evidence and development of a shorter version. In: Brink TL (ed) *Clinical gerontology: a guide to assessment and intervention*. The Haworth Press, New York. pp. 165–73.

Polypharmacy

- Polypharmacy is defined as the prescribing of four or more drugs to an individual. It is often one of the main causes of emergency admissions.
- Adverse drug events are more likely to occur in older patients and account for ~6.5% of all hospital admissions.
- Inappropriate prescribing is not uncommon, and it includes the prescription of drugs that are contraindicated or that are not likely to be beneficial, and also over-prescribing a drug in terms of dose and duration.
- Taking a detailed drug history is absolutely essential in the older patient, and nurses should always consider the likelihood of an adverse drug reaction being a contributing factor to the PC.
- Likewise, when administering analgesia under PGDs, nurses should be judicious and bear in mind that older patients often have impaired renal function and may not tolerate medications as well as younger patients.

Nursing assessment and interventions

Nursing assessment

- Follow the ABC approach.
- Patients presenting with polytrauma need to be managed according to ATLS principles, bearing in mind they do not respond well to prolonged immobilization (➔ see Chapter 15).
- Assess pain as a priority. Consider using the Abbey Pain Scale in patients with cognitive impairment (➔ see Fig. 20.1).
- Record vital signs and an ECG. EWS must be undertaken for all frail older patients.
- Obtain a urine sample for urinalysis, as a UTI is common in the elderly and is a cause of confusion and delirium.
- Measure CBG levels to exclude conditions such as hyperosmolar non-ketotic hyperglycaemia.
- Older people have impaired homeostasis, and so are more vulnerable to environmental stressors such as extreme cold or heat.
- Exposure should be considered if the person has been found lying on the floor for a long period.
- Assess cognition, using the AMT4 as a crude assessment of cognitive impairment (➔ see Fig. 20.3).
- Assess nutritional and hydration status.
- Assess and document sensory loss (hearing impairment, poor vision).
- Assess and document skin condition (Waterlow score). Document and report any pressure ulcers.
- Assess mood. Depression is treatable but is commonly overlooked in the elderly.
- Assess mobility where possible.
- Assess continence.

Nursing interventions

Be sensitive to the fact that patients with cognitive impairment or sensory deprivation may become distressed by interventions such as cannulation or urinary catheterization.

If the patient is confused, always have two nurses to perform tasks, one to distract and comfort the patient whilst the other completes the task.

Screening tools

The Abbey Pain Scale (⮞ see Fig. 20.1), ISAR screening tool (⮞ see Fig. 20.2), and AMT4 screening tool (⮞ see Fig. 20.3) can assist emergency care clinicians in the initial assessment of elderly patients.

Abbey Pain Scale

For measurement of pain in people with dementia who cannot verbalize.

How to use scale: While observing the resident, score questions 1 to 6

Name of resident: ....

Name and designation of person completing the scale: ....

Date: ....Time: ....

Latest pain relief given was...at ....hrs.

Q1. **Vocalization**
eg. whimpering, groaning, crying   Q1 ☐
Absent 0   Mild 1   Moderate 2   Severe 3

Q2. **Facial expression**
eg: looking tense, frowning grimacing, looking frightened   Q2 ☐
Absent 0   Mild 1   Moderate 2   Severe 3

Q3. **Change in body language**
eg: fidgeting, rocking, guarding part of body, withdrawn   Q3 ☐
Absent 0   Mild 1   Moderate 2   Severe 3

Q4. **Behavioural change**
eg: increased confusion, refusing to eat, alteration in usual
patterns   Q4 ☐
Absent 0   Mild 1   Moderate 2   Severe 3

Q5. **Physiological change**
eg: temperature, pulse or blood pressure outside normal
limits, perspiring, flushing or pallor   Q5 ☐
Absent 0   Mild 1   Moderate 2   Severe 3

Q6. **Physical changes**
eg: skin tears, pressure areas, arthritis, contractures,
previous injuries.   Q6 ☐
Absent 0   Mild 1   Moderate 2   Severe 3

Add scores for 1–6 and record here ☐ ⮕ **Total Pain Score** ☐

Now tick the box that matches the
Total Pain Score ⮕

0–2	3–7	8–13	14+
No pain	Mild	Moderate	Severe

Finally, tick the box which matches
the type of pain ⮕

Chronic	Acute	Acute on Chronic

Dementia Care Australia Pty Ltd
Website: www.dementiacareaustralia.com

Abbey, J; De Bellis, A; Piller, N; Esterman, A; Giles, L; Parker, D and Lowcay, B.
Funded by the JH & JD Gunn Medical Research Foundation 1998–2002
(This document may be reproduced with this acknowledgment retained)

Fig. 20.1 Abbey Pain Scale screening tool.

(Reproduced from Abbey, J., De Bellis, A., Piller, N., Esterman, A., Giles, L., Parker, D., and Lowcay, B. Funded by the JH & JD Gunn Medical Research Foundation 1998–2002.)

ISAR screening tool (Identification of Seniors At Risk) *Ask carer if patient unable to answer*

Before the illness or injury that brought you to the Emergency Department, did you need someone to help you on a regular basis? ☐ No ☐ Yes

Since the illness or injury that brought you to the Emergency Department, have you needed more help than usual to take care of yourself? ☐ No ☐ Yes

Have you been hospitalized for one or more nights during the past 6 months (excluding a stay in the Emergency Department)? ☐ No ☐ Yes

In general, do you have serious problems with your vision, that can't be corrected by glasses? ☐ No ☐ Yes

In general, do you have serious problems with your memory? ☐ No ☐ Yes

Do you take more than three different medications every day? ☐ No ☐ Yes

A score greater than 1 suggests increased risk of severe functional impairment, frequent hospitalization and depression over the following six months; in this case please

Number of questions answered with YES

• *Ask a Primary Care Coordinator to review (if one is available)*

• *Inform GP*

Fig. 20.2 ISAR screening tool.
(Reproduced from McCusker J., Bellavance F., Cardin S., Trepanier S., Verdon J., Ardman O. Detection of older people at increased risk of adverse health outcomes after an emergency visit: the ISAR screening tool. *Journal of the American Geriatrics Society*, 1999; **47**: 1229–1237. With permission of John Wiley and Sons.)

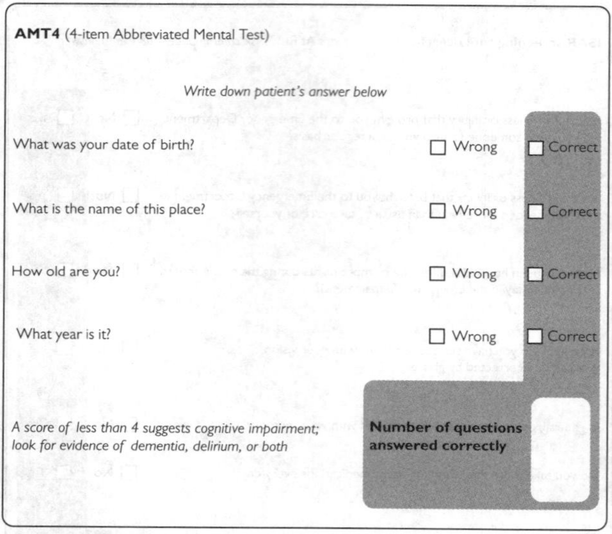

AMT4 (4-item Abbreviated Mental Test)

Write down patient's answer below

What was your date of birth?   ☐ Wrong   ☐ Correct

What is the name of this place?   ☐ Wrong   ☐ Correct

How old are you?   ☐ Wrong   ☐ Correct

What year is it?   ☐ Wrong   ☐ Correct

A score of less than 4 suggests cognitive impairment;
look for evidence of dementia, delirium, or both

Number of questions answered correctly

Fig. 20.3 AMT4 screening tool.
(Reproduced from Swain D.G., Nightingale P.G. Evaluation of a shortened version of the
Abbreviated Mental Test in a series of elderly patients. *Clin Rehabil* 1997;**11**:243–8.)

Occupational health and physiotherapy

The ED is often the first port of call for an older person who is becoming increasingly frail and struggling to cope alone. This may be the perfect opportunity to identify older people at risk who may be in need of greater support to live safely in their own home.

These patients should be referred for physiotherapy and occupational health assessment, especially for those who are not deemed to need medical admission and are therefore being discharged from the ED.

Introduction

This chapter aims to provide a quick reference guide to the numerous skills that are used every day in emergency care settings. It is not meant to be a definitive guide for the uninitiated, but a quick clinical reminder that can be used in practice. Where relevant, you will find information about the following: rationale for the skill/procedure, equipment needed, nursing role, how to perform the procedure, patient assessment and monitoring, and any special considerations.

This chapter aims to provide a quick refresher for skills not routinely used. It could also be used by the experienced nurse when teaching junior/inexperienced staff unfamiliar with various procedures.

❶ An assumption has been made that safe sharps disposal and the correct level of infection prevention and control will be undertaken when any clinical skill is performed. For this reason, the repeated mention of sharps disposal, handwashing, eye protection, and sterile gloves, gowns, and aprons has been omitted from each of the skills in this chapter.

There are many skills in emergency care that are transferrable between adults and children. Where there are specific 'paediatric considerations' (➔ see Symbols and abbreviations, p. xiii) to a particular skill, this is denoted by the following ❹.

Airway management

Ensuring that all patients have an adequate and secure patent airway is, in most cases, the highest priority of care and an essential lifesaving procedure. All nursing assessments should start with the 'ABC' of CPR. Without a patent airway, any further patient assessment is futile, and irreversible brain damage will occur within minutes.

The talking and fully conscious patient with a GCS score of 15 is demonstrating the following:

- a patent airway;
- ventilation is intact;
- the brain is being adequately perfused.

▶ Remember that a conscious patient with a GCS score of 15 may still have debris or secretions in the airway that must be assessed.

- Any reduction in GCS will reduce airway muscle tone; this can cause the tongue to partially or completely occlude the airway and allow secretions to gather, with a risk of aspiration.
- Following facial trauma, there may also be blood, swelling, and/or FBs, such as teeth, in the airway.

Nursing role

- Assess the airway for patency.
- Use manual methods to open an obstructed airway.
- Use basic airway adjuncts to intervene if the airway is compromised, e.g. suction, oral airway.
- Assist in the maintenance of the airway using advanced airway adjuncts, e.g. intubation, surgical airway.
- Deliver O_2, when required, using appropriate methods.
- Continually assess airway patency and ventilatory status of the patient using clinical observation and relevant monitoring.
- Explain procedures clearly to the patient and any family members.

Look, listen, feel

This is the standard assessment approach that should be used when assessing the airway of any unresponsive patient.

- Look for chest rise and fall.
- Listen for breathing and any abnormal airway sounds.
- Feel for breath.

Manual airway opening manoeuvres

Any patient who is not able to open their mouth, when asked, should have it manually opened and inspected for actual or potential obstruction. Any abnormal finding following the 'look, listen, feel' assessment (➋ see Airway management, p. 641) also requires further intervention. The tongue is the commonest cause of airway obstruction in a patient with a reduced GCS. Manual airway opening techniques are a simple and effective way of lifting the tongue from the oropharynx in many situations.

Head tilt/chin lift

(➋ See Fig. 21.1.)
- Place the palm of one hand on the patient's forehead.
- Gently extend the neck by lifting the chin in an upward direction with the thumb and/or fingers of the other hand.

❶ Not to be used following trauma, in case the C-spine is injured. In these instances, a jaw thrust is required.

Jaw thrust

(➋ See Fig. 21.2.)
Must be used in injured patients and is also an alternative if a head tilt/chin lift is unsuccessful.
- Stand behind the patient.
- Place the tip of the index finger of each hand on the angle of each mandible (the heel of the hand can rest on the patient's cheek if there is no sign of facial injury).
- Lift the jaw upwards, towards the ceiling.

▶ Following any airway intervention, the patient must be reassessed for signs of airway patency and/or effective breathing. Continuous monitoring of vital signs is mandatory at all stages of airway management.

Airway opening manoeuvres in children

⊕ The upper airway anatomy in infants and children differs from that of the older child and adult. ∴ There are some slight differences in management.

Head tilt/chin lift
- In an infant: neutral position with slight chin lift. This might require a pad under the shoulders.
- In a small child: slight head tilt/chin lift.

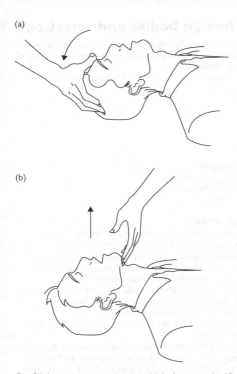

Fig. 21.1 (a) Performing a head tilt. (b) Performing a chin lift.

(Reproduced with permission from Thomas, J. and Monaghan, T. (eds.) (2014). *Oxford Handbook of Clinical Examination and Practice Skills*, 2nd edn, fig. 18.3, p. 603. Oxford University Press, Oxford.)

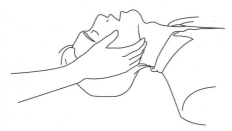

Fig. 21.2 Performing a jaw thrust.

(Reproduced with permission from Thomas, J. and Monaghan, T. (eds.) (2014). *Oxford Handbook of Clinical Examination and Practice Skills*, 2nd edn, fig. 18.3, p. 603. Oxford University Press, Oxford.)

Removal of foreign bodies and secretions

Once the tongue has been manually lifted from the oropharynx, the airway needs further assessment for the presence of FBs. The airway is at risk of aspiration if protective reflexes are lost.

The airway must be assessed for the presence of the following:
- vomit;
- secretions;
- blood;
- teeth;
- FBs;
- swelling.

- Gurgling suggests liquid FBs.
- Snoring suggests tongue obstruction.
- Stridor suggests FB obstruction.

Removal of foreign bodies
- Liquid FBs (blood, saliva, vomit, secretions) should be removed by gentle suction under direct vision, using a rigid Yankauer sucker.
    - ⚠ Care must be taken to ensure the Yankauer is not advanced to the back of the throat, which may stimulate the gag reflex or cause laryngospasm and compromise the airway further.
    - Fine-bore flexible suction catheters can also be used and are ideal when an airway adjunct is *in situ*, as they can be fed though the airway to reach secretions in the oropharynx.
- Solid FBs should be removed from the mouth/oropharynx under direct vision, using suitable forceps.
    - ⊕ ⚠ Care must be taken not to push the object further into the trachea, as this may result in the need for a surgical airway. This is of particular relevance in children who have a 'cone-shaped' larynx, so that FBs are most likely to become wedged.

Simple airway adjuncts

Simple airway adjuncts should be inserted to relieve airway obstruction by the tongue. When inserted properly, the health-care professional may no longer need to manually maintain the airway through head tilt/chin lift or jaw thrust. However, simple airway adjuncts are not a definitive means of airway protection, as the aspiration of blood, vomit, and other secretions can still occur.

Oropharyngeal airway

An oropharyngeal airway (also known as an OPA, a Guedel airway, or an oral airway) is a curved and flattened plastic tube with a reinforced flange at the outer end. OPAs come in four adult sizes (5, 4, 3, 2) and three (1, 0, 00) for children. They must be measured to ensure the correct size is inserted.

- Indications: patients with tongue obstruction and an absent gag reflex.
- Contraindications: presence of a gag reflex, as the patient may vomit or develop laryngospasm; in this case, a nasopharyngeal airway (NPA) is preferred.

Sizing

Place the OPA along the side of the face, with the flange at the incisor. The tip should end at the angle of the mandible.

Insertion

For adults, do the following.
- Open the patient's mouth.
- Insert the OPA upside down into the mouth (the tip should point to the roof of the mouth).
- Once the tip reaches the end of the hard palate, rotate the OPA 180°.

▶ This method of insertion ensures that the OPA does not push the tongue further into the oropharynx.

Alternatively, the OPA can be inserted under direct vision, using a tongue depressor to anchor the tongue forward, allowing the OPA to be inserted the right way up.

⚕ ▶ This alternative method is the advised method in children and infants.

Considerations

- Improper sizing may cause trauma and bleeding in the airway.
- If the OPA is too large, it may close the glottis and thus occlude the airway.
- A patient having a seizure with clenched teeth will not tolerate an OPA.

Nasopharyngeal airway

A nasopharyngeal airway (also known as an NPA) is a flexible tube designed to be inserted into the nasal passage to secure an airway. It has a bevel at the insertion end and a flanged end to which a safety pin is attached prior to insertion. The NPA is also curved along its length to allow easy placement within the nasal passage. An NPA can be used when a gag reflex is present

and is often used in the post-ictal patient. NPAs come in several preset sizes (6.0–9.0). (Smaller sizes are available for children.)
- Indications: patients with airway obstruction ± a gag reflex.
- Contraindications: suspected base of skull fracture.

Cautions
- Known history of nasal polyps.
- Known history of epistaxis.

Sizing
There are several approved methods for sizing.
- Measure from the tip of the patient's nose to the tragus of the ear.
- Does the tip easily insert into the nostril without causing it to blanch? This will be the right size.

Insertion
- Insert a safety pin into the flanged end, if necessary.
- Lubricate the NPA with a water-based gel.
- With the concave aspect facing upwards, the NPA is inserted posteriorly into the nostril, using a gentle rotating motion (a small clockwise motion, followed by a gentle anticlockwise motion), until the flange rests against the nostril.

If there is difficulty inserting the NPA, consider using the other nostril. Do *not* force the NPA into the nasal passage. If well-lubricated and of the right size, it should slide fairly easily into place.

Considerations
- Improper sizing can cause trauma and bleeding to the nasal passage.

▶ Following any airway intervention, the patient must be reassessed for signs of airway patency and/or effective breathing. Continuous monitoring of vital signs is mandatory at all stages of airway management.

Laryngeal mask airway

A laryngeal mask airway (LMA) provides an alternate airway adjunct for use with BVM ventilation. It comprises a tube with an inflatable cuff that is inserted into the pharynx and, when inflated, sits tight over the larynx. Although not the gold standard for airway management in cardiac arrest, LMA insertion is increasingly used when there is no one immediately available with intubation skills. An LMA may not fully protect the airway from aspiration. In difficult intubation situations, when the C-spine is not at risk, an LMA can be a useful airway adjunct.

- Indications:
  - GCS score of 3/15 to ensure an absent gag reflex;
  - inability to maintain a patent airway with simple airway opening manoeuvres;
  - can be used as a temporary alternative in difficult endotracheal intubation.
- Contraindications:
  - Trauma.

Sizing

An LMA can be selected based on the size and weight of the patient requiring airway support (➲ see Table 21.1). Clinical studies have shown that a better seal is obtained by using a larger-size LMA with less air volume inserted into the cuff. Therefore, start by choosing the largest size you think will fit, and inflate with the smallest volume required to obtain an adequate seal. Using too small a mask and overinflating the cuff will ↓ compliance and may result in a poor fit within the laryngeal space.

Equipment required

- BVM.
- Selection of LMAs.
- Lubricating jelly.
- Syringe with adequate volume for the LMA cuff.
- Pulse oximeters.
- Catheter mount and ventilator, if required.

Insertion

- Oxygenate the patient prior to insertion.
- Lubricate the cuff.
- Push the apex of the mask with the open end pointing downwards toward the tongue into the back of the mouth. The tube follows the natural bend of the oropharynx and rests over the larynx.
- Once you are unable to push the tube further back, inflate the cuff to achieve a good seal.
- Connect the BVM, and auscultate the lung fields to ensure good air entry.
- Connect a catheter mount and ventilator, if required.
- Check SpO_2 and CO_2.

Table 21.1 Sizing an LMA

LMA size	Suitable patient	Maximum cuff inflation volume
1	Neonates/infants <5kg	4mL
1.5	Infants 5–10kg	7mL
2	Infant/child 10–20kg	10mL
2.5	Child 20–30kg	14mL
3	Child 30–50kg	20mL
4	Adult 50–70kg	30mL
5	Adult 70–100kg	40mL
6	Adult >100kg	50mL

Endotracheal intubation

Endotracheal intubation involves the insertion of an ETT into the trachea. It is the definitive method of airway control, as the airway is protected from aspiration and the ETT provides a means of mechanical ventilation. In emergency situations, an ETT is usually passed through the oral route. Prior to transfer, the nasal route may be used.

During cardiac arrest, intubation is performed without the need for anaesthetic drugs. However, in most other situations, it will be performed as part of an RSI where induction agents, muscle relaxants, and anaesthetic agents are required. ⚠ An RSI checklist must be used prior to and during the procedure.

Indications for intubation

• High aspiration risk.
• Apnoea.
• GCS score <9.
• Sustained seizure activity.
• Unstable midface trauma.
• Airway injuries.
• Large flail segment.
• Respiratory failure.
• Inability to otherwise maintain an airway or adequate oxygenation.
• Ventilation.

Endotracheal tube sizes

• For women: 7.0, 7.5, or 8.0.
• For men: 8.0, 8.5, or 9.0.
• ⊕ For infants and children, ⮕ see Table 21.2.

Nursing role

The nurse must assemble and check the equipment (⮕ see Box 21.1).
▶ The patient must receive full monitoring before, during, and after the procedure.

Cricoid pressure will be required in all intubations using RSI and may also be requested during cardiac arrest intubations. The correct and sustained application of downward pressure supplied by the thumb and forefinger over the cricoid cartilage will protect the airway from aspiration. This

Table 21.2 Endotracheal tube sizes for infants and children

	Uncuffed	Cuffed
Premature neonates	Gestational age in wk/10	Not used
Full-term neonates	3.5	Not usually used
Infants	3.5–4.0	3.0–3.5
Child 1–2y	4.0–4.5	3.5–4.0
Child >2y	Age/4 + 4	Age/4 + 3.5

Maconochie I, Bingham R, Eich C, et al. (2015). European Resuscitation Council Guidelines for Resuscitation 2015. Resuscitation 95, 222–47. Available at: ℘ http://www.cprguidelines.eu/.

Box 21.1 Endotracheal intubation: equipment needed and checks required

- ETT with 10mL syringe of air and lubricating gel.
  - Inflate the ETT cuff with 10mL of air, and check for leaks.
  - Deflate the cuff.
  - Lubricate with gel.
- Laryngoscope × 2.
  - Check that it is the correct blade, as requested.
  - Use straight blades in children: size 1, infant; size 2, older children.
  - Check that the light bulb is working.
- Suction. Check that it is turned on and working effectively.
- BVM with a connecting catheter mount, filter, and O_2.
  - Check that O_2 is turned on at 15L/min and the reservoir is full.
  - Prior to intubation, a face mask will be used.
- Ribbon gauze to tie in the ETT. Check that it is of suitable length.
- Bougie or stylet (for difficult intubation; acts as a guide through narrow airways). Ensure that it is clean and the type requested.
- Stethoscope. Use to check bilateral air entry.
- SpO$_2$ monitoring. Check that there is good placement and signal strength.
- Waveform capnography. Connect to the monitor.
- Emergency procedure for failure to oxygenate or ventilate should be immediately available.

technique can also assist in the visualization of the vocal cords and ↑ the ease of inserting the ETT. Cricoid pressure must be applied and removed only following the instruction of the intubating clinician.

▶ Cricoid pressure should only be undertaken by clinicians trained and experienced in its application.

Considerations prior to/during intubation
- The patient must be pre-oxygenated with high-flow O_2 delivered by BVM for at least 15s.
- The intubation should take no longer than 30s. After 30s (which the nurse should time), the intubation should stop, and pre-oxygenation should resume.

Checking tube placement following intubation
- Observe for bilateral chest rise and fall.
- Observe O_2 saturations.
- Attach to capnography, and observe recordings. EtCO$_2$ monitoring plays an important role in establishing tube placement, monitoring ventilation rate during CPR, and identifying ROSC.
- Chest auscultation for bilateral air entry.
- Auscultation over the epigastrium for gurgling indicating oesophageal intubation.

Surgical airway

A surgical airway is described as 'the technique of failure', as it should only be used in situations where all other methods of securing the airway have been attempted and failed. All techniques require knowledge of the regional anatomy and should only be performed by, or under the instruction of, an experienced and skilled clinician.

Cricothyroidotomy

This procedure provides a temporary emergency airway in situations where there is obstruction at or above the level of the larynx, such that oral/nasal, endotracheal intubation is impossible. It is a relatively quick procedure, taking <2min to complete.

There are two main techniques (for more information, ➔ see Percutaneous needle and surgical cricothyroidotomy, pp. 654–5).

- Percutaneous needle cricothyroidotomy punctures the cricothyroid membrane and enables oxygenation through a fine-bore cannula.
- Surgical cricothyroidotomy creates a surgical incision through which a tracheostomy tube is passed.

Indications

Need for an emergency airway when:

- standard endotracheal or nasotracheal intubation cannot be achieved or failed attempts;
- need to avoid C-spine manipulation;
- severe facial trauma;
- excessive haemorrhage obscuring the view of the vocal cords;
- oedema of the throat tissues preventing visualization of the cords;
- FB in the upper airway.

Contraindications

- Inability to identify landmarks.
- Underlying anatomical abnormality.
- Tracheal transection.

⊕ In young children, needle cricothyroidotomy, followed by a tracheostomy, is the preferred method.

Complications of a surgical airway

- Aspiration.
- Cellulitis.
- Haemorrhage/haematoma.
- False passage.
- Mediastinal emphysema.
- Subglottic stenosis.

Percutaneous needle and surgical cricothyroidotomy

Percutaneous needle cricothyroidotomy

(➔ See Fig. 21.3.)
- This technique can result in significant hypercarbia and should only be used for 30–40min.
- Needle cricothyroidotomy will provide oxygenation but will not ventilate; there will be no chest rise and fall.
- An ABG sample should be monitored.

Equipment
- 12–14 Fr cannula.
- 'Y' connector.
- Syringe.
- O_2 delivery at 15L/min.
- Vitals observation monitoring.
- Jet insufflator kits are available in some hospital EDs and theatre areas. Please familiarize yourself with your own hospital's difficult intubation equipment.

Procedure
- The skin over the cricothyroid membrane is pierced by the cannula, which is then inserted into the trachea.
- The cannula is aspirated to confirm its position.
- The O_2 supply is connected via the Y connector.
- Deliver 15L/min for an adult. In a child, set the gas flow to the age of the child in years.
- Oxygenate by covering the patent port of the Y connector with a thumb to allow O_2 to flow for 1s (transtracheal insufflation). Remove the thumb to allow expiration for 4s via the upper airway. Jet insufflation devices are also available to deliver the O_2.

Surgical cricothyroidotomy

(➔ See Fig. 21.4.)

Equipment
- Skin cleansing solution.
- Scalpel.
- Curved forceps.
- Plastic cuffed tracheostomy tube or cuffed ETT (size 6–8 in an adult).
- Gauze.
- Syringe to inflate the cuff.
- Tracheal suction catheter.
- Catheter mount.
- Ventilating device.
- Securing device.

Procedure
- The skin is dissected overlying the cricothyroid membrane, and an incision made in the membrane so that the tracheostomy tube can be inserted.
- Once inserted, the cuff should be inflated, and the tube secured and attached to a ventilating device.

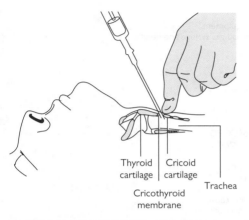

Thyroid | Cricoid
cartilage | cartilage
        Trachea
Cricothyroid
membrane

Fig. 21.3 Percutaneous needle cricothyroidotomy.
(Reproduced from Wyatt, J. et al., *Oxford Handbook of Emergency Medicine*, 4th edn, 2012, p.327, with permission from Oxford University Press.)

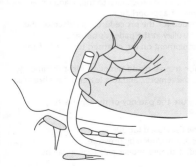

Fig. 21.4 Surgical cricothyroidotomy.
(Reproduced from Wyatt, J. et al., *Oxford Handbook of Emergency Medicine*, 4th edn, 2012, p.327, with permission from Oxford University Press.)

Arterial blood gas sampling

ABG sampling allows for immediate analysis of the patient's acid–base balance by sampling arterial blood. Most resuscitation rooms and critical care areas have an ABG machine.

Equipment
- Two-tier trolley—cleaned.
- Gloves and apron.
- Skin cleansing equipment.
- Appropriate blood gas syringe and needle.
- Gauze and tape.
- 1% LA.

Indications
- Post-cardiac arrest.
- Shock.
- Sepsis.
- Suspected PE.
- Exacerbation of COPD.
- Asthma if SpO_2 <93%.
- DKA.
- Respiratory distress.
- Multiple trauma.
- Head injury.
- Hypoxia from any cause.
- Acute confusional state.
- Following intubation and ventilation for whatever reason.

Procedure
- Identify that you have the correct patient.
- If the patient is conscious, explain the procedure to them, and obtain consent. Explain to the relative, if appropriate.
- Assemble the equipment needed for the procedure, and place on the bottom level of the two-tier trolley at the patient's bedside.
- Assemble the appropriate equipment on the cleansed top level of the trolley.
- Select the appropriate site for arterial blood sampling. Most commonly, the radial artery is used, but the femoral, and to a lesser extent brachial, artery can also be used.
- Perform an Allen's test to ensure the patency of the ulnar artery.

Allen's test
1. The hand is elevated with the fist closed for 30s.
2. The ulnar and radial arteries are occluded by pressure.
3. The elevated hand is opened. It should appear pale (pallor can be observed at the fingernails).
4. Pressure over the ulnar artery is released, and the colour should return in 7s. This suggests that the ulnar artery supply is sufficient, and it is safe to puncture the radial artery.

If colour does not return or returns after >7s, then the ulnar artery supply to the hand is not sufficient, and ∴ the radial artery cannot be safely punctured.

- Expose the selected site, and palpate for the radial pulse. This is helped by hyperextending the wrist and resting it on a pillow.
- Palpate the radial artery, and cleanse the skin with appropriate swab.
- Administer 1% LA to the SC area to reduce the pain. This is rarely done routinely in emergency care settings but reduces the amount of pain experienced by the patient considerably. LA also enables the patient to remain still during the procedure.
- Expel any bubbles and the heparin from the blood gas syringe.
- Introduce the needle at an angle of 60°, passing through the artery.
- Withdraw the needle, whilst simultaneously pulling the plunger back slightly; carry on until blood begins to fill the syringe.
- When the syringe has filled to the appropriate level, withdraw the needle, and apply pressure over the puncture site with gauze for 5min.
- Remove the needle from the syringe, and apply the cap provided in the packaging. Label the syringe with Trust-approved identification. Send the sample for ABG analysis.
- Dispose of all the equipment.

Risks

- Introduction of infection.
- Leakage of blood and formation of haematoma.
- Pain.
- Needle-stick injury.
- Contamination to the clinician.

Arterial line insertion and invasive blood pressure monitoring

▶ This should only be carried out in a closely monitored environment such as critical care, ED resuscitation area, or theatre.

Indications

- When continuous BP monitoring is required in critical injury or illness.
- An arterial line also allows easy convenient access to the arterial circulation for ABG analysis.

Equipment

- Monitoring equipment.
- Pressure bag.
- 500mL bag of normal saline or heparinized saline.
- Transducer cable, arterial giving set (with red stripe running through to indicate arterial, if available).
- Appropriately sized arterial catheter, long for femoral or short for radial. Smaller sizes for young children.
- Sterile dressing field, gloves, and apron.
- Suture pack.
- Appropriate sutures.
- Lidocaine 1%.
- Variety of syringes.
- Skin cleansing equipment.
- Transparent dressing, arterial catheter label.

Procedure

- If the patient is not unconscious or sedated, explain the procedure to the patient and/or relatives.
- Place the saline/heparinized saline bag into the pressure bag.
- Run the saline/heparinized saline through the arterial line set, using the flush device to prime the line, and ensure there are no bubbles.
- Inflate the pressure bag to 300mmHg. This ensures that the infusion is under higher pressure than the patient's systolic BP and the fluid maintains the patency of the arterial catheter.
- Prepare the equipment, ensuring that there is a sterile field around the chosen arterial insertion site.
- Following insertion of the arterial catheter, connect the arterial line set aseptically. Ensure that all cannula connections are securely fastened.
- Secure the cannula with transparent dressing, and label the line.
- Connect the transducer cable to the arterial line set.
- Zero the transducer device.
- Turn the three-way tap distal to the patient 'off' to the patient, and then open the port to air.

- Zero the monitoring equipment. Once zeroed, close the port, and turn the three-way tap 'off' to the port.
- Secure the transducer device (level with the RA) with tape to the upper arm.
- The arterial line should produce a waveform on the monitor, and the patient's BP and MAP are displayed on the monitor screen. An MAP of >65mmHg indicates adequate perfusion.

Complications

- Massive blood loss.
- Infection.
- Loss of blood supply to the hand.
- Injection of medications directly into the artery by mistaking it for venous access.

Bag–valve–mask ventilation

A BVM or 'Ambu' bag is a hand-held device that provides mechanical ventilation. A BVM consists of a self-inflating bag, a one-way valve, and a face mask. When a reservoir with supplemental high-flow O_2 is attached, 80–90% O_2 concentrations can be delivered. When the self-inflating bag is squeezed, the device forces air via a one-way valve into the patient's lungs. When the bag is released, it self-inflates, drawing in ambient air and any supplied O_2, whilst the patient's lungs deflate through the one-way valve.

Indications

- Respiratory arrest.
- Inadequate RR.
- Inadequate respiratory effort.

Complications

- Overinflating the lungs can damage delicate tissues.
- Air leak into the stomach causes gastric distension and possible vomiting.

Equipment

- Correct-sized BVM with a reservoir.
- ⓘ Appropriate-sized face mask (0, 1, 2 for children; 3, 4, 5 for adults).
- Suction.
- Airway adjunct, if required.
- Pulse oximeter.

Ventilating with a bag–valve–mask

- The correct-sized BVM needs to be selected. An adult BVM can be used for any age, but, if the BVM is too small, there will be inadequate ventilation.
- Ensure an adequate jaw thrust is employed.
- A good face mask seal must be achieved; this may require a 'two-person' technique (➔ see Fig. 21.6). One person uses both hands to secure the face mask. The second person operates the self-inflating bag.
- ⓘ In children, a one-person technique should use the following hand position (➔ see Fig. 21.5). The thumb and index finger form a 'C' shape and provide anterior pressure over the mask; the middle, ring, and little fingers form an 'E' on the line of the jaw and create the seal.
- Airway opening manoeuvres or an airway adjunct may be required.
- ⓘ A self-inflating bag should be squeezed to deliver 5–6mL/kg of air (e.g. 50mL in a 10kg child; ~500mL in an adult).
- The patient's chest should visibly rise with each ventilation.
- A rate of 10–12 ventilations/min should be adequate for an adult.
- ⓘ A rate of 20–30 ventilations/min is adequate for a child, and 30–40 ventilations/min for an infant.

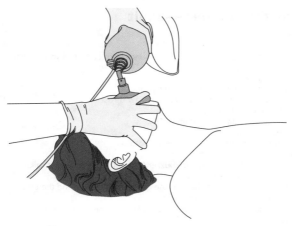

Fig. 21.5 ⊕ One-person BVM technique.

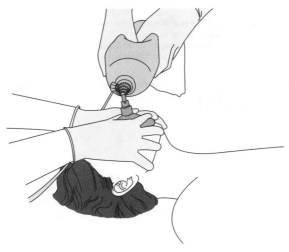

Fig. 21.6 Two-person BVM technique.

Basic life support—adult

(➲ See Fig. 21.7.)

- Unresponsive?
  - Shake the shoulders, and ask loudly into both ears, 'Are you all right?'
- Shout for help.
- Open the airway.
  - Use the head tilt and chin lift technique.
  - If possibility of C-spine injury, use a jaw thrust.
- Not breathing normally?
  - Look, listen, and feel for up to 10s.
  - Feel for a carotid pulse.
  - If breathing, place in the recovery position.
- Call 999 if out of hospital.
- In hospital, pull the emergency buzzer/put out a cardiac arrest call.
- Give 30 chest compressions.
  - Place the heel of one hand in the centre of the chest and the other hand on top, interlocking fingers.
  - Press down on the sternum 4–5cm, keeping the arms straight.
  - Repeat at a rate of ~100–120 times a minute.
- Two rescue breaths:30 compressions.
  - Use a BVM or pocket mask, if available, with high-flow supplemental O_2.
  - If not, take a normal breath, and place the lips around the patient's mouth, ensuring a good seal. Blow steadily into the mouth, whilst watching for the chest to rise.
  - As soon as an automated external defibrillator (AED) arrives, attach it to the patient, switch it on, and follow instructions.

▶ Stop to recheck the patient only if they start to breathe normally. Otherwise, do not interrupt resuscitation. Continue until medical help/ advanced life support arrives.

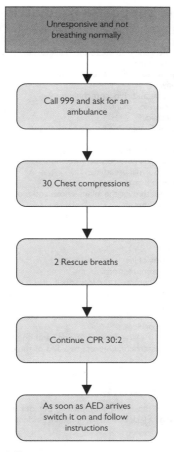

Fig. 21.7 Adult basic life support.
(Reproduced with the kind permission of the Resuscitation Council (UK). 2015 Guidelines.)

❶ Basic life support—paediatric

(➔ See Fig. 21.8.)
- Unresponsive?
  - Shake the child gently; speak to the child. Is there any age-appropriate response?
- Shout for help—in hospital, get senior help.
- Open the airway.
  - Use the head tilt and chin lift technique.
  - Neutral position for an infant.
  - Sniffing for a child.
  - If possibility of C-spine injury, use a jaw thrust.
- Breathing normally?
  - Look, listen, and feel for up to 10s.
  - If breathing, place in the recovery position.
- If in doubt about normal breathing:
  - Give five rescue breaths.
  - Infant: your mouth over the infant's nose and mouth.
  - Child: mouth to mouth.
  - Blow steadily for about 1s, enough to see a visible chest rise.
- Feel for a pulse:
  - infant: brachial;
  - child: carotid.
- If there are no signs of life:
  - Give 15 chest compressions.
  - For all children, compress the lower half of the sternum.
  - Depress the chest 1/3 of its anterior/posterior diameter.
  - Infants: the tips of two fingers can be used if one rescuer. If two rescuers, use the hand encircling technique. Depress a third of the chest diameter or 4cm.
  - Children over 1y: place the heel of one hand one finger breadth above the xiphisternum. Depress to a 1/3 of the chest diameter or 5cm.
  - Repeat at a rate of ~100–120 times a minute.
- Give two ventilations, and continue at 15:2 ratio.
- Give CPR for 1min; then call 999.

▶▶ In hospital, pull the emergency buzzer/put out a paediatric cardiac arrest call as soon as a lack of normal breathing is identified.

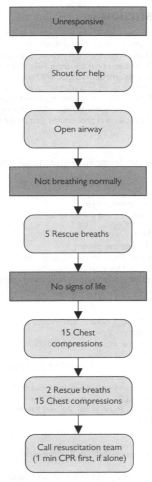

Fig. 21.8 Paediatric basic life support (health-care professionals with a duty to respond).

(Reproduced with the kind permission of the Resuscitation Council (UK). 2015 Guidelines.)

Blood transfusion

The transfusion of blood and blood products is a fairly common occurrence in emergency settings. In the resuscitation room, the procedure usually has to be carried out urgently; a full patient history may not be known, and there may not have been time to order fully cross-matched blood. In less critical situations, cross-matched blood will have been ordered, and the transfusion can be administered in a planned way. Whatever the method of administration, the following principles must be followed, as transfusion errors can have serious consequences. The administering clinician must also be familiar with local policies and procedures that relate to transfusion.

Indications
- Replacement of RBCs.
- Replacement of clotting factors/other blood products.

Equipment
- Blood/blood product.
- Blood giving set with integral filter.
- Blood warmer should be used if >50ml/kg/h.

Patient preparation
- Explain the procedure to the patient.
- Ensure the patient is wearing an identity bracelet that documents their name, date of birth, and hospital number.
- Ensure all patient identification checks have been carried out according to local policy.

Procedure
- Collect the blood/blood products, ensuring all the checking processes are completed correctly.
- When in the clinical area, ensure the blood/blood products are checked again according to hospital policy.
- Ensure that the blood has been prescribed, with reasons for transfusion clearly documented in the patient's notes.
- Transfusion must be commenced within 30min of the blood/blood product being collected from the hospital fridge.
- Record baseline temperature, pulse, BP, and RR immediately before starting the transfusion.
- Document the transfusion start time and date on the compatibility form and drug chart.
- Record temperature, pulse, BP, and RR 15min after commencement of transfusion.
- If vital signs within normal range at 15min, subsequent observations can be recorded at hourly intervals.
- Vital signs should be recorded at the end of the transfusion, and the finish time documented on the compatibility form.
- Urine output must be monitored throughout the transfusion.
- Transfusion should be completed within 4h.

- All medications should be given as charted and in a timely way.
- If any transfusion adverse reaction occurs, stop the transfusion immediately, record vital signs, and ask the medical team to urgently review the patient.
- Notify the lab.
- Keep the bag and giving set to which reaction has occurred, and return to the lab. Keep IV line patent with saline.
- No meds to be given through the blood giving set/line.

Cannulation

▶ Cannulation is a routine emergency care skill. However, there is a danger, because it is done so frequently that important assessment steps are not taken.

Prior to cannulation, considerations should be given as to why the cannula is being inserted and for what it will be used. This will allow the clinician to decide if a cannula is even needed and then to select the right-sized cannula and the right site (➋ see Table 21.3).

Equipment
- Sterile field/tray.
- One appropriately sized cannula.
- Skin cleaning product (as per Trust policy).
- One adhesive cannula dressing (check patient allergies).
- 10mL syringe with 5mL of normal saline.
- PPE, i.e. gloves and apron.
- Tourniquet.
- Kidney dish and sharps bin.

Procedure
- Introduce yourself to the patient, explain the procedure, and gain informed consent.
- Select a site for the cannula, based on why it is being inserted.
  - If rapid transfusion of large amounts of blood/fluid is anticipated, a large vein is needed. The antecubital fossa (ACF) is widely used for this purpose.
  - If a cannula is needed for medication or maintenance fluid, a smaller vein can be used and is often better tolerated by the patient. The dorsum of the hand or cephalic vein, as it runs over the radial aspect of the wrist, can be used for this purpose.
  - The veins of the ankle/foot should be avoided due to the risk of DVT development.
  - Ideally, the patient's non-dominant arm should be used.
- Look for a suitable vein, and apply a tourniquet to assess it further.
  - Palpate the selected vein to assess its suitability. It should be bouncy and prominent, refill easily when depressed, and be fairly straight to accommodate the length of the cannula.
  - ✪ Several sites should be assessed, particularly in children. This will ensure that the best vein has been selected and will minimize the number of attempts required.
- Clean the skin with an appropriate agent/product according to Trust policy.
- Anchor the chosen vein by applying traction to the skin distal to the cannulation site, so it becomes taut. Do not release traction until the cannula is *in situ*.
- Puncture the skin over the vein at a 30–45° angle. Observe for blood in the flashback chamber—the cannula is in the vein. Decreasing the angle, guide the cannula a little further into the vein 1–2mm. Gradually slide the cannula off the needle all the way into the vein.

Table 21.3 Cannula sizes and uses

Colour	Gauge	Indications
Yellow	24	Paediatric
Blue	22	Paediatric
Pink	20	Paediatric, 2–3L of fluid/24h
Green	18	Larger volumes
White	17	Rapid infusion, viscous solution
Grey	16	Rapid infusion, viscous solution
Brown	14	Rapid infusion of blood

- Discard the needle in a sharps bin.
- Apply the cap to cannula end or other appliance, as per local policy.
- Secure with adhesive dressing.
- Flush the cannula as per local policy.

Risks associated with cannula insertion

- Introduction of infection (including methicillin-resistant *Staphylococcus aureus*, MRSA).
- Haematoma formation.
- Thrombosis of the vein.
- Pain.
- Allergy to device/dressing.
- Phlebitis.
- Cellulitis.

Capnography

Capnography is the measurement of $EtCO_2$ and should be measured in all intubated and ventilated patients. Capnography measures the CO_2 content in the expired breath. The establishment of an $EtCO_2$ measurement confirms that the ETT is in the airway. A continuous trace enables the clinician to optimize the ventilator settings and tailor them to the patient's condition.

There are two principal ways of monitoring $EtCO_2$. The CO_2 level can be transduced through an airway adapter and then via a cable out to the monitoring equipment, giving a continuous trace. Alternatively, a disposable device can be attached to the breathing circuit. This will change colour, confirming the presence of CO_2. The disposable device will not give a continuous trace.

Equipment

- CO_2 airway adapter and transducer cable compatible with monitoring equipment.
- Disposable CO_2 detector.

Procedure

- After intubation, ensure the ETT is held securely.
- Connect the airway adapter between the ETT filter and breathing circuit (it usually will only fit one way round).
  - Disposable $EtCO_2$ detector. The colour of the detector changes according to CO_2 levels. If using these devices, refer to the manufacturer's instruction about the interpretation of the colour change.
  - Transduced $EtCO_2$ monitors. Attach the transducer cable to the airway adapter; it will only attach one way. Connect the cable to the appropriate monitor (some machines need to be warmed up before use).
- With transduced $EtCO_2$ monitoring, a continuous waveform will be present on the monitor and give a numerical reading in either kPa or mmHg.
- With the disposable devices, there will be a colour change in the presence of CO_2.

Caution

If the patient has drunk carbonated drinks or ingested antacids before intubation, there can be CO_2 in the oesophagus. This could lead to a false reading if a misplaced oesophageal intubation occurs. Ordinarily, CO_2 should not be detected in the oesophagus.

Capnography for sedation

Patients in the ED are quite often sedated to reduce fractures or dislocations. Nasal capnography cannulae are available to monitor CO_2.

Cardiac pacing

Temporary transcutaneous cardiac pacing is an emergency procedure that is required when a patient has symptomatic bradycardia. Transcutaneous pacing enables the patient's condition to be stabilized until a temporary pacing wire can be inserted.

Indications

- Third-degree heart block.
- Ventricular standstill.
- Symptomatic bradycardias: hypotension; altered level of consciousness; chest pain; breathlessness. See ℘ http://www.resus.org.uk.

Equipment

- Defibrillator with pacing facility.
- Pacing pads.
- Razor.
- Alcohol skin prep if the patient is clammy.
- Sedation.

▶ It is vital that the operator has a detailed knowledge of the defibrillator to be used—machines vary in their pacing capabilities and parameters.

Patient preparation

- Explain the procedure to the patient and family. There will be some discomfort felt, as the machine delivers each paced beat, and the patient may 'jolt'.
- Explain that this is a temporary procedure and that pain relief and sedation can be given.
- Ensure adequate pain relief.
- Ensure sedated, if appropriate.

Procedure

- Prepare the chest skin, and clip hair if there is time. If not, shave chest hair, taking care not to cause skin abrasions. If the skin is clammy, wipe with alcohol skin prep.
- Ensure the patient is monitored through lead II via the three chest leads.
- Disconnect the defibrillator paddles, if not already, and connect the pacing cable.
- Connect a set of multifunction electrodes.
- Apply the pads (there is a diagram on each pad indicating where it should be placed)—one pad to the right of the sternum, just below the clavicle; the other to the fifth/sixth ICS in the left anterior axillary line (➋ see Fig. 21.9).
  - This pad position is quick and easy to perform. However, the anterior/posterior position (front and back of the patient's chest) may be more effective in obtaining mechanical and electrical capture.
- Ensure the pads are well adhered.
- Plug the pacing pads into the pacing cable.

- Turn the pacer on.
- Using the other pacing buttons, select the required:
  - mode ('demand' or 'fixed'). Demand is usually used;
  - paced pulses per minute (ppm). Start at 70ppm;
  - milliamperes (mA). Start at the lowest setting.
- Your selection will be displayed in the pacing dialogue box on the screen.
- When ready to start pacing, press the start/stop button once. (Pressing this button again will stop pacing.)
- Establish electrical capture (a QRS complex should immediately follow a pacing spike). The mA will need to be slowly ↑ until electrical capture is achieved.
- Establish mechanical capture (check the patient's pulse).
- Once pacing is established, monitor BP and HR, and palpate for a pulse every 5min.
- Prepare for transfer to coronary care for immediate transvenous cardiac pacing.

▶ If patients are symptomatic and an external pacing machine is not available, you can perform external cardiac percussion using a clenched fist. With blows (more gentle than a precordial thump) delivered at a rate of 100/min, you can produce a QRS complex.

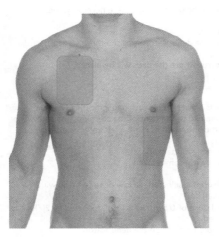

Fig. 21.9 Correct position of the gel pads or AED electrodes on the patient. Ensure that they are not touching or overlaying any wires, O_2 tubing, or any other conducting material. Ensure that the patient's chest is dry and shaved if particularly hairy.

(Reproduced with permission from Thomas, J. and Monaghan, T. (2007). *Oxford Handbook of Clinical Examination and Skills*, fig. 17.41, p. 639. Oxford University Press, Oxford.)

Cardioversion

Cardioversion is a procedure that delivers a synchronized electrical current at a specified moment in the cardiac cycle. It is used to terminate an abnormally fast heart rhythm in an unstable patient, e.g. VT. Cardioversion should be carried out by an appropriately trained clinician and only when indicated. The nurse has a vital role in monitoring the patient and preparing them and their relatives for the procedure, which often has to be carried out rapidly.

▶ The nurse and clinician delivering the cardioversion *must be* familiar with the defibrillator and how to operate it for cardioversion and defibrillation.

Equipment
- Defibrillator.
- Adhesive conductive pads.
- Razor.
- Appropriate sedation.
- Full monitoring:
  - cardiac monitoring;
  - non-invasive BP;
  - continuous pulse oximetry;
  - RR.

Patient preparation
- Explain the procedure to the patient and, where necessary, their relatives.
- Obtain informed consent.
- Connect the patient to the defibrillator using the three standard cardiac monitoring chest leads.
- Shave away any chest hair where the pads will be placed.
- Dry the skin.

Procedure
- Apply the pads (there is a diagram on each pad indicating where it should be placed)—one pad to the right of the sternum, just below the clavicle; the other to the fifth/sixth ICS in the left anterior axillary line (➔ see Fig. 21.9).
- Ensure all other monitoring is attached.
- Administer O_2, if not already commenced.
- Administer sedation.
- The energy to be delivered is selected—a low dose to begin with, usually 50–100J. This can be ↑.
- 🔆 In children, an initial dose of 0.5–1J/kg is used, followed by 2J/kg if a second shock is required.
- Activate the synchronized function on the defibrillator.

- All staff are instructed to 'stand clear'.
- The shock is delivered.
- The rhythm is reassessed. If the tachycardia has not been reverted, a second highly synchronized shock can be delivered.
- If a second shock is administered, *ensure* the synchronized function is activated.
- When the rhythm is stabilized, record the patient's vital signs.

Catheterization—female

Urethral catheterization is the introduction of a catheter into the bladder for the collection and/or measurement of urine. The catheter may remain *in situ* for a period of time or can be removed once the bladder is drained.

Indications

- To relieve obstruction to the outflow of urine.
- To accurately monitor urine output.
- To protect the skin when its integrity is compromised through incontinence.

Equipment

- Bladder scanner.
- Two-tier trolley—cleaned.
- Catheterization pack.
- Sterile gloves—two pairs.
- Disposable apron.
- Sodium chloride 0.9% for cleansing.
- Lidocaine local anesthetic gel.
- ♂ ♀ catheters: sizes 10 and 12 (shorter in length) with 10mL of water for injection (usually included in the pack). ♂ ➔ See Table 21.4 for paediatric sizes.
- Drainable urine bag ± urometer if hourly measurements required.
- Clinical waste bag.

Patient preparation

- Explain the procedure to the patient.
- Obtain informed consent.
- Undress, if not already undressed.
- Ensure privacy by performing the procedure in an area that will not have any interruptions.
- Position the patient supine with their hands by their side. Do not expose the perineum until necessary.
- Scan the bladder, and document the results.

Procedure

- Place bed protection under the patient in case of any spillages.
- Ask the patient to bend their knees, bringing both heels together. Ask the patient to let their knees flop apart, exposing the perineum.
- Apply both pairs of sterile gloves.
- Place sterile towels on either side of the perineum. Using a saline-soaked swab, clean from the top of the labia down towards the patient's anus until clean.
- Remove the outer pair of gloves.
- Bring the sterile kidney dish and catheter. Rest them on sterile towels.
- Dip the catheter tip into the anaesthetic gel to provide lubrication.
- Open the labia, and insert the catheter into the urethra; urine should appear in the tube. Continue to insert the catheter ~10cm, keeping the open end in the kidney dish.

- Attach the drainage bag.
- Insert the water for injection into the additional port.
- Gently retract the catheter tube slightly, until stopped by the inflated balloon.
- Dispose of waste, and wash hands and trolley.
- Measure the amount of urine drained.
- Assist the patient to dress, and maintain their dignity.
- Document on the catheter care pathway the catheter inserted, water used to inflate the balloon, and urine drained.

Table 21.4 Paediatric sizing for catheters (both ♂ and ♀)

🛈 Age of child	Catheter size (Fr)
Neonate	5*
0–2y	6
2–5y	6–8
5–10y	8–10
10–16y	10–12

* It is common practice to use 5 Fr feeding tubes in this age group.

Catheterization—male

Rationale

- To relieve obstruction to the outflow of urine.
- To accurately monitor urine output.
- To protect the skin when its integrity is compromised through incontinence.

Equipment

- Bladder scanner.
- Two-tier trolley—cleaned.
- Catheterization pack.
- Sterile gloves—two pairs.
- Disposable apron.
- Sterile anaesthetic lubricating jelly.
- Sodium chloride 0.9% for cleansing.
- ♂ catheters × 2 size 14 and 16 (longer than ♀) with 10mL sterile water for injection (included in pack) (➲ see Table 21.4 for paediatric sizes).
- Drainable urine bag ± urometer if hourly measurements required.
- Clinical waste bag.

Patient preparation

- Explain the procedure to the patient.
- Scan the bladder, and document findings.
- Obtain informed consent.
- Undress, if not already undressed.
- Ensure privacy by performing the procedure in an area that will not have any interruptions.
- Position the patient supine with their hands by their side. Do not expose the perineum until necessary.

Procedure

- Place bed protection under the patient in case of any spillages.
- Ask the patient to expose their genitals.
- Apply both pairs of sterile gloves.
- Place a sterile towel over the genital area, with a tear in the middle to expose the penis.
- Place a sterile swab around the penis, retracting the foreskin, and clean the glans with a saline-soaked swab.
- Remove the outer pair of gloves.
- Insert a small amount of lubricating gel to the opening of the urethra; wait a few minutes.
- Bring the sterile kidney dish and catheter. Rest them on sterile towels.
- Hold the penis in a vertical position.
- Insert the tip of the anaesthetic gel tube into the urethra, and administer the rest of the gel. (Wait ~3–5min, so that the gel is able to coat the urethra and anaesthetize it.)
- Continue to hold the penis vertically. Insert the catheter all the way into the urethra (if any obstruction is felt, gently insert the catheter whilst asking the patient to cough).

- Attach the drainage bag.
- Insert the water for injection into the additional port.
- Gently retract the catheter tube slightly, until stopped by the inflated balloon.
- Ensure the foreskin (if present) is pulled forward again over the glans.
- Dispose of waste, and wash hands and trolley.
- Measure the amount of urine drained.
- Assist the patient to dress, and maintain their dignity.
- Document the catheter inserted on the catheter care pathway, water used to inflate the balloon, and urine drained.

For paediatric catheter sizes, see Table 21.4.

Central venous pressure line insertion and monitoring

CVP lines are often inserted into critically ill or injured patients, as they provide direct access to the central circulation. Central access enables drugs and/or fluids to be given rapidly and to act immediately, and also allows close monitoring of pressures within the central venous system. CVP lines can accurately monitor intravascular volume, and assess hydration and levels of hypovolaemia. It is a common procedure prior to transfer to intensive care.

Indications for insertion and CVP monitoring

- Shock.
- Inotrope infusion.
- Fluid resuscitation.
- Cardiac arrest.
- Multiple trauma.

Equipment

- Central venous catheter pack with appropriate number of lumens.
- Sterile dressing field, gloves, and gown/apron.
- Pressure bag.
- 500mL bag of normal saline or heparinized saline.
- Transducer set (with blue stripe to indicate venous, if available).
- Suture pack.
- Appropriate sutures.
- 1% lidocaine.
- Variety of syringes.
- Heparinized flush.
- Skin-cleansing equipment.
- Transparent dressing; CVP line label.

Patient preparation

- Explain the procedure to the patient and/or family.
- Help position the patient, usually flat with 10° head down tilt.
- Support the patient during the procedure.

Procedure

- Place the saline/heparinized saline bag into the pressure bag.
- Run the saline/heparinized saline through the transducer set, using the flush device to prime the line, and ensure there are no bubbles.
- Inflate the pressure bag to 300mmHg. This ensures that the infusion is under higher pressure than the patient's systolic BP and the fluid maintains the patency of the line.
- Prepare the equipment, ensuring that there is a sterile field around the chosen insertion site.
- Following insertion of the catheter, connect the set aseptically. ▶ Ensure that all cannula connections are securely fastened.
- Secure the cannula with transparent dressing, and label the line.

- Connect the transducer giving set to the distal port if more than a single lumen (this should be labelled clearly on the catheter).
- Connect the transducer cable to the transducer giving set, and connect to the monitor. CVP transducers are usually connected to the P1 connection on the monitor.
- Tape the transducer device to the upper arm, in line with the heart.
- Ensure that a CXR has been ordered post-insertion. This is to check the position before administering drugs through the central line.

Complications

- Haemothorax.
- Pneumothorax.
- Cardiac arrhythmias.
- Thoracic duct trauma.
- Brachial plexus injury.
- Air embolism.
- Haemorrhage.
- Misdirection or kinking.

Measurement of CVP using a transducer

In resuscitation rooms, the CVP measurement is transduced to monitoring equipment to give a continuous reading. CVP measurements can be undertaken manually using a pressure manometer. This is usually done in non-critical care areas.

- Position the patient.
- Turn the 3-way tap off to the patient; open to the air, and remove the cap.
- 'Zero' the monitor, and wait for calibration.
- When 'zeroed', replace the cap, and turn the 3-way tap on to the patient.
- The CVP trace should produce a waveform on the monitor, associated with right atrial contraction, and a measurement displayed as a number on the monitor screen. Document the measurement.

Normal CVP ranges are 5–10mmHg or 4–8cmH$_2$O.

Nursing role

- Monitor the CVP readings, and document the measurements.
- Report any changes.
- Ensure the site is observed for haemorrhage or loose connections.
- Monitor for complications.
- If a multi-lumen line is being used, ensure no drugs are given via the distal port where the CVP is being monitored. This lumen often gets flushed or primed, and the patient may receive a sudden injection of a drug, which could have a dramatic effect.

Cervical collar application

Cervical collars are devices used to immobilize the necks of patients whose mechanism of injury may have caused a C-spine injury. Patients need to stay immobilized in a cervical collar until their C-spine has been 'cleared' of possible injury (→ see C-spine assessment, pp. 688–9).

Indications

→ See C-spine assessment, pp. 688–9.

Equipment

- Selection of different sizes of hard collar.
- Measuring device (optional).
- Two people to apply the collar (person 1 to hold and stabilize the neck; person 2 to apply the collar).
- Head blocks and straps.

Application

- Explain the procedure to the patient and/or relatives.
- Check motor and sensory function of the hands and feet prior to collar application.
- Prior to collar application, the patient should be positioned with the spine in alignment. Using your hands to support the neck, slowly move the head until the neck is straight and the head faces forward.
- Person 1: ideally approach the patient from behind, placing both hands on either side of the face and neck. Spread the fingers out along the occipital ridge, and hold firmly. Maintain this position until both the collar and head blocks are in place.
  - ▶ *Do not let go until procedure is completed.*
- Person 2: measure the patient for the correct size of collar, following the manufacturer's instructions.
  - ▶ It is important that you are familiar with the types of collars available, how they are sized/measurement for the correct fit, and how they are put together.
  - Ensure the chin support is folded out on the collar.
  - Before applying the collar, remove any earrings and necklaces to ensure no metal will obscure X-rays or scanned images.
- Person 2: slide the back of the collar under the back of the neck, taking care not to move the head or neck. Sweep the front of the collar under the chin, so that the chin sits on the chin rest, and fasten securely.
- Person 1: as the collar is applied carefully, move the hands out over the collar, so that, when the collar is secured, your hands are not inside.
- If the patient has been sitting during collar application, they can be sat on a trolley with the backrest upright. Gradually move the backrest to a flat position.
- At this stage, the neck is stable in the collar, but not fully immobilized until the head has been secured with some form of immobilization device, e.g. head blocks and tape, spinal board.

- In patients who are cooperative, the care of the immobilized C-spine is usually uncomplicated. They should be managed in a well-observed area with O$_2$, suction, and a call bell to hand.

Considerations

- ⚡ ❗ In adults or children who are uncooperative/combative for whatever reason, the continuous presence of a nurse is mandatory.
- The airway is at risk from vomiting or secretions, and the adult/child may try to remove immobilization devices.
- ⚡ ❗ The combative adult/child should be managed in whatever way is possible, without using forcible restraint, as this ↑ the risk of further injury to the C-spine. Children may be most settled on a parent's knee, with a collar *in situ*.

Chest drains

A chest drain is used to drain or 'decompress' the contents of the pleural space. Most commonly, air occupies the pleural space. Following trauma, blood is more likely. Occasionally, other fluids may be present such as chyle, pus, or gastric/oesophageal contents. As contents fill the pleural space, the underlying lung expansion is restricted, and the lung 'collapses'. Pneumothoraces are classified as:

- spontaneous/simple pneumothorax—a non-expanding collection of air around the lungs/pleural space, caused by an injury to the lung tissue or spontaneous rupture of a pleural bulla;
- tension pneumothorax—an expanding collection of air in the pleural space, which can be life-threatening if left untreated;
- open pneumothorax—caused by penetrating trauma, as air allowed into pleural space via a wound—classically an 'open sucking chest wound';
- haemothorax—a collection of blood in the pleural space, usually caused by blunt or penetrating trauma or occasionally through the erosion of pulmonary vessels by a tumour.

Indications Symptoms vary, depending on the amount of air/fluid in the pleural space. A small pneumothorax may have relatively few symptoms. The larger the area of 'collapse', the more significant the respiratory distress and the need for intervention with a chest drain ± needle thoracocentesis. Presenting symptoms may include:

- respiratory distress: breathlessness; tachypnoea; confusion;
- ↑ work of breathing, accessory muscle use;
- pleuritic chest pain;
- pallor, greyness progressing to cyanosis;
- reduced air entry on the affected side;
- unequal chest rise;
- reduced SpO_2;
- hyper-resonance to percussion on the affected side in pneumothorax;
- dullness to percussion on the affected side in haemothorax;
- sucking chest wound in an open pneumothorax;
- deviated trachea, distended neck veins, hypotension/shock in tension pneumothorax.

Equipment

- Two-tier trolley.
- Sterile dressing field, gloves, and gown/apron.
- Chest drain insertion pack: scalpel, instrument for blunt dissection.
- Hand-held suture (e.g. 1.0 silk).
- 1% lidocaine.
- Syringes.
- Needles: green and orange.
- Skin-cleansing equipment.
- Transparent dressing.

- Chest drain. Size depends on whether air or fluid needs to be drained and on the weight of the patient. Wider-bore tubes are needed to drain blood. To drain blood/fluid in an adult, use a size 28 Ch tube or larger. It is increasingly common to use smaller-bore Seldinger chest tubes (usually size 12 Ch) to drain air. In children, the smallest possible tube should be used. ❶ Use ➔ Table 21.5 as a guide for tube sizes in children.
- Bottle of sterile water.
- Chest drainage system with tubing.
- Transparent dressing to secure the drain. A large dressing is not necessary.

Preparation
- Prepare the chest drain bottle. Connect to the chest drain when inserted.
- Using sterile technique, open the chest drainage system.
- Pour sterile water into the drainage bottle until it reaches the prime level.
- Connect one end of the tubing to the drainage system.
- The other end of the tubing is inserted into the chest drain.

Patient preparation
- Explain the procedure to the patient and/or relatives.
- Obtain patient consent.
- Assist with positioning the patient. This depends on the site of the chest drain.
- Ensure SpO_2, HR, and BP are monitored.
- Ensure pain is scored, and analgesia is given.
- Ensure O_2 therapy is administered, as required.
- Ensure the patient has patent IV access and IV fluids as required.

Table 21.5 Paediatric chest drain sizes (for draining blood/fluid)

Weight of patient (kg)	Chest tube size (Fr)
<3	8–10
3–5	10–12
6–10	12–16
11–15	17–22
16–20	22–26
21–30	26–32
>30	32–40

Care following insertion of the chest drain

- Continue monitoring cardiovascular/respiratory status. Record observations.
- Rescore pain, and give further analgesia as indicated.
- Check the chest drain is bubbling (swinging) at regular intervals. (Air and water in the chest drainage system move with each inspiration/expiration.)
- Bubbling chest tube only to be clamped under specialist supervision.
- Do not allow the chest drain or tubing to 'kink'.
- Ensure the chest drainage system is protected from accidentally being knocked over by securing on a stand to the ED trolley.
- Do not allow the chest drain to be lifted higher than the insertion site.
- Ensure a repeat CXR is ordered.
- Monitor and record any fluid drainage every 15min for the first hour, every half hour for the next 2h, and hourly thereafter.

▶▶ Alert the clinician for the patient if >500mL of blood drained. May need: urgent cross-match; rapid IV infusion of warmed fluids/blood; ABG.

C-spine assessment

The assessment, protection, and clearance of a potential C-spine injury is critical, as poor management can lead to significant morbidity and mortality. Most patients who require C-spine protection and clinical assessment are already immobilized with appropriate devices in the prehospital setting. However, patients will often self-present with a significant injury that must be suspected in the first instance and then managed correctly.

▶ There are potential pitfalls, especially when the mechanism is unclear or the patient is vague about their symptoms.
- *Always* have a high index of suspicion in the elderly or where a significant mechanism has been involved.

Indications for assessment and possible imaging of the C-spine

Step 1
- Clinical suspicion of a neck injury and GCS score of 15.
- Is there any paraesthesiae in the extremities?
- Are they ≥65y?
- Is there a potentially dangerous mechanism?
  - fall from ≥1m or five stairs;
  - axial load to the head;
  - high-speed motor vehicle collision (>60mph);
  - rollover or ejection from vehicle;
  - bicycle collision or motorized recreational vehicle.
- Are there any prior neck problems (making the neck more vulnerable)?
  - ankylosing spondylitis;
  - rheumatoid arthritis;
  - spinal stenosis;
  - previous cervical surgery.

Yes
If the answer is yes to any of the queries in Step 1, apply a hard collar, and use an immobilization device. A C-spine X-ray will be required as a minimum.

Equipment
- Appropriately sized collar.
- Immobilization device.

Patient preparation
Explain the procedure to the patient, ensuring they understand the need to remain still whilst the assessment takes place.

Collar application
➔ See Cervical collar application, pp. 682–3.

No

If the answer is no to all of the queries in Step 1, the assessment continues to Step 2, to identify if there are any 'safe assessment features'.

Step 2: are there any safe assessment features?

- Simple rear-end collision.
- Comfortable in a sitting position.
- Ambulatory since the time of injury and no midline C-spine tenderness.
- Delayed onset of neck pain.

No safe assessment features

⚠ Apply a hard collar, and use an immobilization device. A C-spine X-ray will be required as a minimum.

One or more safe assessment features

The presence of one 'safe assessment feature' indicates that it is safe to assess the range of movement of the neck as in Step 3.

Step 3: range of movement assessment

Has the patient got 45° left and right lateral rotation?

- If the answer is *yes*, the patient does not require C-spine immobilization.
- ⚠ If the range of movement is limited or painful, apply a hard collar, and use an immobilization device. A C-spine X-ray will be required as a minimum.

Further reading

See National Institute for Health and Care Excellence. Available at: ℘ http://www.nice.org.uk.

Defibrillation—manual

Indications

Defibrillation is used in the treatment of VF and pulseless VT. Prompt defibrillation offers the greatest chance of survival in cardiac arrest.

Equipment

- Defibrillator.
- Appropriate adhesive defibrillation pads.
- Towel to dry the chest.
- Razor for any chest hair.

Safety

⚠ Safety during defibrillation is of paramount importance. The clinician who delivers the shock has ultimate responsibility for the safety of the patient and the team. When delivering defibrillation, the aim is to have minimal interruption to CPR. The person doing cardiac massage continues cardiac massage, whilst the defibrillator is being charged, and only stands clear when shock is about to be delivered.

Procedure

- Call for help.
- Ascertain that it is safe to approach.
- Confirm cardiac arrest: the loss of consciousness with the absence of a carotid or femoral pulse.
- Switch on the defibrillator, and select the appropriate energy level (this will be dependent on the monitor).
  - In adults, the biphasic energy is 150J.
  - ⊕ In children, the biphasic energy is 4J/kg.
- Prepare the chest. Ensure that it is dry, that any chest hair that may prevent the adhesive pads from having good contact is removed, and that any jewellery or metal-based patches are removed.
- Ensure the monitor is reading the rhythm through 'pads'. Apply the pads (there is a diagram on each pad indicating where it should be placed)— one pad to the right of the sternum, just below the clavicle; the other to the fifth/sixth ICS in the left anterior axillary line.
  - ▶ Pads must be placed at least 12.5cm away from a pacemaker (➔ see Fig. 21.9).
- Once the pads are in place, check the monitor, and confirm the cardiac arrest rhythm. If the rhythm is pulseless VT or VF, prepare to shock the patient.
- In a loud, clear voice, inform all other clinicians, except the person carrying out cardiac massage, to 'stand clear' and that you are 'charging the defibrillator'.
- Simultaneously, perform a visual check of the immediate area and all the staff, ensuring that no one is in direct or indirect contact with the patient.

- Instruct the person managing the patient's airway to 'take the oxygen away' if it is not a sealed unit. Ensure that this is done.
- As you are about to deliver the shock, shout 'stand clear'. The person carrying out cardiac massage should now stand clear.
- Perform a further visual sweep of the patient and bed area to confirm that there is no direct or indirect contact with the patient.
- Finally, confirm that the patient remains in a shockable rhythm, and deliver the shock.
- Immediately after the shock is delivered, start/resume BLS.

Defibrillation—using an automated external defibrillator

Indications

For use in cardiac arrest in and out of hospital. Prompt defibrillation offers the greatest chance of survival in cardiac arrest.

Equipment

- AED.
- Appropriate adhesive defibrillation pads.
- Towel to dry the chest.
- Razor for any chest hair.

Safety

⚠ Safety during defibrillation is of paramount importance. The clinician who delivers the shock has ultimate responsibility for the safety of the patient and the team. When delivering defibrillation, the aim is to have minimal interruption to CPR. The person doing cardiac massage continues cardiac massage, whilst the defibrillator is being charged, and only stands clear when shock is about to be delivered.

Procedure

- As soon as the AED is available, switch it on, and attach the pads. Ensure the chest is bare and dry.
- Ensure CPR is interrupted and nobody is touching the patient, whilst the AED assesses the rhythm.
- Follow the spoken instructions.
- If a shock is indicated, deliver it. Fully automated AEDs will deliver the shock automatically.
- Immediately re-start CPR.
- Continue to follow spoken prompts.

Diagnostic peritoneal lavage

Diagnostic peritoneal lavage (DPL) is the introduction of a catheter into the peritoneum, so that fluid can be instilled into the peritoneal cavity and drained out. DPL is infrequently performed in resuscitation rooms, with the advent of bedside USS and the ↑ availability of CT scans. However, there may be occasions when USS and CT care are not available and an injured patient requires an urgent diagnosis of any intra-abdominal pathology. Alternatively, peritoneal lavage with warmed fluids is indicated in the rewarming of hypothermic patients (➔ see Hypothermia, pp. 574–5).

Indications
- Rewarming in hypothermia.
- Blunt abdominal trauma. DPL is 98% sensitive, but with a low specificity.

Equipment
- Peritoneal catheter.
- Scalpel.
- LA.
- Skin-cleansing solution.
- Gloves, mask, gown, apron.
- Sterile drapes.
- 1L bag of warmed saline plus giving set.
- Catheter drainage bag.

Patient preparation
- Explain the procedure to the patient.
- Ensure the patient has adequate IV access.
- Assist the patient into a comfortable lying position, and expose the abdomen when the procedure is about to start.
- Obtain consent.
- NG tube: it is important to decompress the stomach.
- Urinary catheter: it is essential that the bladder is empty.

Procedure
DPL is usually performed by a surgeon.
- The skin is cleaned; LA is used to infiltrate the area, and a scalpel is used to make a small incision below the umbilicus.
- The surgeon identifies the peritoneum and makes a small incision into it to introduce the peritoneal catheter. At this stage, blood may ooze from the incision site, giving a positive result.
- If no obvious blood is seen, a giving set primed with warmed fluid is attached, and 1L of saline is infused via the catheter into the peritoneum.
- The empty fluid bag can then be placed lower than the patient's abdomen, and the fluid drains back into the bag.
- The fluid that has drained from the peritoneum is then observed for blood, bile, or faeces.
- If the DPL is negative, the incision will be closed in layers, and a dressing applied.
- If the DPL is positive, the patient is likely to go to theatre for a laparotomy.

Special considerations

- DPL will not diagnose a ruptured diaphragm or retroperitoneal haemorrhage.
- In the obese, it is technically difficult to perform.
- During the procedure, air can be introduced to the peritoneal cavity. X-rays of the chest or abdomen may have air visible on them.

DPL for active rewarming in hypothermia

- The peritoneal catheter is inserted.
- A volume of 500–1000mL of warmed fluid is infused into the peritoneal cavity and left *in situ* for 10–20min.
- The fluid is then drained out and replaced with more warmed fluid.

Donway splint

The Donway splint is a pneumatic traction splint for use in patients with a fractured shaft of femur. It is washable and reusable, and X-rays can be taken to demonstrate the position of the fracture after the splint is applied.

Indications

Early splinting of a femur fracture has several benefits: pain relief; stabilization of the fracture site (which can help prevent the development of a fat embolism); prevention of further damage to muscle, vessels, and soft tissue from the fractured bone ends; and a reduction in blood loss.

Equipment

- An appropriately sized splint comprising:
  - one extended U-shaped ring;
  - one ischial ring (black padded semicircle with strap and buckle);
  - two leg supports (broad black perforated plastic straps);
  - one knee strap;
  - one foot plate;
  - one heel stand;
  - one ankle strap;
  - one pneumatic pump;
  - one pressure gauge.

Application of the splint

- Explain the procedure to the patient and/or relatives.
- Check the pedal pulse is present and distal sensation is intact.
- Ensure the patient has received adequate analgesia, including a femoral nerve block. Entonox® may be required when the splint is fitted.
- Lie the patient on a trolley, exposing the injured leg.
- Place the ischial ring around the uppermost part of the injured leg, and secure using a belt.
- Place the affected limb in the U-shaped frame, resting the limb on the leg supports.
- Ensure the patient's foot rests on the foot plate, and secure the ankle tightly using the straps. Finish strapping the ankle with a figure of eight over the back of the foot plate. It is important to spend time applying the ankle strap correctly and tightly, or the splint will be ineffectual.
- Secure the ischial ring into the side arms of the U-shaped frame, and ensure the screw-lock caps are released.
- Gently extend the splint by pumping air in, using the pump, to a pressure of 10–14 pounds/square inch (green area of the pressure gauge). Once the splint has been extended, the patient's pain should diminish.
- Once the required traction has been achieved, lock the screw caps, and release the pressure by pressing the air release valve (orange valve beside the pressure gauge). The heel stand can be used but may cause the splint to topple over.
- Recheck the pedal pulse and distal sensation.
- Document the splint application and neurovascular status of the limb.

ECG recording

Equipment needed

- ECG machine with ten leads and clips for the adhesive tabs.
- Adhesive tabs.
- Clippers.
- Towel.

Preparation

- Check the ECG machine is set to the standard mode of recording, 25mm/s, and the standard calibration of 10mm/mV.
- Explain the procedure to the patient and/or relatives.
- Inform the patient that the best recording will be obtained when relaxed and still.
- Ensure the patient's privacy and dignity are maintained, as the chest needs to be exposed.
- Position the patient reclined, either on a trolley or bed.
- There needs to be access to the skin of the chest, arms, and lower legs to allow correct placement of adhesive tabs. To maintain dignity, the patient's chest can be covered once the leads are attached correctly.
- Remove any excess chest hair with clippers.
- Dry any damp skin with a towel. This gentle exfoliating motion also improves the contact of the adhesive tabs.

Placement of adhesive tabs and ten leads

Limb leads

(➔ See Fig. 8.2.)

- Place the tabs on the four limbs, e.g. shins or ankles, shoulders or inner wrists.
- Attach the limb leads which are either labelled or colour-coded:
  - red lead—right arm (RA);
  - yellow lead—left arm (LA);
  - green lead—left leg (LL);
  - black lead—right leg (RL).

Precordial or chest leads

(➔ See Fig. 8.1.)

The correct position for the placement of the chest leads is as follows.

- V1: fourth ICS, right sternal border;
- V2: fourth ICS, left sternal border;
- V3: midway between V2 and V4;
- V4: fifth ICS, left mid-clavicular line;
- V5: left anterior axillary line at the same horizontal* level as V4;
- V6: left mid-axillary line at the same horizontal* level as V4 and V5.

---

* At right angles to the mid-clavicular line.

Attach the chest leads, labelled V1–V6. When recording an ECG on a ♀ patient, it is conventional to place electrodes V4–V6 under the left breast. Although it is acknowledged that attenuation of the signal does not change when electrodes are placed over the breast, there is insufficient published evidence to support this.

Right-sided leads

Are mirror images of normal left-sided leads and may be requested when ST segment elevation in V1 and V2 is noted on standard ECG. Right-sided leads can more accurately determine an RV infarction.

- The limb leads are placed in the standard position;
- V1r: fourth ICS, left sternal border;
- V2r: fourth ICS, right sternal border;
- V3r: midway between V2r and V4r;
- V4r: fifth ICS, right mid-clavicular line;
- V5r: right anterior axillary line at the same horizontal* level as V4;
- V6r: right mid-axillary line at the same horizontal* level as V4 and V5.

*At right angles to the mid-clavicular line.

⚠ The ECG machine does not usually recognize that leads are not in the standard position. Therefore, the labelling needs to be clearly changed on all chest leads. The right-sided leads are usually labelled with an 'r'.

Posterior leads

Indicated when there is a tall 'R' wave in V1, ST segment depression in V1 and V2, and tall upright T waves are noted on standard ECG. Posterior leads more accurately determine a posterior infarct.

- The limb leads are placed in the standard position.
- All the chest leads are removed.
- Ask the patient to lean forward, as three tabs have to be placed on the posterior chest.
- Place the first tab at the same horizontal* level as V6 in the posterior axillary line—this is V7.
- Place the next tab between V7 and V9—this is V8.
- Place the final tab at the same horizontal* level as V6 next to the vertebral column—this is V9.

*At right angles to the mid-clavicular line.

⚠ The ECG machine does not usually recognize that the leads are not in the standard position. Therefore, the labelling needs to be clearly changed. There will only be three chest leads on this ECG, and they should be relabelled V7, V8, and V9.

✪ Paediatric considerations

Use paediatric tabs. Pad position same as in adult.

Recording the ECG

- Enter the patient's details, name, and other identifiers into the ECG machine.
- Ensure the patient is relaxed and still.
- Press the 'record' button.
- Avoid using any filter buttons, unless interference from muscle movement makes it difficult to interpret the ECG.
- Ensure the ECG is a good trace; disconnect the leads, and maintain patient dignity.
- If any cardiac signs or symptoms, document them on the ECG.
- The ECG should be shown to a clinician able to interpret it, to ensure any urgent medical treatment can begin.
- Ensure the equipment is cleaned and tidied away, ready for next use.
- Inform the patient of the results.

Troubleshooting

- AC interference/artefact. Remove any electrical equipment, if possible; ensure the leads are untangled; check the adhesive tab contact, and ensure the patient is not touching metal.
- Wandering baseline. Check the adhesive tab contact; check the patient is not moving or that there is no 'pull' on the leads.
- Tremor. Usually due to patient movement. Ensure the patient is not cold and is as relaxed as possible.

Eye irrigation

Eye irrigation is an urgent procedure and is indicated when there is any chemical splash in the eye/s. Patients with any chemical in their eye/s will be allocated a high triage priority for immediate irrigation. The commonest irrigating fluid is normal saline (0.9%), but sterile water is also appropriate. When neither of these fluids is immediately available, tap water is an adequate substitute and is often used in the prehospital setting.

Equipment

- pH paper.
- Irrigation fluid, bag of IV 1L of normal saline 0.9%.
- IV giving set.
- Gloves.
- Receiver.
- Towels.
- Anaesthetic drops (reduce pain and enable the patient to cooperate).

Procedure

- Protect the patient's clothing with a towel. It may be easier for the patient to remove their top clothes and wear a gown.
- If immediately available, use pH paper to ascertain the pH of the chemical.
- Remove contact lens.
- Instil LA eye drops, and repeat, as necessary, during the irrigation.
- Position the patient with the head inclined to the affected side.
- Prime your giving set with your fluid, bringing the roller clamp close to the end of the line to ensure better control.
- Ask the patient to hold the receiver close to their eye to collect the irrigation fluid.
- Alternatively, if appropriate and a sink is available, the patient can lean over the sink.
- Hold the patient's eye apart, using your first and second fingers against the orbital ridge.
- Direct the fluid from the nasal corner outwards, and ask the patient to move their eye in all gaze directions.
- Evert the lid to ensure that any particles have been removed. Remember to examine the lower fornix.
- To thoroughly cleanse, a minimum of 1L of fluid should be used.
- Recheck the pH.
- Dispose of the equipment.
- Check the patient's VA.
- Document the procedure and pH measurements in the patient's notes.
- If the pH does not return to normal after irrigation with 2L of saline, an ophthalmologist must be consulted immediately.

❶ All, but the most trivial of, injuries should be referred to an ophthalmologist.

❻ Eye irrigation can be impossible in young children. Tap water is a reasonable substitute.

Eyelid eversion

Upper eyelid eversion is a routine procedure when examining a patient with an eye injury. It should also be done during eye irrigation, especially if there is particulate matter in the eye, as some may remain under the lid despite copious irrigation. Lid eversion is a simple procedure, once mastered, and can be practised on willing colleagues or relatives. If the upper lid is very swollen, lid eversion is much more difficult—document any failed attempts clearly in the notes.

Equipment
- Cotton bud.
- LA eye drops, if needed.
- Good lighting.

Patient preparation
Some patients become very anxious if you describe the procedure in detail, and, in those cases, it may be wiser just to inform them you are checking under their upper eyelid.

Procedure
(➔ See Fig. 21.10.)
- Wear gloves. However, if the patient has very short eyelashes, it can be difficult to feel them with gloves on.
- Instil LA eye drops if the eye is painful.
- Instruct the patient to 'look down' with their eyes, as if trying to see their shoes. Keep the head in a neutral position.
- Dry the eye/eyelashes with a swab if they are wet.
- Grasp the eyelashes in the middle of the upper eyelid, and pull outwards, stretching the lid away from the globe.
- With the tip or side of the cotton bud, gently press down on the middle of the upper lid, and 'flip' the tarsal plate over the bud.
- Inspect under the lid.
- Remove any FB with the cotton bud.
- Release the lashes, and return the lid to the normal position.

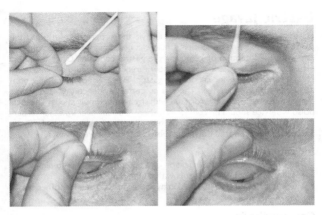

Fig. 21.10 Eyelid eversion.

Gastric lavage

Gastric lavage is the passage of a tube via the orogastric route into the stomach, so that small amounts of fluid can be administered and siphoned out, with the intention of removing the gastric contents. Once a routine procedure in EDs, gastric lavage is now rarely performed. Following toxicology research, the indications for gastric lavage in accidental and non-accidental ingestion are few. There is no certain evidence that it improves clinical outcome, and it is associated with significant complications. The local poisons service should be contacted if there is doubt over whether to perform gastric lavage. If lavage is indicated, 50g of activated charcoal may be indicated. This is poured down the tube just before its removal.

Indication
- The only indication is the ingestion of a potentially life-threatening amount of poison that presents within 60min of ingestion.
- The instillation of warmed fluid in hypothermia (➔ see Hypothermia, pp. 574–5).

Contraindications
- Loss of protective airway reflexes, unless intubated and ventilated.
- Ingestion of a corrosive material.
- Patients with oesophageal varices or other pre-existing medical or GI problem that may be adversely affected by lavage.

Complications
- Laryngospasm.
- Aspiration.
- Oesophageal perforation.
- Hypoxia.
- Hypercarbia.
- Trauma to the throat and larynx.
- Bradycardias.

❶ Combative patients are more at risk of complications.

❶ Because of possible serious complications, two members of staff with advanced airway management skills and experience of performing lavage *must* carry out the procedure.

Equipment
- Gastric lavage tube with funnel-type attachment and mouthpiece airway.
- Two large buckets: one empty, the other with lukewarm water.
- pH paper.
- Jug.
- O_2.
- Suction.
- Lubricating jelly.
- Continuous monitoring. Ideally, the procedure should be performed in a resuscitation room.
- Gloves, aprons, floor protection (sheets, towels), and shoe covers.

- 50g of activated charcoal, if prescribed.
- Towels to protect the patient, patient gown.

Patient preparation

The procedure must be explained to the patient, and verbal consent gained. If consent is refused, the procedure must not be performed; uncooperative patients are at significant risk, and performing a procedure without consent is assault. Explain to the patient that a plastic tube will be passed into their stomach through their mouth, so that the 'tablets' can be washed out with warm water. The procedure is not painful but is uncomfortable. Patients often feel that they cannot breathe. Reassure them that the tube will be immediately removed if any problems are encountered.

The patient should be undressed and put in a gown, as their clothing is likely to become wet. Transfer the patient to an appropriate area with O_2, suction, and monitoring. Position them in the left lateral position with a 20° head down tilt; their left arm should be behind their back.

⚠ If the patient has an altered level of consciousness or loss of protective airway reflexes, they *must* be intubated prior to the procedure.

Procedure

- One member of staff performs the procedure; the other has responsibility for holding the patient's head/neck, managing the airway, and observing the vital signs. The patient is likely to vomit during the procedure, as he/she 'gags' on the orogastric tube—airway management is vital.
- Protect the floor with towels/sheet, so that staff do not slip if spillages.
- Protect the patient's bed sheet. Place a plastic-backed pad under the head/neck.
- Hold the tube to the patient's nose, and measure the approximate length to the epigastrium. This is the approximate length of the tube that should be inserted.
- Ensure the bed is at a reasonable height, so that gravity assists in the drainage of the gastric contents.
- Insert the mouthpiece. This prevents the patient from biting down on the orogastric tube and occluding it.
- Lubricate the end of the tube with jelly.
- Insert the tube through the mouthpiece and into the patient's mouth. Tell them to swallow the tube when they feel it at the back of their throat.
- Push the tube into the mouth/throat. Once the patient swallows, continue to push the tube into the stomach until you reach the measured length.
  - ⚠ Force must *not* be used.
- Once tube in place, hold the 'funnel' end into an empty bucket, and wait until gastric secretions drain out. Drop a pH paper into the bucket; ensure it changes colour and confirms a pH <4 to indicate gastric secretions. Alternatively, air can be instilled, whilst listening over the stomach with a stethoscope. 'Gurgling' over the stomach confirms correct placement.

- Once correct placement of the tube confirmed, the lavage can begin. Slowly instil 200–300mL of warm water down the tube; tip the funnel end into the bucket, and allow the water to siphon out. Repeat until the lavage fluid runs clear. This may take 5–10 instillations of water.
- Instil charcoal, if prescribed.
- Remove the lavage tube.
- Help the patient into a comfortable position, and assist with hygiene needs.

⚠ If the patient shows any sign of airway compromise or respiratory difficulty, the tube should be immediately removed.

Inhaler technique

When adults and young people are discharged home after receiving emergency asthma treatment, their inhaler technique should be checked. Poor technique and lack of knowledge about the importance of regular inhaled therapies can contribute to a worsening of symptoms and the need to seek emergency care.

There are many inhalers available and as many spacer devices. However, a metered dose inhaler (MDI) is the device most commonly used and stocked in emergency care areas to be given out at discharge.

Step-by-step use of an MDI

- Remove the cap, and shake the inhaler.
- Breathe out gently.
- Place the mouthpiece in the mouth, and, as you begin to breathe in, press the canister down, and continue to inhale steadily and deeply.
- Hold your breath for 10s (or as long as comfortable).
- Wait for 30s before taking any additional doses, and follow the above steps again.
- ▶ Only use the inhaler for the number of doses stated on the label; then start a new inhaler.

ⓘ If a patient has difficulty using an MDI, a spacer can be used. This is routine in younger children.

Further reading

Asthma UK. Available at: ℜ http://www.asthma.org.uk.

● Intraosseous insertion

An IO needle is an alternative to IV access and is most commonly used in cardiac arrest and critical illness in children. There is ↑ use in adult practice. In cardiac arrest (unless IV access is already established), the IO route should be used. In other situations, when a child is critically ill or injured, do not waste time trying to establish an IV line; an IO needle should be used. IO needle insertion is not a skill limited to medical staff. ED nurses can learn and use it in an emergency (● see Fig. 21.11).

Equipment

- IO needle.
- Skin-cleansing solution.
- 3-way tap with a short 10cm extension.
- Fluid giving set.
- 20mL/50mL syringes.
- 500mL normal saline.
- Saline flush.
- First-line resuscitation drugs, fluid bolus.
- Splint for the limb, if required.
- Tape.

Site selection

- The commonest site is the proximal tibia 2.5cm below the knee (or one finger breadth) on the flat anteromedial surface.
- Other sites include the distal tibia, proximal humerus, and sternum in adults.
- Limbs where there is a fracture above the chosen site must not be used.

Patient preparation

- Expose the site for insertion.
- LA can be used if the child is not unconscious.
- Clean the skin.
- Explain the need for the procedure to parents/carers.

Complications

- Infection.
- Fracture.
- Extravasation—if IO placed in proximal tibia, ensure limb observations are recorded. Compartment syndrome is a risk in the event of extravasation.

Procedure

- Flush a 3-way tap and 10cm extension with saline. Have a 5mL syringe available and first-line resuscitation drugs.
- Support the limb, but do not hold it underneath the site for insertion.
- Hold the IO needle firmly, with the butt of the needle in the palm of your hand and with 'gloved' fingers close to the tip of the needle. Holding the needle too near to the butt reduces tactile control.

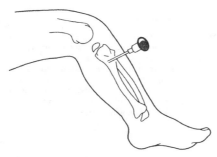

Fig. 21.11 Tibial intraosseous access.
(Reproduced with permission from Wyatt, J. et al. (2012). Oxford Handbook of Emergency Medicine, 4th edn, fig. 15.1, p. 641. Oxford University Press, Oxford.)

- Place the needle onto the bone, aiming at 90° or at an angle away from the knee if the flat anteromedial surface of the tibia is your chosen site. Insert with a twisting action (or a rotating action if the IO needle is based on a screw design). The twisting action resembles the 'bevelling' of a hole.
- There are a number of mechanical devices available—ensure you are trained and competent to use them.
- Continuous pressure is required until there is a loss of resistance as the IO needle enters the cortex.
- Remove the stylet. Attach a 5mL syringe, and aspirate a 'bone marrow' sample. Often this proves impossible. If sample obtained, send for U&E, FBC, or cross-match.
- Flush the needle with 10mL of saline (use the previously prepared 3-way tap with extension). Observe for leaking around the insertion site and/ or swelling of local tissues.
- Attach the fluid giving set to the 3-way tap. Fluid boluses can be administered from the IV fluid via the tap.
- The IO needle is typically 'stable' within the cortex of the bone. The use of a 3-way tap with a 10cm extension reduces the risk of accidental removal of the IO needle by reducing local movement as syringes are attached or removed. Application of tape and a splint can improve stability.
- All drugs can be administered via an IO needle.
- Insertion of an IO needle with a power drill (e.g. EZ-IO) is similar to that described above but is generally easier and faster to achieve.

Nursing care of the IO needle
- Examining the site and local tissues to identify leaking reduces adverse risk.
- Remove the needle once IV access is reliable. This is the best risk reduction strategy.

Minor injury treatments

There are numerous 'minor' treatments that are completed each day in emergency care. The treatment of 'minor' injuries may seem very simple and sometimes even mundane. However, the injury may have a significant impact on the patient's daily life. The time taken to give a clear explanation of the injury, the expected recovery, and the important features of self-care are essential in shortening the recovery phase and preventing unplanned follow-up. Ideally, all verbal advice should be given in written form, so that it can be referred to at a later date. ⏻ The following minor treatments apply equally to adults and children.

Neighbour/buddy strapping

Indications

For fractures, or sprains of fingers and lesser toes. NB. The great toe should not be strapped to the second toe. Injuries to the great toe can be treated with a toe spica.

Equipment

- Gauze.
- Adhesive tape (non-elasticated).
- Scissors.

Patient preparation

- Explain the procedure to the patient.
- Strapping toes can be painful.

Procedure

- Expose injured fingers or toes.
- Fold one piece of gauze, and cut to the length and width of fingers/toes.
- Cut two lengths of tape; use one piece of tape to strap the proximal phalanx together, the other to strap the middle phalanx.
- Ensure strapping is comfortable and not too tight; check capillary refill.

Discharge advice

- Advise the patient to keep the fingers/toes strapped for as long as the injury requires; most strains/sprain need early mobilization.
- If the digit is swollen, advise about the importance of elevation.
- Advise about pain relief.
- Advise about work/school, contact sport, and other activities that the patient may regularly undertake.
- Advise about follow-up, and how and when to seek further help if problems persist.

Slings

Broad arm sling

Indications

To support an injured shoulder or arm, or to elevate a swollen upper limb.

Equipment
- Triangular sling.
- Tape or nappy pin.

Patient preparation
- Explain the procedure to the patient.
- Place the arm in the correct position, usually with the shoulder and elbow at 90°.

Procedure
- Locate the 90° angle on the sling. Holding this with one hand, slide the sling under the injured arm, so that the 90° angle is at the patient's elbow.
- Put the uppermost corner of the sling over the opposite shoulder.
- Bring the lower corner of the sling over the injured arm, and tie the two ends behind the neck.
- Secure the elbow in the sling with tape or a safety pin.

Discharge advice
- Advise the patient about whether to wear the sling under or over their clothes (this will depend upon the injury).
- Patients do not usually have to sleep in a sling.
- Advise about the importance of elevation, especially if the limb was swollen.
- Advise about pain relief.
- Advise about work/school, contact sport, and other activities that the patient may regularly undertake.
- Advise about follow-up, and how and when to seek further help if problems persist.

High arm sling

Indications

To reduce swelling of the hand, wrist, forearm, or fingers, or to help control haemorrhage.

Equipment
- Triangular sling.
- Tape or nappy pin.

Patient preparation
- Explain the procedure to the patient.
- Place the arm in position, with the shoulder and elbow at 90°.

Procedure
- Locate the 90° angle on the sling. Holding this with one hand, slide the sling under the injured arm, so that the 90° angle is at the patient's elbow.
- Put the uppermost corner of the sling over the opposite shoulder.
- Bring the lower corner of the sling over the injured arm, and tie the two ends behind the neck.
- Secure the elbow in the sling with tape or a safety pin.
- Place the hand of the injured arm on the opposite shoulder.
- Fold the now loose sling up and over the arm, and secure with a nappy pin.

Discharge advice
- Advise about the importance of elevation.
- Advise about pain relief.
- Advise about work/school, contact sport, and other activities that the patient may regularly undertake.
- Advise about follow-up, and how and when to seek further help if problems persist.

Collar and cuff

Indications
- Fracture of the humerus.
- Elbow injury/fracture.
- Post-reduction of a dislocated shoulder.

Equipment
- Collar and cuff.
- Tie fastener.
- Elastic adhesive tape.
- Scissors.

Patient preparation
- Explain the procedure to the patient.
- Place the arm in position, with the shoulder and elbow at 90°.

Procedure
- Cut the required length of collar and cuff foam by measuring against the patient.
- Encircle in a figure of eight around the neck and wrist of the injured arm.
- Secure with a tie fastener; cut the unused end off.
- Cover the tie fastener with elastic adhesive tape, so no sharp edges are exposed.
- Check for circulation by checking the radial pulse and observing the colour and sensation of the hand.
- Ensure the patient can slip the collar over the head and hand.

Discharge advice
- Advise the patient about whether to wear the collar and cuff under or over their clothes (this will depend upon the injury).
- Patients may have to sleep in the collar and cuff. Wearing a snug fitting T-shirt over the collar and cuff will help keep the arm secure by the patient's side.
- Advise about pain relief.
- Advise about work/school, contact sport, and other activities that the patient may regularly undertake.
- Advise about follow-up, and how and when to seek further help if problems persist.

Splints and thumb spica

Wrist splint

Indications
- Soft tissue injuries.
- Tenosynovitis.

Equipment
- Correct-sized splint (small, medium, large, or extra large, and in right or left).

Patient preparation
- Explain the procedure to the patient.
- Expose the patient's forearm and wrist.

Procedure
- Position the wrist brace with a metal bar running along the palmar aspect of the wrist.
- Place Velcro™ straps across the dorsum of the wrist and between the thumb and index finger.
- Ensure the wrist brace fits snugly around the wrist, allowing full movement of the fingers and thumb. The patient may be able to adjust the fit more easily.

Discharge advice
- Advise the patient about when to wear the splint and for how long (this will depend upon the injury).
- Advise about pain relief and NSAIDs, if appropriate.
- Advise about work/school, contact sport, and other activities that the patient may regularly undertake. If the patient has been prescribed the wrist brace for tenosynovitis, they may have to wear it for prolonged periods.
- Advise about follow-up, and how and when to seek further help if problems persist.

Thumb spica

Indications
- Fractures of the thumb.
- Soft tissue injuries of the thumb.

Equipment
- 5cm crêpe bandage.
- Adhesive tape.
- Beware of possible allergy.

Elastoplast® tape can be used for a thumb spica, but there is no evidence to support the use of crêpe over Elastoplast®. Elastoplast® is more difficult to apply and painful to remove. Therefore, crêpe should be used when there is no clear rationale for Elastoplast®.

Patient preparation
- Explain the procedure to the patient.
- Expose the patient's wrist, hand, and thumb.
- Ask the patient to hold their wrist in a neutral position and extend their thumb.

Procedure
- Anchor the bandage around the wrist several times.
- Place the bandage, from the wrist to around the tip of the thumb, in a figure of eight.
- Continue the figure-of-eight bandaging down the thumb until all the thumb and thenar eminence are supported.

Discharge advice
- Advise the patient about wearing the spica and for how long (this will depend upon the injury).
- Advise about pain relief and NSAIDs, if appropriate.
- Advise about work/school, contact sport, and other activities that the patient may regularly undertake. Advise about follow-up, and how and when to seek further help if problems persist.

Mallet splint

Indications
- Mallet deformity ± a fracture.

Equipment
- Gauze.
- Non-elastic tape.
- Mallet splints of various sizes.

Patient preparation Explain the procedure and the role of the mallet splint to the patient.

Procedure
- Wrap a thin layer of gauze around the finger. This provides padding and absorbs perspiration.
- Fit the appropriate-sized splint. The splint should force the DIPJ into 10–15° extension and not be too tight. If there is swelling at the DIPJ, the rest of the splint may appear loose. Several sized splints may need to be fitted until the 'best fit' is found.
- Tape in place around the base of the splint over the middle phalanx.

Discharge advice
- Advise the patient about continually wearing the splint.
- Arrange follow-up, and refer for splint care. Advise how to remove the splint, and to keep the DIPJ in extension to wash the finger and then to reapply the splint.
- Advise about work/school, contact sport, and other activities that the patient may regularly undertake.

Trephining

Indications

Recent subungual haematoma causing pain and discomfort. Old haematomas that have clotted under the nail will not drain.

Equipment

- Gauze.
- Trephining tool. Most tools generate intense heat to burn through the nail.
- Dressing.
- Eye protection is essential.

Patient preparation

Explain the procedure to the patient, reinforcing that it is not painful and will immediately relieve symptoms.

Procedure

- Lay the patient down.
- Place the hand/foot on a flat, hard surface.
- Gently apply the trephining tool until a give is felt and blood escapes. This should be done in the centre of the nail, not over the nail bed.
- Apply gentle pressure to the pulp of the digit until all the blood has been released.
- Apply a dressing.

Discharge advice

- Advise the patient about pain relief.
- Advise the patient about elevation of the limb, if appropriate.
- Advise about work/school, contact sport, and other activities that the patient may regularly undertake.

Mobility assessment

Many patients who have accessed emergency care will require an assessment of their mobility prior to discharge. A comprehensive mobility assessment is usually done by a physiotherapist or occupational therapist. However, there are many instances when a brief assessment of mobility is made by the emergency care clinician.

Indications

- Prior to discharge in any patient who is known to have a mobility problem.
- Prior to discharge in any patient with an injury that has the potential to affect their mobility.

To assess

- Is the patient safe to mobilize independently (with or without the use of walking aids)?
- Is the patient safe to transfer from sitting/lying to standing position independently (with or without the use of mobility aids)?
- Is the patient able to stabilize themselves and walk around the cubicle/bed area with no assistance needed (with or without walking aids)?

If there is doubt about the need for a comprehensive mobility assessment, request physiotherapy/occupational therapy input.

Tips for observation

- Observe the patient transfer from bed/trolley to standing position.
- Observe the patient sitting down and standing up from an appropriately sized chair.
- Observe the patient mobilize around the bed area for a distance of at least 2m.

▶ Two health-care professionals should perform a mobility assessment. Both assessors should stand close to the patient to allow for support and stabilization, if needed.

Key questions

What is the patient's existing mobility? Confirm this with relatives or carers. Patients often overestimate their usual level of function.

- Will the patient be safe at home alone or with family members?
- Will the patient need a new walking aid? If so, the patient must be trained on the appropriate use of such an aid.

Nasal packing

Indications

Nasal packing is frequently performed in emergency settings when simple first aid measures and/or cautery fail to stop an epistaxis. Both nostrils must always be packed, so that pressure is applied to the septum from both sides. It is rare to have to perform this procedure on children.

Equipment

- Two-tier silver trolley.
- 2 × expanding foam tampons.
- Apron and sterile gloves.
- Sufficient light.
- LA spray: lidocaine.
- Dressing pack or sterile field and gauze.
- Receiver.
- 2 × syringes with 10mL of sterile water.
- Naseptin® or other antibiotic nasal cream.
- Tape.

Patient preparation

This is an unpleasant procedure for the patient. Whilst not usually painful, it can be distressing, and some patients are not able to tolerate it. It is crucial that what needs to be done, why, and what it will be like is clearly explained, so the patient knows what to expect. Reassure them that it will be over quickly and, in almost all cases, is successful in stopping the bleeding.

Depending upon how much the patient is able to cooperate with the procedure, a second person may be required, i.e. to hold the receiver.

Procedure

- Position the patient sitting upright, either in a chair or on a trolley.
- Have a light positioned, so that patient's face is well lit.
- Prepare the trolley, dressing pack, and gauze.
- Prepare each tampon, coating each side liberally with antibiotic cream. This eases insertion and prevents infection.
- Ask the patient to blow their nose. This will remove any clots and allow the tampons to be more easily inserted.
- Ask the patient/second person to hold the receiver at the patient's mouth, so that blood and/or clots can be spat out.
- Spray each nostril with LA spray.
- Insert the first tampon into the nostril that is bleeding. Push (the end without the cotton) horizontally along the floor of the nostril. This has to be done firmly and may cause the patient some distress. Push until it will not go any further; the end with the cotton should be just visible. (How much of the tampon is inserted will depend, to some extent, on the size of the patient's nose.)

- Put the tip of a water-filled syringe directly on the exposed tampon, and soak the tampon. The tampon will swell and fill the nostril.
- Insert a second tampon into the other nostril as above.
- Tape the cotton to each side of the face.
- Help the patient wash and clean their face.
- Prepare the patient for admission.

Nasogastric tube insertion

Indications

NG tube insertion is usually indicated in the following emergency situations: perforated peptic ulcer; bowel obstruction; multiple trauma; pancreatitis; and in some cases of persistent vomiting. Ventilated adults and children also need an NG tube to decompress the stomach, which can improve ventilation. ❸ Some adults and children are managed at home with an NG tube for feeding and may attend the ED if the tube 'falls out'.

Contraindications

- Severe mid-face trauma.
- Recent nasal surgery.
- Recent banding of oesophageal varices.

Equipment

- Apron and gloves.
- NG tube (select an appropriate size).
- 50mL catheter tip syringe.
- Drainage bag and spigot.
- Lubricant.
- pH indicator strips.
- Cup of water.
- Tape.

Cooling the NG tube in a fridge for 20min can sometimes ease its passage, as it stiffens the tube.

Patient preparation

This is an unpleasant procedure. It makes the patient retch and feel as if they cannot breathe. Many patients cannot tolerate the procedure and may stop you proceeding. Gain verbal consent. Explain the procedure to the patient and the reasons why an NG tube is required. Assist the patient into a comfortable position, ideally sitting upright on a trolley. Explain to the patient their role in the procedure, which is:

- to signal by raising their hand if they want the procedure to stop;
- to drink water and swallow when they are instructed to; this will be when they feel the tube at the back of their throat.

Procedure

- Measure the approximate length of the NG tube. Take the tip of the tubing, and place at the epigastrium; place the tubing up the patient's chest, over the ear, and to the bridge of the nose. Note the point on the tubing at the level of the nose; the tubes have centimetre markings on them. This is the length of the tube that should be passed.
- Ensure the patient is ready to proceed and understands the procedure.
- Lubricate the tip of the NG tube.

- Insert the tip of the tube into the nostril. Pass the tubing along the floor of the nostril, ensuring there is no resistance. If resistance occurs, withdraw the tubing slightly, and advance again carefully at a slightly different angle. Rotating the tube slowly whilst advancing can help. Do not force.
- As the tubing advances and the patient feels it at the back of their throat (which is when you may feel some slight resistance), offer them water to drink. This should enable them to swallow the NG tube and ease its passage into the stomach.
- The patient may cough and retch. This is normal, and you should continue to try to pass the tube. However, if the patient is distressed, raises their hand, or appears to have difficulty breathing, remove the tube immediately.
- Continue to pass the tube until the marker you have noted is at the nostril.
- Secure the tube with tape to the nostril and side of the face.
- Check for correct insertion into the stomach by aspirating the NG tube and measuring the pH of the aspirate to make sure it is <5.5.
- Ensure that a CXR is ordered to check the exact site of the tube.
- Spigot the tube, or apply a drainage bag.

Complications

- Inadvertent passage down the trachea and into the pulmonary tree.
- Failure to pass into the stomach (sometimes the tube can coil up at the back of the throat).
- Epistaxis.

Needle thoracocentesis

Needle thoracocentesis is the initial procedure used to correct a tension pneumothorax. A tension pneumothorax is a life-threatening condition and needs to be dealt with rapidly by this method. A needle thoracocentesis is a temporizing measure and must be followed up by an immediate chest drain (➔ see Chest drains, pp. 684–6).

Signs and symptoms of a tension pneumothorax

- Respiratory distress: breathlessness; tachypnoea; confusion.
- ↑ work of breathing, accessory muscle use.
- Pallor, greyness progressing to cyanosis.
- Little or no air entry on the affected side.
- Little or no chest rise on the affected side.
- Reduced SpO_2.
- Hyper-resonance to percussion on the affected side.
- Deviated trachea.
- Distended neck veins.
- Hypotension/shock.

Patient preparation

This is an immediately life-threatening situation, and the procedure has to be performed rapidly. The patient is critically hypoxic and, in many cases, comatose. A quick and brief description of the procedure should be given when and if appropriate.

Equipment

- Skin-cleansing product as per local protocol.
- A 14G cannula.
- Chest drain equipment.

The clinician will clean the skin and insert the cannula into the second ICS, mid-clavicular line on the affected side. As the cannula needle is removed, air will be released, and a 'hiss' should be heard. A chest drain then needs to be inserted.

Nursing role

- To continuously monitor ABC.
- To monitor vital signs, especially O_2 saturations and RR, and inform the treating clinician of improvement or deterioration.
- Apply high-flow O_2.
- Ensure adequate analgesia has been provided.
- Prepare for a chest drain.

Neurological assessment: the Glasgow Coma Score

The GCS is a key component of a neurological assessment and, together with an assessment of the pupils, limbs, and vital signs, can provide a bedside assessment of cerebral function. GCS assesses and monitors the conscious level in patients who have an actual or potential neurological problem. It assesses the integrity of normal brain functioning and, when repeated at regular intervals, can identify if the patient's neurological function is improving or deteriorating. The GCS was developed for assessing the conscious level of adults. A modification has been developed for use in children—the 'Children's Glasgow Coma Score' (CGCS).

The GCS assesses and scores three parameters:
- eye opening;
- verbal response;
- motor response.

How to record GCS

Eye response
- Score 4. Eyes open spontaneously. The patient is seen to be awake with eyes open. The patient should be aware of your presence.
- Score 3. Eyes open to verbal command. Do not touch the patient. Speak to the patient in a normal voice first. Then, if necessary, gradually raise the volume of your voice.
- Score 2. Eyes open to painful stimuli. Initially, to avoid distress, touch or shake the patient's shoulders. If there is no response to this, inflict a painful stimulus (➋ see Box 21.2).
- Score 1. No eye opening. There is no response to painful stimuli. Only score when satisfied that sufficient stimulus was applied.

Verbal response
- Score 5. Orientated. The patient is orientated to time, place, and person.
- Score 4. Confused. The patient is unable to say who they are, where they are, and why, and the current year and month.
- Score 3. Inappropriate words. Words that are not understandable or things said in an incorrect context.
- Score 2. Incomprehensible sounds. More often making sounds in response to a painful stimulus, rather than conversation. Moaning, groaning, or crying sounds, instead of formed words.
- Score 1. No verbal response. Unable to produce any speech sounds in response to a verbal or painful stimulus.

Box 21.2 **Painful stimuli**

- Supraorbital pressure. Just below the inner aspect of the eyebrow is a small notch through which a branch of the facial nerve runs. The nurse should use their thumb to press this area for a maximum of 30s.
- Trapezium squeeze. Hold the trapezium muscle between the thumb and forefinger, and apply, gradually increasing the pressure, for a maximum of 30s.

Motor response
- Score 6. Obeys commands. The patient accurately responds to instructions, e.g. stick your tongue out.
- Score 5. Localizes to pain. The patient will move their hand to the point of stimulus, in an obvious coordinated attempt, to remove the cause of the pain.
- Score 4. Withdrawal from pain. The patient will move in a purposeful way away from the stimulus, but the response is not specific to the site of stimulus.
- Score 3. Flexion (decorticate posturing). The patient flexes their elbows and rotates their wrists inwards.
- Score 2. Extension (decerebrate posturing). The patient straightens their arms at the elbow and internally rotates their shoulders. Often the legs are also in extension with the toes pointing down.
- Score 1. No motor response. No movement at all.

▶ Important considerations
- Sometimes it is difficult to accurately assess the GCS, e.g. in patients with learning disabilities. If you are unsure of the assessment, double-check the GCS score with a colleague.
- Sleeping patients should always be woken, e.g. it should never be presumed that a child with a head injury is 'just sleeping'.
- Ideally, the same person should perform the GCS assessment; this ensures consistency in assessment.
- The painful stimuli used should be documented and consistently used in each assessment.
- When the patient is handed over to another nurse or transferred out of the emergency care area, there should be formal handover of the GCS and agreement between the two clinicians as to what the GCS is at that time.
- Establishing and documenting a normal baseline in patients who already have some degree of neurological abnormality are vital. Assessing the GCS in patients with dementia and cerebral palsy, for example, can be difficult. Relatives and carers can give vital information about what is 'normal' for the patient and if they perceive any change in behaviour or functioning.

Neurological assessment: other tests

Assessing pupil reaction

Pupil size and reactivity are a measure for the function of CN III, the oculomotor nerve. Any rise in ICP will eventually put pressure on this nerve, causing its function to be impaired and pupil reactions altered.

- Use a bright light. Covering one eye and shining the light in the other assess pupillary response. Repeat for the other eye.
- The light should be brought in from the side of the patient's face twice.
- The two eyes should then be compared at the same time for pupil equality.

In intubated patients who have been paralysed and sedated (by anaesthetic drugs), this is one of the only ways of monitoring neurological status and any ↑ in ICP.

A sluggish pupillary response can indicate some CN III compression. A fixed and dilated pupil indicates CN compression on the affected side. When both pupils are fixed and dilated, this indicates significantly raised ICP and brainstem herniation.

⚠ Be aware of the effects of drugs on pupillary response, e.g. drugs such as opiates or recreational drugs.

Limb response

Assessment of limb movement identifies if there is any upper or lower, unilateral or bilateral limb weakness. Each limb should be assessed separately.

- Arms. Tell the patient to hold the arms out in front. Look for signs of weakness or drift.
- Legs. Ask the patient to push and pull the feet towards the assessor, or ask the patient to raise their legs off the bed and to hold them there for a short amount of time.
- If a limb does not move, then a painful stimulus needs to be applied to that limb to assess if this elicits any response.

Vital signs

Hypertension, bradycardia, and respiratory irregularity are the cardinal signs of significantly raised ICP. Patients with a GCS <15 should have their observations recorded half-hourly for 2h, then 1-hourly for 4h, and then 2-hourly after that if no significant changes occur.

❶ Neurological assessment in children

A neurological assessment, including GCS, has to be performed in children in emergency care areas frequently, most commonly in head injury. For children aged ~5y and over, the standard adult GCS assessment can be performed. However, in preverbal-/preschool-age children, the verbal and motor assessment elements have to be modified.

GCS in children <5y

Eye response
- Score 4. Eyes open spontaneously. The child is seen to be awake with eyes open. The child should be aware of your presence.
- Score 3. Eyes open to verbal command. Do not touch the child. Speak to the child (or ask a parent/carer to do so) in a normal voice first; then, if necessary, gradually raise the volume of your voice.
- Score 2. Eyes open to painful stimuli. Initially, to avoid distress, touch or gently shake the child's arm or shoulders. If there is no response to this, inflict a painful stimulus (➐ see Box 21.2).
- Score 1. No eye opening. No response to painful stimuli. Only score when satisfied that sufficient stimulus was applied.

Verbal response
- Score 5. Smiles. An alert infant, contented with their parent.
- Score 4. Cries. A child who will not settle with a parent.
- Score 3. Inappropriate cries. At times, cries out; not related to being disturbed.
- Score 2. Occasional whimper. Less frequent cries; may be associated with occasional whimper.
- Score 1. No verbal response. Unable to produce any sounds in response to verbal or painful stimulus.

Motor response
- Score 6. Obeys commands; spontaneous movement. Spontaneous, normal movements for the child.
- Score 5. Localizes to pain. Withdraws to touch.
- Score 4. Normal flexion. Withdraws from pain.
- Score 3. Abnormal flexion (decorticate posturing). The child flexes their elbows and rotates their wrists inwards.
- Score 2. Extension (decerebrate posturing). The child straightens their arms at the elbow and internally rotates their shoulders. Often the legs are also in extension with the toes pointing down.
- Score 1. No motor response. No movement at all.

Oxygen delivery

O_2 delivery is integral to many aspects of emergency care treatment in adults and children. Selecting the correct device to deliver supplemental O_2 ensures that the patient's O_2 needs are met.

Head box oxygen

Used for supplemental O_2 in neonates and infants. Supplemental O_2 fills a Perspex™ box placed over the baby's head. A gauge measures the concentration of O_2 in the box, which can be titrated against O_2 saturations.

Nasal cannulae

Can deliver 24–40% O_2 at flow rates of 1–5L/min. They are often used for patients who have O_2 at home. Nasal cannulae can also be useful for patients who only require low concentrations of O_2 and cannot tolerate a face mask. Flow rates >4L/min are very drying to the nasal passages and can be uncomfortable.

Oxygen (Venturi) mask

A Venturi mask mixes room air with O_2 through a flow valve and can deliver settings of 24%, 28%, 35%, 40%, and 60%, depending on which valve is attached. Venturi masks are particularly useful when there is concern about CO_2 retention.

Simple face mask

A simple face mask (often used in prehospital settings) delivers 40–60% O_2 at flow rates of 5–10L/min.

Non-rebreathing face mask with reservoir

If patients require >40% O_2, the use of a non-rebreathing mask should be considered. With a tight-fitting mask and the reservoir bag inflated, 85–90% O_2 concentrations can be delivered with a flow rate of 10–15L/min.

Bag–valve–mask ventilation

For patients who require more active respiratory support, a BVM, with a reservoir, good face mask seal, and flow rates of 10–15L/min, delivers ~90% O_2.

Paediatric considerations

Forcing O_2 therapy on a child should be avoided, as this ↑ their work of breathing and O_2 demand. Various techniques using play and turning the therapy into a game can be used to gain a child's trust and cooperation. Parents are often key in enabling O_2 to be administered. Holding free-flowing O_2 in the general direction of the child's face may be the only compromise possible in a distressed child.

▶ Routine O_2 should be prescribed.

Pain assessment and management

Pain assessment and its subsequent management are an integral part of every clinical assessment in emergency care and should be regularly reassessed. There are few emergency care presentations that do not have a painful element. Failure to adequately manage pain can have serious consequences: ↑ anxiety; violence; aggression; distress for the patient or relatives; dissatisfaction with care; and physiological deterioration.

There are many challenges to be faced when managing pain, the first being appropriate assessment, which is not an easy task. Pain assessment must take the following variables into consideration: age; culture; previous pain experiences; level of anxiety; ability to use pain assessment tools; and activity disruption.

The four 'As' of effective pain management in emergency care are:
- assess: pain score;
- administer: give pain interventions promptly;
- appropriate: ensure the interventions are appropriate;
- assess again: reassess after a period of time.

Pain assessment

The effectiveness of pain management cannot be assessed without a baseline measurement, which is most commonly represented as a score out of 10: 0/10 = no pain, and 10/10 = the worst possible pain. A pain assessment tool that combines a behavioural tool, verbal descriptor tool, and visual analogue scale can be used for adults and children in emergency care settings (➔ see Fig. 21.12a). ❸ Face scales are also valuable for assessing pain in younger children (➔ see Fig. 21.12b). ❸ Assessing pain in children and those with cognitive problems is particularly challenging. Parents and carers are especially valuable in assisting with pain assessment in these situations.

Pain intervention

The 3 'Ps' for pain intervention are:
- practical: splinting; elevation; slings; pillows; wound dressings; relocation of dislocation; treatment of the cause, e.g. acute retention;
- psychological: distraction; explanation; reassurance; play;
- pharmacological: simple analgesia; compound analgesia; NSAIDs; opiate analgesia; local/regional anaesthetic; Entonox® nerve blocks.

Severity of pain Pain can be classified as mild (0–3/10), moderate (4–6/10), or severe (7–10/10). Linking pain scoring to triage priorities ensures that moderate/severe pain is dealt with swiftly.

All severities of pain will require practical and psychological interventions. For pharmacological intervention, ➔ see Table 21.6.

Pain reassessment

This is the final element of pain management. It must never be assumed that pain interventions have been successful. The clinician must reassess the patient's pain after an appropriate time interval and provide further intervention if and when necessary.

Table 21.6 Pharmacological interventions in pain management

Severity of pain	Analgesia
Mild	Simple
Moderate	Simple/compound ± NSAID
Severe	Opiate

(a)

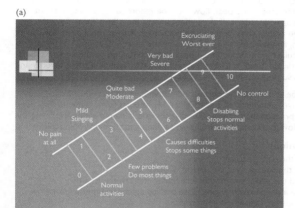

(b)

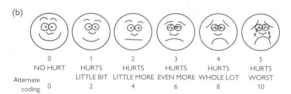

0	1	2	3	4	5
NO HURT	HURTS LITTLE BIT	HURTS LITTLE MORE	HURTS EVEN MORE	HURTS WHOLE LOT	HURTS WORST
Alternate coding 0	2	4	6	8	10

Fig. 21.12 (a) Manchester pain ladder.

(Adapted with permission from Manchester Triage Group (2005). *Emergency triage*, 2nd edn. Wiley–Blackwell Publishing, Oxford.)

(b) Face scale.

(Reproduced with permission from Hockenberry, M.J., Wilson, D., and Winkelstein, M.L. (2005). *Wong's essentials of pediatric nursing*, 7th edn, p. 1259. Mosby, St. Louis.)

Peak flow measurement

Peak flow is an objective measure of lung function and is predominantly used for assessing patients with new onset of asthma or to monitor patients with known asthma. Patients with established asthma should regularly record their peak flow, as a reduction can indicate early deterioration in lung function. Often patients do not know their baseline peak flow when well or the 'best' peak flow they have ever performed.

Measuring peak flow is a crucial assessment parameter in diagnosing the severity of an asthma attack and then in monitoring the response to inhaled or IV therapies. The peak flow *must* be recorded on arrival in all patients attending with asthma. If the patient knows their 'best' peak flow, the percentage against their best can be calculated. If their usual peak flow is not known, an estimate can be made using the chart in ➔ Fig. 21.13.

Calculating the reduction in peak flow, compared to the patient's 'best' or predicted 'best', is a key element in the diagnosis of asthma severity and guides subsequent treatment.

❸ A peak flow can be performed, depending on individual ability, usually from age 6 upwards (➔ see Fig. 21.14), though some patients may need more practice than others. Good technique is essential in performing the peak flow for accurate recording, and a demonstration may help achieve this.

Technique

- Put the pointer to zero.
- Ask the patient to stand upright, if possible.
- Hold the peak flow mouthpiece horizontally to the mouth.
- Take a deep breath in, and close the lips tightly around the peak flow mouthpiece, making a good seal.
- Blow into the peak flow meter hard and fast. It should be like blowing out a candle, rather than blowing up a balloon.
- Three attempts should be made, with a check on the technique each time. The best (highest) reading should be recorded.

Poor technique is common. Often patients either fail to make a tight seal around the mouthpiece with their lips or do not 'blow' quickly enough or hard enough.

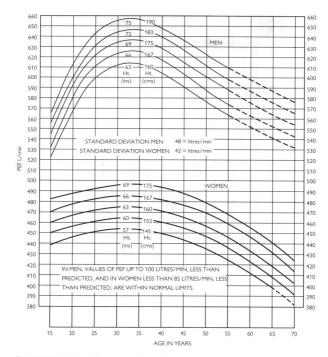

Fig. 21.13 Adult peak expiratory flow chart.

(Reproduced with permission from Wyatt, J., *et al.* (2012). *Oxford Handbook of Emergency Medicine*, 4th edn, p. 105. Oxford University Press, Oxford.)

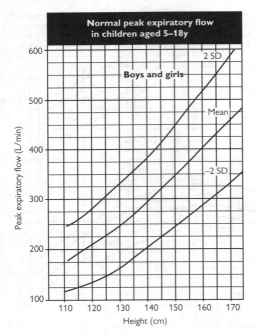

Fig. 21.14 Paediatric peak expiratory flow chart.

(Adapted from Godfrey, S., Kamburoff, P.L., and Nairn, J.R. (1970). Spirometry, lung volumes and airway resistance in normal children aged 5 to 18 years. *British Journal of Diseases of the Chest* **64** (1), 15–24. © 1970, with permission from Elsevier.)

Pelvic fixation

Major pelvic fractures are a true orthopaedic emergency. They are often associated with massive blood loss, which can be life-threatening if the fracture is unstable. If an unstable fracture is suspected, an external pelvic binder should be applied. The patient's ankles/feet should also be brought together, as this helps to rotate the hips and stabilize the pelvis. Patients with suspected pelvic fractures often have an external pelvic binder applied in the prehospital setting. If already applied, these should not be removed in the ED, unless a pelvic fracture has been excluded. Pelvic binders should be applied in the ED if a pelvic fracture is suspected.

External fixation can control any further haemorrhage by preventing the movement of the pelvis but is rarely applied in the ED—it is more likely to be done in theatre. If an unstable fracture is suspected, an orthopaedic surgeon must be involved early in the patient's care.

Indications
- Uncontrolled hypovolaemic shock from a pelvic fracture.
- Unstable pelvic ring fracture.

Equipment
- External pelvic fixator set.
- Scalpel.
- LA.
- Skin-cleansing solution.
- Mask, gloves, gown/apron.
- Sterile drapes.
- Skilled operator, usually an orthopaedic surgeon.
- An image intensifier, if available.

Patient preparation
- Explain the procedure to the patient and/or relatives.
- Obtain consent.
- Expose the pelvis.
- Continuous vital sign monitoring.
- Ensure adequate fluid resuscitation.
- Ensure adequate pain relief.
- Assess and document the femoral and popliteal pulses.

Procedure
- The skin is cleansed, and LA infiltrated into the proposed sites for insertion.
- Small incisions are made into the skin at the insertion sites.
- The metal frame is inserted into the sites on the pelvis, under an image intensifier, if possible.
- The frame is then coupled together, and the various pieces tightened together until the frame is complete and secure.

Considerations

If the patient does not require external fixation or a device is not readily available, a sheet can be used. Place a sheet under the patient's pelvis, and tie the ends together. There are various manufactured 'pelvic binders' available that can also be used.

Pericardiocentesis

Pericardiocentesis (also called pericardial tap or percutaneous pericardiocentesis) is used to remove excess fluid from the pericardial sac. When a pericardial effusion has developed over some time, the procedure can be performed electively. In emergency situations, the haemopericardium has to be drained immediately. The pericardial sac has filled rapidly with blood, and cardiac filling and emptying are grossly impaired.

↑ amounts of pericardial fluid may result from:
- trauma (penetrating and non-penetrating): can result in life-threatening amounts of blood in the pericardial sac (cardiac tamponade)—a resuscitative thoracotomy should be considered;
- MI, CCF;
- pericarditis caused by chest trauma, MI, infection, inflammation;
- surgery or other invasive procedures performed on the heart;
- cancer producing malignant effusions;
- renal failure.

In emergency care, the procedure is most commonly performed to remove blood from the pericardial sac and relieve the cardiac tamponade.

Signs and symptoms of acute pericardial effusion
- Beck's triad. Distant heart sounds, neck vein distension (due to compression on RA/RV), and hypotension.
- Tachycardia usually occurs due to ↑ venous pressure and ↓ BP, which indicates haemodynamically significant pericardial effusion.
- Tachypnoea will develop in acute situations.
- Narrow pulse pressure can occur in patients with significant pericardial effusion.
- Cardiac arrhythmias and PEA can occur if large effusions.
- Elevated CVP occurs from ↑ pressure in the pericardial space and the ventricles. This condition is usually associated with hypotension.

▶ In the busy resuscitation room, clinical signs can be hard to isolate. An echocardiogram is an invaluable diagnostic tool.

Indications
- Cardiac tamponade due to trauma—a resuscitative thoracotomy should be considered.
- Haemodynamic compromise due to large/rapidly developing pericardial effusion.
- Management of large pericardial effusion (>20mm separation of pericardial membranes on echocardiography).
- In cardiac arrest as a possible reversible cause of PEA.

Contraindications
- Small effusions do not require emergency needle pericardiocentesis.
- Haemodynamically stable patients can be managed conservatively.
- Aortic dissection as a cause for the pericardial effusion.
- Uncorrected bleeding disorder.
- Posteriorly located pericardial effusion.

Equipment

- Two-tier procedure trolley.
- 18–20G cardiac/spinal needle.
- A 3-way stopcock.
- Syringes (10mL, 20mL, and 60mL).
- Antiseptic skin-cleansing solution.
- ECG monitor and defibrillator.
- Specimen collection tubes for fluid analysis and cultures.
- Small-gauge needle for LA and lidocaine.
- Sterile gloves, mask, gown, dressing materials, and gauze.
- Resuscitation drugs.
- Sedating medications, if required.
- There are manufacturers who produce pericardiocentesis kits with the correct needles and drains needed.

Patient preparation

- This emergency procedure has to be performed rapidly. Patients are critically ill with profound haemodynamic compromise. Explain the procedure clearly to gain consent if the patient is conscious.
- Sedation may be administered if the patient is restless or anxious.
- Position the patient upright at ~45° angle.
- Tell the patient to remain still, and support throughout if conscious.
- Cardiac monitoring and vital signs are recorded throughout the procedure.

Nursing role

- Support the patient during the procedure. The patient may experience a sensation of pressure, as the needle enters the membrane.
- Monitor vital signs and cardiac rhythm during pericardiocentesis. If the myocardium is stimulated by the needle, ST segment elevation will be noted on the ECG, and the needle will need to be withdrawn slightly.
- When the needle is in the correct position, the clinician will withdraw blood from the pericardial sac with a syringe.
- A pericardial catheter may be attached to the needle to allow for continuous drainage of blood.
- After the cardiac needle is removed, pressure is applied to the puncture site for ~5min, and the site is then dressed.
- Continuous vital signs and cardiac monitoring.

▶ It is often reported that the blood aspirated from a haemopericardium does not clot in the syringe, as the fibrin has been inactivated by the movement of the heart.

Patients often make a dramatic recovery immediately after pericardiocentesis; their conscious level, BP, and cardiovascular status improve.

Complications

- Laceration of coronary artery/vein.
- Acute LVF with pulmonary oedema.
- Puncture or laceration of any cardiac chamber.
- Bleeding.
- Ventricular/atrial ectopic beats.
- Arrhythmias.
- Hypotension.
- Pneumothorax.
- Pulmonary oedema.

Plastering skills

Applying a POP or fibreglass cast is commonly done to immobilize a limb, following a fracture or other significant injury. Plastering is one of the commonest skills used in emergency care, and a large range of casts may need to be applied. You may find that there are several ways of applying the same plaster, and each clinician may have a slightly different approach. This section describes the general principles for applying common casts in adults and children.

Patient preparation

- Check you have the right patient, and identify the correct limb.
- Check the patient notes and X-rays, and ensure the plaster prescribed is appropriate for the injury.
- Inform the patient of the procedure and rationale for applying the plaster.
- Obtain the patient's consent.
- Identify any allergies or sensitive skin conditions.
- Ensure adequate pain relief. This is crucial to enable the limb to be positioned correctly.
- Assist the patient into the most comfortable, appropriate position.
- Remove clothing, as appropriate, from the affected limb.
- Make sure you are at a comfortable height, and have assistance to hold the limb, if necessary.
- Remove rings, watches, and bracelets from the limb to be plastered.
- Check the skin is intact. If there are any wounds, ensure they are cleaned, ± closed and dressed, as appropriate.
- Protect the patient's clothing from the wet plaster.
- Assess and document the neurovascular status of the limb (colour, sensation, capillary refill).
- Formal assessment of VTE risk should be undertaken.

Plaster application—general principles

- Collect the correct-sized stockinette, padding, plaster, and bandages if a back slab is being applied.
- Apply adequate padding smoothly and evenly.
- Each plaster bandage should be soaked individually.
- Water should be lukewarm, and the patient informed that, when the plaster is applied, it will feel warm and that this is normal (due to the thermogenic reaction of the setting plaster).
- Roll on the plaster bandage, starting from one end of the limb. Cover 50% of the previous turn, keeping the bandage smooth and without applying tension.
- When the required number of bandages has been applied, smooth with water, so that each layer bonds together.
- Clean the patient's skin where any plaster has come into contact.

Discharge assessment and information

- Assess the ability to perform ADLs, social circumstances, and available support. Refer to social services/intermediate care, if necessary.
- Patients should be advised of the importance of elevation in reducing swelling, pain, discomfort, and complication.
- Give written and verbal 'plaster care instructions' (➜ see Box 21.3).
- Ensure adequate discharge analgesia.
- Arrange follow-up.
- Supply necessary walking aids.

Fibreglass casts

These are often used after the initial swelling has settled or if a below-knee walking cast is required. The principles for application are similar to those for POP, with several important caveats.

- Gloves must always be worn, as the adhesive resin within the fibreglass does not wash off skin.
- Clothing must be protected, as the resin will not wash off clothing.
- Great care should be taken around the edges of the cast, and extra padding applied. As there is no 'give' in a fibreglass cast, the edges remain hard and can be rough, causing skin irritation, blistering, and even cuts.
- The importance of elevation should be emphasized, as fibreglass is a rigid structure and can quickly become too tight.

▶ Back slab casts are most commonly applied in the ED as the first cast because of the risk of swelling. Full casts are often applied a few days later.

Box 21.3 Plaster care instructions

- Do not get the plaster wet.
- Keep the limb elevated.
- Do not walk on a lower-limb plaster, unless instructed to do so.
- Keep the fingers/toes moving.
- Return if your fingers/toes become painful, blue, numb, or difficult to move, or you experience pins and needles—the plaster may be too tight.
- Return if the plaster becomes loose, cracked, or damaged in any way.

Upper limb casts

Below-elbow back slab

This plaster provides support yet allows for any swelling in the initial period post-injury.

Equipment
- Stockinette.
- Wool padding.
- POP (cut to reach from 1cm proximal to the metacarpal phalangeal joint (MCPJ) and 2cm from the elbow; folded to give 6–8 layers).
- Bandage.
- Scissors.
- Warm water (25–35°C).
- Gloves.
- Apron.
- Sling.

Application
- Apply the stockinette to the limb, cutting a hole for the thumb.
- Apply padding from the knuckles to the elbow crease, overlapping each previous layer by 50%.
- Trim the plaster slab to round the corners, and cut out a triangle at one end to allow movement of the thumb.
- Ensure the patient's elbow is resting on a firm surface, the wrist in a neutral position, and the fingers and thumb outstretched.
- Wet the plaster slab, and apply to the forearm; the wrist should be in a neutral position.
- Smooth to the contours of the arm, and fold over the stockinette to a neat edge.
- Secure with pre-soaked bandage, including securing through the first web space.
- Finish with a small extra strip of plaster slab to secure a final layer of bandage on top of the slab.
- Apply a broad arm sling, and advise the patient on elevation.

Below-elbow full cast

This cast is used to immobilize the upper limbs, usually for fractures in the distal third of the forearm bones. This cast should extend from just above the knuckles at the back of the hand to allow full flexion/extension of the MCPJs to just below the elbow, allowing full movement at the elbow joint. The thumb should be completely free.

Equipment
- Stockinette.
- Wool padding.
- POP bandage.
- Warm water.
- Gloves.
- Apron.
- Sling.

Application
- Apply the stockinette to the limb, cutting a hole for the thumb.
- Apply padding from the knuckles to the elbow crease, overlapping each previous layer by 50%.
- Position the limb in the required position for the type of fracture.
- Begin bandaging with the wetted plaster bandages at the elbow and down the arm towards the hand.
- Bring the bandage up through the first web space; fold down the stockinette, and catch with the second layer of bandage.
- Mould the cast into the palm to allow the layers to bond.
- Ensure there is adequate room for the thumb to move, without rubbing on the plaster.
- Apply a broad arm sling, and advise the patient on elevation.

Scaphoid cast

This is a below-elbow full cast but includes the thumb to the level of the interphalangeal joint (IPJ), whilst allowing movement of this joint.

Equipment
- Stockinette in two sizes.
- Wool padding.
- POP bandage.
- Warm water.
- Gloves.
- Apron.
- Sling.

Application
- Apply the stockinette to the limb, cutting a hole for the thumb. Cover the thumb with a slimmer length of stockinette.
- Apply padding from the knuckles and around the thumb to below the elbow crease, overlapping each previous layer by 50%.
- Position the limb in the required position for the patient (ask them to maintain a circle with the tips of the thumb and forefinger). The wrist should be in a neutral position.
- Begin bandaging with the wetted plaster bandages at the elbow and down the arm towards the hand.
- Bring the bandage up through the first web space, and go around the thumb.
- Fold down the stockinette on the hand and thumb and at the elbow, and catch with the next layer of plaster. The tip of the thumb from the level of the IPJ should be exposed, and the patient should be able to flex and extend the IPJ.
- Mould well into the palm and around the thumb.
- Apply a broad arm sling, and advise the patient on elevation.

Lower limb casts

Below-knee back slab

This cast provides support and immobilization, whilst allowing for any initial swelling post-injury.

Equipment
- Stockinette.
- Wool padding.
- POP bandage.
- Bandage.
- Warm water.
- Gloves.
- Apron.

Application
- Apply the stockinette to the limb, so that it extends beyond the toes and above the knee.
- Apply padding from below the knee joint to the base of the toes, overlapping each previous layer by 50%.
- Cut a plaster slab of eight layers that extends from the back of the knee to the base of the toes.
- If applying the plaster without any assistance, it will be easier to position the patient prone, with their ankle bent over the edge of the trolley, so it is at a 90° angle.
- Wet the plaster slab, and apply to the lower limb. It should go posteriorly just below the knee, over the ankle, and to the base of the toes. The ankle should be at 90°.
- Smooth to the contours of the leg, and fold over the stockinette to create a neat edge.
- Secure with pre-soaked bandages.
- A long U-shaped slab called a stirrup may need to be added if the cast is immobilizing an unstable ankle fracture. The stirrup is applied down one side of the leg above the ankle, under the heel, and up the other side of the leg to the ankle. This is held in place with a pre-soaked stretch bandage.
- Finish with a small strip of plaster slab to secure the final layer of bandage over the slab.

Below-knee cast

This cast immobilizes the leg for lower limb injuries.

Equipment
- Stockinette.
- Wool padding.
- POP bandage.
- Bandage.
- Warm water.
- Gloves.
- Apron.

Application

- Apply the stockinette to the limb, so that it extends beyond the toes and above the knee.
- Apply padding from below the knee joint to the base of the toes, overlapping each previous layer by 50%.
- Soak the plaster bandage, and apply to the lower limb, starting just below the knee and extending to the base of the toes. The ankle should be held at 90°.
- Smooth to the contours of the leg, and fold over the stockinette to create a neat edge.
- Catch the edges in with a second layer of plaster bandage.
- Smooth to allow the layers to bond together.
- Advise the patient on elevation.

Cylinder cast

This type of cast is used for leg injuries where the ankle does not need to be immobilized. It is usually used for injuries to the knee.

Equipment

- Stockinette.
- Wool padding.
- Felt padding.
- POP bandage.
- Stretch bandage.
- Warm water.
- Gloves.
- Apron.

Application

- Apply a 2in wide strip of orthopaedic felt around the ankle, just above the malleoli.
- Apply the stockinette to the limb, so that it extends from the level of the ankle to the groin.
- Apply padding from the top of the thigh to the ankle, overlapping each previous layer by 50%.
- The leg should be supported, and the knee flexed at 10°.
- Soak the plaster bandage, and apply to the limb. It should start distally just above the bottom edge of the felt padding.
- Smooth to the contours of the leg, and fold over the stockinette to create a neat edge.
- Catch the edges in with a second layer of plaster bandage.
- Smooth to allow the layers to bond together, especially around the medial and lateral sides of the thigh.
- Advise the patient on elevation.

Pulse oximetry

Pulse oximetry is a routine monitoring tool used in most, if not all, emergency care areas. It measures the amount of O_2-saturated Hb in the blood, giving a bedside picture of O_2 requirements.

- ✚ Probes are available for all ages and weights of children and neonates, and can be attached to fingers, hands, toes, feet, or earlobes, depending on their design.
- ► For an accurate reading, it is vital that the correct probe is used and it is attached to the right site.
- In health, O_2 saturations should be >95%; 93–95% is often recorded in patients who smoke.

Equipment needed

- Pulse oximeter.
- Appropriately sized and type of probe.
- O_2 and delivery devices, if required.

Procedure

- Explain the need for pulse oximetry to the patient and/or parent.
- Remove any nail varnish, as this may interfere with the reading.
- Ensure the probe is clean; attach to the patient's finger, ear, or toe, depending on the probe design.
- Observe the trace on the monitor. A poor trace may give a falsely low reading.
- When the trace and signal are of good quality, record the O_2 saturation level.

► Reminders

Pulse oximetry is a quick, non-invasive method of measuring O_2 saturation. However, it has many limitations.

- It is unable to differentiate between Hb that is saturated with O_2 and Hb that is saturated with CO. In CO poisoning, pulse oximetry is of little value in establishing O_2 requirements.
- As the O_2 saturation falls, there is a disproportionate fall in PaO_2. When saturations fall below 90%, there is a dramatic fall in PaO_2.
- If the patient is cold, hypovolaemic, or peripherally vasoconstricted, there may be an artificially low reading.
- In severe anaemia, saturations may be 100%. This is because all the available Hb is saturated with O_2. The probe does not identify when Hb levels are low.
- The pulse oximeter does not detect the retention of CO_2; this is measured by ABG sampling.

Rapid infuser

The rapid infuser enables the rapid infusion of warmed IV fluids and requires *one* dedicated member of staff to operate it. This is a commonplace piece of equipment in resuscitation rooms and other critical care areas. There are many different models in use; it is essential that staff are familiar with how to operate the model in their resuscitation room.

Indication for use

To provide rapid flow of warmed fluid, such as crystalloid or blood product, including RBCs, as volume replacement for patients suffering from blood loss due to trauma or surgery.

Operation

Please refer to the operator's manual for in-depth instructions and alarms.

Equipment

- Disposable rapid infuser set.
- IV fluid.
- Fluid balance recording chart.

Set-up

- Power off.
- Install disposable set.
- Prime disposable set.
- Power on.
- Fluid begins to warm.
- Activate pressure chambers.

Use of fluid warmer

- Ensure set-up has been completed.
- Load the pressure chambers. Ensure the solution bag is hanging on an appropriate hook inside the door.
- Pressurize the pressure chambers.
- Connect to the patient, and begin infusion.
- Change the fluid bag.
  - Release the pressure in the chamber.
  - Close the clamp under the empty bag.
  - Open the door, and remove the used fluid bag.
  - Spike a new bag.
  - Hang the new bag, and close and latch the door.
  - Pressurize the chamber.
  - Open the clamp.
- Record times, types, and volumes of fluid delivered accurately.

After use

- Discontinue infusion.
- Turn the fluid warmer off.
- Release the chamber pressure.
- Remove the disposable set.
- Discard the set in a biohazard container/sharps bin.
- Visually check the condition of the device, and report any problems.
- Clean with warm soapy water.

Sengstaken tube insertion

Sengstaken–Blakemore tubes are used as a salvage procedure. The tube acts as a temporary tamponade for any severe or life-threatening oesophageal bleeding. The tube has three lumens: one to inflate a gastric balloon; one to inflate an oesophageal balloon; and the third to aspirate the stomach.

Indication
• Severe/life-threatening haemorrhage from oesophageal bleeding.

Equipment
• Sengstaken–Blakemore tube (from the fridge).
• Lubricant.
• Manual sphygmomanometer.
• 50mL catheter tip syringes.
• 1L of normal saline.
• Cushioned clamps.
• White ETT tie.
• LA throat spray.

Patient preparation
• Explain the procedure to the patient. It can be unpleasant but is vital in the attempt to control the bleeding.
• Assist the patient into the left lateral position (unless intubated), or sat up to protect the airway.

Procedure
• Check all the balloons inflate and do not leak.
• Hold the tube to the patient's nose, and measure the approximate length to the epigastrium. This is the length of the tube that should be inserted; note the marker on the side of the tube (usually to the 50cm mark).
• Spray the throat with LA, if not intubated.
• The tube is inserted through the mouth. It can also be inserted through the nose.
• Lubricate the tube.
• Insert ~10cm past the marker noted on the side of the tube when it was measured.
• Inflate the gastric balloon with 50mL of air. Then clamp the gastric port. An X-ray is usually done at this point to confirm the position of the balloon is below the diaphragm. The gastric balloon may then be inflated more (up to another 250mL of air). Withdraw the tube until resistance is felt. The tube should be sat below the oesophageal sphincter.
• The oesophageal balloon is not normally inflated, unless the patient continues to bleed. If it is inflated, it should not be inflated with a pressure higher than 45mmHg of air. This should be measured by attaching a 3-way tap to a manual sphygmomanometer at the gastric port and inserting 50–70cc of air.
• The stomach can be aspirated to remove any residual blood. This is done via the aspiration port.

- The tube is then attached to a weight (1L of saline). Using some white ETT tape, this helps to ensure the tube remains *in situ*. The weight can be suspended over the edge of the bed. At this point, the patient's mouth edge should be protected by gauze.
- Support the patient during the procedure, as it can be very distressing, if not intubated.
- Monitor vital signs continuously.
- Give mouth care.
- *Administer fluids or drugs necessary to support the patient's haemodynamic state.*

Complications
- Oesophageal rupture.
- Gastric rupture.

Skin traction: application

Skin traction is always applied prior to the use of a Thomas splint (➔ see Thomas splint application, pp. 758–9) or prior to Gallows traction in children <2y ❶.

Rationale for use of skin traction

- To immobilize and maintain bone alignment by pulling the limb into a straight position.
- To reduce a fracture.
- To relieve muscle spasms.
- To relieve pain.
- To take pressure off the fractured bone ends by relaxing the muscle.
- To prevent further vessel or soft tissue injury.

Equipment

- Correct skin traction pack (adult or child).
- Razor.
- Scissors.
- Bandages.
- Tape.

How to apply leg skin traction

- Both sides of the limb should be shaved, so that the fabric tape can adhere firmly to clean, dry skin.
- Follow steps in Figs. 21.15–21.19.
- Once the bandage is secured, traction can be applied, using standard 5–7lb weights. The pull of the cord must be level with the fabric tape (➔ see Fig. 21.19).
- Assess the distal colour, sensation, and movement of the limb, once the traction has been applied.

Precautions for use

- Avoid creases and wrinkles of the fabric tape, as these could lead to pressure problems and cause ulcers.
- Patients with allergies to tape or Elastoplast® may have a reaction, and their skin should be observed regularly.
- Avoid traction weight greater than that which can be applied through the skin, i.e. not exceeding 7lb.

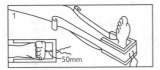

Fig. 21.15 With the foot in dorsiflexion (toes pointing towards the ceiling), place the spreader plate with foam padding inwards towards the sole of the foot. It should be placed at a distance of ~50mm from the sole of the foot. This allows free movement of the ankle joint and protects the ankle and the side of the foot from pressure.

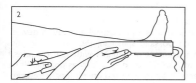

Fig. 21.16 Remove the backing material, and unroll the full skin traction kit up either side of the patient's leg, keeping the spreader plate 5cm from the foot. Smooth the adhesive surfaces of the fabric tape firmly up the leg.

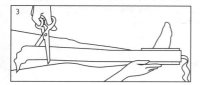

Fig. 21.17 The correct length of the adhesive tape can be determined and cut, as desired, depending on the fracture site. Repeat the procedure for the opposite side of the limb.

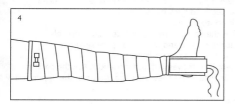

Fig. 21.18 Maximum adhesion can be obtained by application of the retention bandage. Commence bandaging at the ankle with one or two turns initially to secure the fabric tape. Use a firm, but even, tension along the length of the limb.

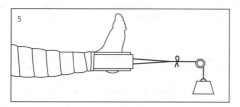

Fig. 21.19 Ensure the patient is on a hospital bed prior to applying the weights, as ED trolleys do not have the correct attachment to attach the weights.

Spinal boards

Spinal boards were originally designed as a prehospital extrication device used to transport patients with possible spinal injuries. They are not designed for the long-term management of patients with spinal injuries, and patients should be taken off a spinal board as quickly as possible. It is increasingly common for patients to be transported on a 'scoop' stretcher and then placed directly onto an ED trolley.

Uses

- The spinal board is a valuable tool for transfer and allows patients to be moved from one place to another without movement of their spine.
- Patients arrive at the ED already on a spinal board. It is rare that patients are put on to a board in the ED.

Equipment

- Hard collar.
- Spinal board and head blocks.
- Three body straps.
- Suction.
- Five persons.

Care of patient who arrives on a spinal board

- Explain to the patient the need to stay on the spinal board until an examination of the neck and back has taken place.
- Instruct the patient not to move.
- Ensure the collar has the correct size and is fitted appropriately.
- Ensure the head blocks, straps, and body straps are secure.
- Ensure O_2 and suction are readily available.
- Assess and document limb movement and sensation. Ask the patient to gently wiggle their fingers and toes; check sensation in the upper and lower limbs.
- Ensure adequate pain relief.
- If the patient is nauseated, arrange for an antiemetic to be given.
- Give the patient and/or relative a call bell, so they can immediately summon help.
- Any patient with GCS score <15 or a potential airway problem, or who is anxious, agitated, or intoxicated should not be left unsupervised.
- Mobilize a log roll team as soon as possible, so that the spinal board can be removed.

Cautions

- Pressure areas are at immediate risk once a patient is placed on a spinal board. Therefore, they should be taken off it as soon as possible.
- Any clothing under the patient can be uncomfortable and may contribute to pressure if it is wrinkled. Remove clothing to smooth out, where possible.
- The airway is potentially at risk on any patient immobilized and strapped to a spinal board. A careful assessment must be made of the risk to their airway, and it must be managed appropriately.

Log rolling on a spinal board

This is undertaken to examine the patient's neck and back.

- Assemble a team: one person to examine the patient, one team leader to take control of the head and neck, and three other people to perform the log roll.
- Ensure there is enough space to perform the log roll and that the trolley is at a comfortable height for the procedure.
- The team leader is responsible for coordinating the whole procedure, and their commands *must* be followed at all times.
- Explain the procedure to the patient, and reassure them that they will not fall.
- Any clothing that needs to be removed should be cut at this stage to enable easy removal when the patient is rolled.
- The team leader takes manual control of the head and neck after the straps and blocks have been removed. At no time is the head/neck left unrestrained. Depending on the patient's injuries and complaints of pain, the collar may also be removed to allow examination.
- The 'log roll' team of three stand along one side of the patient. The patient should be rolled on to the side of least injury.
- The clinician examining the patient's neck and back stands on the opposite side from the team.
- The body straps are removed.
- The 'log roll' team position themselves. Person 1 stands at the level of the patient's shoulder, with one hand over the far shoulder and the other over the far hip. The second person places one hand over the far hip next to person 1's hand, and their second hand under the far knee. The third person places both hands under the far leg.
- On the team leader's instruction (the team all have to be clear on what the instruction is), the patient is rolled on to their side towards the team.
- The examining clinician removes the clothing and examines the back and/or neck.
- Once the examination is complete, the spinal board and any clothing are usually removed.
- The team leader gives the command to roll the patient back on to their back.
- The collar, head blocks, and straps may be reapplied.
- Depending upon the examination findings, the patient may have to stay flat on the ED trolley, with their neck immobilized until further investigations have been done.
- Movement and sensation of the limbs should be checked at the end of the procedure.

Thomas splint application

Indications

A Thomas splint is a traction splint, most commonly used to manage fractured shaft of femurs in adults and children >2y ⊕. A Thomas splint provides:
- immobilization and stabilization;
- reduction of pain from muscle spasm.

Equipment

- Thomas splint (correct size, and one size above and below).
- Tape measure.
- Calico slings.
- Safety pins (large).
- Skin traction kit.
- Crêpe bandages.
- Padding (cotton wool rolls).
- Strong stretch tape (Elastoplast®).
- Two-tongue depressors.
- Pillows.

Patient preparation

- Explain the procedure to the patient.
- Gain consent.
- Ensure adequate pain relief, ideally with a femoral nerve block. Use Entonox®, as required.

Procedure

▶ This procedure requires at least three people to ensure the comfort and safety of the patient.

- Identify that you have the correct patient.
- Assemble the equipment needed for the procedure.
- Identify the affected limb by confirming with the notes/X-rays and the patient.
- Measure the affected limb to determine the correct size of splint. Measure obliquely around the thigh at its highest point, allowing an extra 1cm. Then measure from the perineum to the heel for the length of the splint, allowing an extra 15–20cm for plantar flexion.
- Choose the appropriate-sized splint and one size above and below.
- Prepare the splint by attaching the calico slings with the safety pins, ensuring that the pins are fastened at the back on the lateral aspect to avoid their contact with the patient.
- Check the status of the limb—pulse, colour, temperature, sensation, and movement—and document your findings.

An appropriately qualified person should apply gentle traction to the affected limb for the remainder of the procedure.
- Apply the skin traction kit (➲ see Skin traction: application, p. 754).
- Gently place the leg through the Thomas splint, ensuring that the Achilles tendon is not lying on the calico slings. If the splint is the wrong size, remove, whilst still maintaining traction, and reapply the correct size. Ensure the splint is not rubbing against the genitalia or surrounding area.
- Place padding under the leg over the calico slings, with extra padding under the back of the knee and, if required, under the site of the fracture.
- Attach the cords to the splint, whilst gentle traction is maintained.
  - Pass the tapes over the left and right bars, one over and one under.
  - Whilst maintaining gentle traction on the leg, pull the traction cords around the splint end, over and under, then under and over.
  - Knot securely.
- Secure the leg to the splint with the crêpe bandages, and secure the bandages with elastic tape.
- Insert two taped-together tongue depressors between the cords, and gently twist to create traction.
- Elevate the leg on pillows.
- Check circulation and neurological function regularly.
- Re-X-ray the leg to determine the level of traction applied.
- Document the application.
- Dispose of the equipment.

Risks
- ↑ pain to the patient.
- Pressure area formation if padding not applied appropriately.
- Damage to the Achilles tendon if it lies over the calico slings.
- Damage to the peroneal nerve if the knee not appropriately padded.
- Potential foot drop if not enough room to plantar flex the foot.
- There are now different types of the Thomas splint available. They are extendable in length and have varying sizes of rings that are then attached.

Transporting the critically ill

Transporting patients to wards, X-ray, theatre, intensive care, and tertiary centres occurs regularly in emergency care. Transferring the critically ill/injured can be fraught with clinical risk if the transfer is poorly coordinated or lacks the right equipment or staff with the requisite training. Transfer-related mortality and morbidity is frequently reported with patients suffering from a wide range of problems, e.g. hypoventilation, hypotension, hypertension, ABG alteration, HR changes, changes in ICP, airway obstruction, disconnected IV lines, and abrupt stopping of medications.

Departmental policies and procedures should be followed to ensure that risk is minimized. Increasingly, 'retrieval teams' from tertiary centres are used to retrieve patients, ensure they are stable, and transport them to their destination.

▶ Regardless of whether a patient is being transferred within the same hospital or across the country, the same levels of preparation, supervision, and care must be ensured.

Preparation for transfer

Careful planning is required prior to transportation, taking into consideration the following:
- pre-transport coordination and communication;
- mode of transport;
- personnel;
- patient stability;
- information for relatives;
- equipment for transport;
- drugs for transport;
- monitoring during transport.

Pre-transport communication

- The clinician responsible for the care for the patient should communicate directly with the receiving area and ensure that all the advice and instructions have been carried out.
- All notes, investigation results, and patient information should be copied for the transfer.
- The receiving area should be informed of the expected time of arrival of the patient.

Mode of transport

Out-of-hospital transfer could be undertaken by ground or air. Consider the following:
- patient problem/s;
- urgency;
- availability of various modes;
- geography;
- weather conditions;
- traffic;
- cost.

Personnel

Clinical staff with appropriate training who are able to manage any eventuality en route should accompany the patient.

Patient stability

Patients must be fully resuscitated and stable prior to transfer in order to minimize any untoward occurrences. The main exception occurs when patients are being transferred to a tertiary centre for emergency surgery, e.g. vascular or neurological.

- Airway secured and maintained.
- Breathing adequately supported; intubation and ventilation may be required prior to transfer.
- Circulation stable, supported, and adequately monitored, e.g. arterial line, several secure venous lines, blood for transport if required, control of external bleeding, urinary catheter to monitor haemodynamic status.
- Neurological status. Maintain normal ICP; control seizure activity; preserve integrity of the spinal cord.
- Musculoskeletal system. Prevent further blood loss; fracture immobilization; wound care; analgesia.
- All lines and tubes, e.g. ETT, chest drain, should be secure and protected from accidental dislodging.
- Care of the patient's clothing and valuables.

Relatives

- Informed of the need to transfer and approximate time span.
- Ensure that they see their relative prior to transfer.
- Give information about how to reach the destination, and advise not to try to follow an ambulance.

Equipment

- Suitable trolley for transfer.
- Ability to keep the patient warm.
- Equipment that is reliable during transfer, with fully charged batteries and an adequate supplemental O_2 supply.
- Additional equipment in full working order should accompany the patient; this is usually in some form of 'transfer bag'.
- When using equipment, technical problems may occur and should be anticipated.

Drugs

Appropriate drugs to treat any eventuality must be available.

Monitoring during transfer

- Secure monitors; easily visible.
- ECG, non-invasive or invasive BP, SpO_2, $EtCO_2$, temperature.
- Unhindered access to the patient during transfer.

Venepuncture

Venepuncture enables the collection of venous blood without the need to insert an indwelling device, e.g. cannula. The most widely used technique is with a closed Vacutainer® system, as this reduces needle-stick injuries and the possible contamination of blood samples.

Equipment

- Needle or butterfly needle (often used in children) for use with Vacutainer® connection.
- Vacutainer® barrel.
- Appropriate blood collection bottles.
- Tourniquet.
- Non-sterile gloves and apron.
- Sharps bin.
- Alcohol-based cleansing swab.
- Gauze.
- Elastoplast® (check patient allergies).

Patient preparation

- Check it is the correct patient before carrying out the procedure.
- Explain the procedure to the patient, obtaining consent.

Vein selection

- Patients are often able to aid in the selection of a vein, as they know which sites have previously been successful. Follow their advice.
- Usually the best site for venepuncture (unless the patient tells you otherwise) is in the ACF. Veins in the ACF have a large lumen and lie close to the surface of the skin, and there is minimal superficial nerve supply.
- Apply the tourniquet to the middle of the upper arm, 7–10cm above the puncture site.
- With the arm in a downward position, palpate the ACF to locate a vein.
- Identify the course and depth of the vein to distinguish nearby structures such as tendons and arteries. The vein should be bouncy, prominent, and refill easily when depressed.
- Release the tourniquet, and observe the vein decompressing. A thrombosed vein will remain raised and should not be used.

Blood collection

- Wear gloves and an apron.
- Reapply the tourniquet.
- Clean the area over the selected vein, and allow to dry. See local policy for product to be used.
- Connect the Vacutainer® to the needle.
- Without touching the chosen area of skin, apply manual traction, with the thumb of the free hand 2–3cm below the chosen site to anchor the vein in position.
- Holding the needle at a 15–30° angle to the vein, with the bevel pointing upwards, advance into the skin. A sensation of resistance may be felt, followed by the needle entering the vein.
- To stabilize the needle within the vein, advance a further 1–2mm.
- Secure the needle by holding the Vacutainer® firmly in place.
- Using the other hand, advance the blood collection bottles into the Vacutainer® and over the rubber-sheathed needle, one after the other.
- Blood will flow until the vacuum within the bottle is exhausted, ensuring an adequate sample size.
- Remove the final bottle, and release the tourniquet.
- Cover the needle puncture site with the gauze, and swiftly remove the needle from the skin at the same angle of insertion.
- Apply gentle digital pressure over the puncture site.
- Dispose of the needle within the sharps collection bin.
- The patient/relative can then apply digital pressure until bleeding stops (~2min).
- Check the puncture site, and apply the plaster.
- Ensure that the patient is comfortable.
- Check the patient's details, name, and date of birth against the notes, and label the blood samples.
- Transport the samples to the laboratory.

Ventilation: mechanical

Invasive mechanical ventilation may be required when a patient is in respiratory failure and adequate improvement is not made with O_2 or NIV therapy. This could be due to ↓ respiratory effort, acute/chronic pulmonary conditions, or cardiovascular or metabolic compromise affecting respiration.

All patients on a mechanical ventilator need close monitoring, ideally one nurse to one patient. The nurse must have training in use of ventilators or immediate access to staff with adequate training.

Equipment
- Mechanical ventilator.
- Bacterial filter/heat and moisture exchanger (HME).
- Monitoring equipment, including capnograph.
- O_2 supply.
- Suction.
- Ambu bag/water circuit (in case of ventilator failure).
- Stethoscope.

Procedure
- Ensure the patient is adequately sedated.
- Secure the ETT to the patient; document the length that it is secured.
- Ensure the ETT has been sited correctly by auscultation of air entry to both lungs and attaching the capnograph. This should then be confirmed by X-ray.
- Suction if secretions are impeding gas exchange.
- Ensure the patient maintains satisfactory body temperature.
- Use a lubricating ointment to protect the patient's eyes.
- The patient should have IV fluids running, and vasopressors should be available.
- Relatives accompanying the patient should be informed of what is happening and why it is necessary. They often will need ↑ support at this time.

Risks
- Hypotension.
- Barotrauma.
- Inadequate ventilation.
- Build-up of secretions.
- Ventilator failure.
- Aspiration.

Ventilating the patient
- Safety checks should have been performed on the ventilator within the previous 24h or as per manufacturer's specification.
- There must be an anaesthetist/experienced ED clinician present who will prescribe the ventilator settings.
- Ensure full monitoring.
- Plug the ventilator into a piped O_2 source and mains electricity. It is good practice for this to be done at all times.

- Connect the breathing circuit with bacterial filter/HME to the ventilator.
- Set the prescribed ventilator settings before attaching to the patient.
- Set the mode of ventilation, e.g. IPPV.
- Set air or non-air mix (60% O_2 and 40% air in mix setting).
- Set the prescribed frequency of breaths (dependent on patient PCO_2)
- Set the maximum pressure (Pmax), which should never be >35cmH$_2$O, unless advised by the anaesthetist.
- Set PEEP (dependent on patient condition).
- Set I:E ratio (dependent on patient condition).
- Set Vt, based on 6-8mL/kg (ideal body weight).
- Connect to the patient.
- Ensure the patient has 15–30min observations, including recording minute volumes (mV). Minute volumes should be Vt × frequency of breaths.
- Take an ABG every hour.
- Hourly assessment of neurological status and sedation level.
- The patient should be nursed with head up at 30°, unless contraindicated.
- Continuous monitoring of capnography, O_2 saturations, HR, and invasive BP.
- Only disconnect the ventilator from piped O_2 and mains electricity immediately prior to transfer. Transfer O_2 cylinder should have a Schrader valve and sufficient O_2 for transfer. On arrival at destination, reconnect to piped and mains supplies.

Glossary of terms
- IPPV, intermittent positive pressure ventilation.
- CMV, controlled mandatory ventilation.
- SIPPV, synchronized intermittent positive pressure ventilation.
- CPAP, continuous positive airway pressure.
- SIMV, synchronized intermittent mandatory ventilation.
- PEEP, peak end-expiratory pressure.
- I:E, ratio of inspiration time to expiration time.
- Pmax, maximum pressure exerted.
- Vt, tidal volume.
- mV, minute volume.

Ventilation: non-invasive

NIV is the delivery of ventilatory support without the need for an invasive artificial airway, i.e. ETT. NIV plays a significant role in the management of acute and chronic respiratory failure in adults and children. NIV often eliminates the need for intubation or tracheostomy, and preserves normal swallowing, speech, and cough mechanisms. The use of non-invasive positive pressure ventilation (NIPPV) in hospital settings and at home has been steadily ↑. The two commonest types of NIV are continuous positive pressure ventilation (CPAP) and BiPAP.

CPAP maintains the alveoli in an 'open' state by applying pressure at the end of expiration. CPAP reduces alveolar collapse, with a resulting improvement in lung volumes and gaseous exchange. CPAP is effective in type I respiratory failure associated with conditions, such as pulmonary oedema or pneumonia, and is generally associated with the provision of high O_2 concentrations.

BiPAP modes IPAP (intermittent positive airway pressure) and EPAP (end-positive airway pressure) provide positive pressure when the patient starts to breathe in until they start to exhale. BiPAP is synchronized with the patient's respiratory cycle (i.e. the machine complies with the patient). IPAP is applied as the patient breathes in and functions by reducing the patient's work of breathing and ↑ the Vt, allowing greater CO_2 removal (normally set at 12–18). EPAP is the background or CPAP pressure that is on constantly, improving alveoli recruitment.

BiPAP is generally administered with controlled O_2 therapy. It is used in patients with type II respiratory failure associated most commonly with COPD/pneumonia/pulmonary oedema.

Absolute contraindications

- Coma.
- Agitation.
- Inability to protect the airway.

Relative contraindications

- Severe acidosis (pH <7.1).
- Excessive bronchial secretions.
- Haemodynamic instability.
- Pulmonary TB.
- Recent upper GI surgery.
- Orofacial abnormalities.

▶ If a pneumothorax is present, a chest drain must be *in situ*, or there is high risk of a tension pneumothorax developing.

Setting up

Assemble the machine/circuit away from the patient, and ensure it is working properly. The initial settings are usually an IPAP of 12 and an EPAP of 4. If higher settings are likely to be required, starting the patient on the lower settings indicated above can help with compliance.

- BiPAP machine.
- BiPAP circuit.
- NIV face mask. Must be measured to fit the patient using the guide provided.

- Filter.
- Attach the circuit to the machine and mask (usually only one way to do this).
- Attach the O_2 tubing to the port on the mask, and set at the prescribed flow rate.
- If transfer (internal or external) on the machine is a possibility, ensure the transfer battery is on charge.

Patient preparation

The patient's first experience of BiPAP can be distressing, but its effective use may be lifesaving and greatly alter patient outcome.

- Explain clearly to the patient and/or relatives what the machine does and how it will help them.
- Let the patient feel air pressures with their hands before applying to the face.
- When applying the mask to the face, hold it gently in place, allowing the patient to become accustomed to the feel of it.
- Gradually apply more pressure to obtain the snug fit required.
- When the patient is ready, apply the straps.
- Avoid strapping too tightly or unequally, but try to minimize leakage (a small amount of leakage may be unavoidable).
- Try to avoid leaks into the eyes, as this may precipitate drying.
- Dressings, such as Granuflex®, may need to be applied to the bridge of the nose and other pressure points if the patient has friable skin.
- Alterations to settings should be prescribed by the clinician responsible and in response to the patient's tolerance and ABG concentrations.
- Provide continued support and encouragement, reminding the patient that the machine works with their breathing to make it easier.
- If necessary, make an agreed time for short breaks if it aids compliance and will not be detrimental to overall respiratory function.
- Ensure suction, BVM, and resuscitation equipment are immediately available.
- Ensure a CXR has been undertaken to exclude a pneumothorax or other pathology.

Continued care

- Full continuous monitoring should be maintained and documented every 15min at the beginning of treatment. The commencement of treatment as positive airway pressure may alter thoracic pressures and venous return to the heart and cause hypotension.
- Observe for any signs of ↑ respiratory effort, cyanosis, distress, anxiety, or reduced consciousness.
- Drying of the mouth and nasal passages may be reduced with petroleum jelly and regular mouth care.
- Nutrition and hydration should be managed by planned breaks and IV fluids where indicated.
- An NG tube and anti-emetics may be required if there is nausea and vomiting. If the patient's airway is at risk, e.g. vomiting, or the patient becomes acutely distressed, use the quick release section to the front of the mask.

Visual acuity

VA is an objective assessment of visual function and *must* be recorded in all patients attending with an eye problem. Normal vision is 6/6, i.e. the eye can see at 6m what a normal eye can see at that distance.

Procedure

- Test the affected/injured eye first.
- Occlude the other eye, using an occluder or the patient's hand.
- Distance glasses should be worn, as the test is of the *best corrected* VA.
- The test should begin at the top of the Snellen chart, with the patient reading down and making an attempt to read all letters.
- The VA should be recorded as [distance at which the eye is being tested (usually 6m)]/[number on the last line read by the patient].
  - The number for the last line read by the patient is indicated on the Snellen chart, just above or just below the letters.
  - If only part of a line is read, this can be recorded as the line above plus the extra letters, or the line below minus the missed letters. For example, if the patient reads the '18' line, except for one letter, at 6m, it should be recorded as 6/(18−1).

Considerations

- If the patient's vision is <6/9, VA should be assessed with a pinhole (a small hole in a card or a commercial pinhole) held in front of the eye. This corrects for reduced VA caused by refractive error.
- If the patient is unable to read the top letter of the Snellen chart, the distance should be reduced until the patient can see the top letter on the chart, i.e. 5/60, 4/60, etc. to 1/60.
- If the top letter cannot be seen at 1m, the next possible level of vision is to count fingers (CF), see hand movements (HM), or perception of light (PL) at 1m.
- Lack of light perception is recorded as NPL.
- It is important to ascertain if the level of subnormal vision is *normal for the patient*.
- Strategies to overcome language difficulties may include: using a recognition chart, so that the patient may match letters or shapes; and obtaining the services of an interpreter or family member to translate for the patient.
- Children are often cooperative if picture tests (such as the Kay picture test) are used and the procedure is made into a game.

⊕ Vital signs in children

Assessing vital signs in children can be challenging for the clinician without specific paediatric training or experience. Normal parameters are vastly different than in adults and alter with ↑ age (⊖ see Table 21.7).

▶ The accurate interpretation of vital signs in children relies on the clinician knowing what is normal for the age of the child, having the right equipment, and, of equal importance, knowing how to undertake an accurate assessment.

Child's behaviour

Parents usually bring their child to an emergency care facility because of a change in behaviour. It is crucial to listen to the parent and document their concerns. An objective assessment should be made of the child's behaviour and if it is normal for them.

Weight

A child's weight should be considered a vital sign. It enables assessment of growth, development, and hydration status. All medications are given according to weight, so an accurate weight in kilograms should be taken at the earliest opportunity. If a child is critically ill and cannot be weighed, a weight formula in different age groups can be used.

- 0–12 months: weight (in kg) = (0.5 × age in months) + 4.
- 1–5y: weight (in kg) = (2 × age in years) + 8.
- 6–12y: weight (in kg) = (3 × age in years) + 7.

Temperature

Parents know when their child has a temperature without the need for a thermometer. An objective assessment of temperature needs to be made, and a device and route appropriate for the age of the child should be used, e.g. axilla, oral, or tympanic. The manufacturer's instructions should be checked to ensure the device is appropriate for the age of the child.

Respiratory rate

Children rely primarily on their diaphragm for breathing, as their intercostal muscles are immature. It is not easy to see a child's chest rise and fall, as the diameter of their thorax does not alter greatly with respiration. What does alter is the degree to which their diaphragm contracts and flattens when their work of breathing is ↑. It is for this reason that a child's chest and abdomen should be exposed when assessing the RR. The movement of the abdomen, as it is pushed down by the diaphragm, indicates the RR. Alternatively, the child's chest can be auscultated, and their RR counted. The child's neck, clavicular area, chest, and abdomen should also be assessed for signs of recession. Recession indicates work of breathing and is significant.

Oxygen saturations

The right sized probe attached correctly to the right site will ensure accurate assessment.

Table 21.7 Normal values of RR and pulse in children at different ages

Age (y)	RR (breaths/min)	Pulse (bpm)	Systolic BP (mmHg)
Infant, <1	30–40	110–160	70–90
Toddler, 1–2	25–35	100–150	80–95
Preschool, 3–4	25–30	95–140	80–100
School, 5–11	20–25	80–120	90–110
Adolescent, 12–16	15–20	60–100	100–120

Heart rate

A term baby's HR is ~160bpm, which would be considered a tachycardia in an adult. A child's HR can be assessed by listening at the apex. Alternatively, the brachial pulse can be easily palpated in children <1y, and, in children >1y, the carotid or radial pulses are ideal sites to use.

Blood pressure

Assessing a child's BP can be a falsely reassuring sign if the clinician is merely assessing it against normal parameters for the age of the child. Children have an amazing ability to maintain a normal BP, despite profound volume losses of up to 45%. A normal BP, in the absence of other assessments such as capillary refill and conscious level, can lead to cardiovascular abnormalities going undetected. Trends in BP measurements can be much more meaningful. The right sized BP cuff is essential for the accuracy of any assessment.

Capillary refill

In early cardiovascular compromise, the capillary refill time can be ↑ beyond 2s. ↑ the capillary refill time, together with the presence of other signs of cardiovascular compromise, e.g. tachycardia, pallor, cool mottled peripheries, and altered conscious level, requires prompt intervention.
- Use a thumb/finger, and depress the skin of the sternum for 5s; let go, and count how many seconds it takes the blanched skin to return to a normal colour.

Further information

Royal College of Nursing (2013). *Standards for assessing, measuring and monitoring vital signs in infants, children and young people. RCN guidance for nurses working with children and young people.* Available at: ℜ https://www2.rcn.org.uk/__data/assets/pdf_file/0004/114484/003196.pdf.

Wounds: stages of healing

A huge variety of acute and chronic wounds presents to emergency care areas each day. There is no single treatment or wound care product that meets all the criteria for the 'ideal dressing' for each different wound type during each phase of healing. This section of the skills chapter provides evidence-based information on the principles of traumatic wound management, which will support the clinician in making clinically effective and cost-effective dressing choices.

▶ When faced with a wound, it is important to assess its stage of healing (➔ see Box 21.4). There are several points to be considered when approaching wound management at each stage.

> ### Box 21.4 Wounds: stages of healing
>
> *Vascular stage* The commonest stage of healing seen in emergency care. A dressing needs to be able to absorb bleeding and help control it. Some wounds bleed profusely (that is why the patient has attended), e.g. skin loss to a fingertip. An alginate dressing is homeostatic and can help promote clotting. Bleeding should be checked to ensure it is not arterial in origin and can usually be controlled simply with a dressing, pressure, and elevation. If wounds are bleeding, a simple dressing is all that is needed, with redressing planned for 2–3 days later.
>
> *Destructive migratory stage* Wounds at this stage may have a lot of exudate, e.g. burns, and will require a dressing that can absorb the wound 'ooze'. Dead/devitalized tissue needs to be removed. A product to remove slough/eschar may be required, e.g. hydrogel.
>
> *Proliferative stage* A very fragile stage of healing, as new tissue is being formed. Cooling a wound by exposing it for long periods or cleansing with cool solutions will slow, or even stop, epithelialization for several hours. Wound care products must not adhere to the wound surface at this stage, as removing an adhered dressing is not only very painful but will tear away new skin cells and blood vessels from the wound bed—the wound could even be returned to the vascular phase, and healing significantly delayed.
>
> *Maturation stage* Advice about scar care and keeping healed burns from the sun is relevant at this final stage of healing.

Wound care

Healing by 'intention'

Wounds heal by either 1° or 2° intention. Wounds that heal by 1° intention, where the skin edges are brought together by suture, glue, or Steri-Strips™, will heal relatively quickly (5–14 days). Wounds that heal by 2° intention are wounds that extend into the dermis with skin loss. They heal, as new cells are formed, and the defect is filled, e.g. burns. These wounds can take 10–21 days to heal.

Ideal dressing criteria

Dressing products in emergency care areas may be limited, and access to specialist treatments difficult. If a more appropriate dressing is required, early wound review, where the dressing is available, is required. There is no one product that has all the qualities of the 'ideal dressing'; compromises always have to be made. Depending on the wound type, characteristics, and stage of healing, some of the following criteria will be more important than others.

- Maintain high humidity at the wound/dressing interface (to keep the wound moist).
- Remove excess exudate and toxic components (to keep the wound moist, but not saturated, and remove contaminants).
- Allows gaseous exchange (to let the wound breathe).
- Provide thermal insulation (to keep the wound warm).
- Is impermeable to bacteria.
- Is free from particulate and toxic contaminants, i.e. does not introduce anything toxic or leave anything behind.
- Allows removal without causing additional trauma; easy to remove.
- Is non-allergenic, so it does not cause allergic reaction.
- Is comfortable, conformable, and protective, i.e. it is comfortable for the patient, protects vulnerable skin, and bends over joints.
- Is cost-effective and available in the right size. It comes in an appropriate size and does not require frequent changes if the dressing is expensive.
- Is acceptable to the patient. Some dressings have an odour; explain to the patient.

Table 21.8 describes the different traumatic wounds encountered in emergency care and suggests what should be taken into consideration when selecting a dressing.

Other wound characteristics at different stages of healing will require a different approach (➜ see Table 21.9).

Table 21.8 Dressing considerations for different types of wounds

Wound	Mechanism/definition	Dressing considerations
Abrasion	Friction force	Varying depth; can be contaminated; painful
Bite wounds	Human; animal; insect	Infection possible; may swell
Burn	Scald; flame; chemical; electrical	May cover large area; may be difficult to dress; painful; heavy exudate during first 72h
Contaminated wounds	Contamination with: soil; gravel; mud; clothing. Industrial; sport/ recreational	Clean to remove contamination prior to dressing, or use product that removes contamination. May need X-ray to rule out radio-opaque FB
Crush wounds	Blunt force	May swell
Cut/incised wounds	Sharp object: glass/knife	Oppose wound edges with sutures/ glue or Steri-Strip™. Heal quickly
Degloving injuries	Tissue torn from underlying attachments	Usually need plastics referral
Flap wounds	Blunt or penetrating	May be contaminated under flap. If poor blood supply to flap, may become necrotic. Undue tension will compromise flap blood supply further
Fingertip wounds	Crush	Painful. Nail bed may be lacerated and need repair
Lacerations	Blunt force causes skin to split	May swell. Possible contused/ devitalized tissue
Pre-tibial lacerations	Wound to pre-tibial area; usually in the elderly	If poor blood supply to flap, may become necrotic. Undue tension will compromise flap blood supply further. In elderly, blood supply compromised further, and healing delayed
Puncture wound	Penetrating injury	Cannot adequately clean base of wound. May be contaminated or have FB
Skin loss/ avulsion	Skin lost due to crush injuries or incised wounds	May bleed profusely. Prolonged healing by 2° intention
Abscess	Pocket of infection: retained FB; infected sebaceous cyst	Painful. After incision, keep open to heal by 2° intention

Table 21.9 Other wound characteristics affecting dressing choice

Type	Characteristics	Considerations
Necrotic	Black, hard, dry	Remove necrosis, or the wound will not heal. Once removed, assess true depth and extent of wound. Use product that rehydrates wound and removes necrotic tissue
Sloughy	Yellow, or green, or grey. Slough may be soft and easily removed	Wound will not heal, as slough prolongs inflammatory phase. Use desloughing agent
Infected	Red, hot, swollen, pus, painful, delayed healing	May have excess exudate. Some products not licensed for use on infected wounds
Granulating	Red, shiny, 'bumpy' in appearance	Fragile; easily damaged by adherent dressing. Bleeds easily. Use a low-adherent dressing
Epithelializing	Pale red/pink areas of new epithelial cell growth	Fragile new epithelial cells easily damaged. Use low-adherent dressing

Further reading

Detailed data card information on all dressings can be found at ♪ http://www.dressings.org, or read the manufacturer's information leaflet that accompanies the dressing.

Wound cleansing

Wound cleansing is an integral part of wound management and is the mainstay of treatment. Emergency care staff often underestimate the importance of this simple skill and how vital it is in preventing infection and promoting healing. All traumatic wounds should be considered contaminated with debris. Some patients may require a general anaesthetic for adequate cleaning of wounds.

▶ An inadequately cleansed wound will have delayed healing, possible wound infection and scarring, and, on occasion, permanent tattooing that may require surgery.

Indications
• All traumatic wounds.

Equipment
• Tap water.
• 20mL syringe.
• Warmed cleansing fluid.
• Gloves.
• Eye protection.
• Apron.
• Scrubbing brush/toothbrush.
• LA.

There are also various commercial devices available to irrigate wounds under pressure.
   The following points are important to note.
• ▶ There is a strong body of evidence to suggest that, when wounds are cleansed with tap water, there is no higher incidence of wound infection.
• ▶ 'Scrubbing brushes' of various types may have to be used. The risk of causing further trauma to the tissues is outweighed by the benefits of removing debris and preventing permanent tattooing of the wound.

▶ Cotton wool or gauze should be avoided in the cleansing of wounds, as fibres can be shed into the wound. This method does not remove debris—it just moves it around the wound.

Patient preparation
• Explain the procedure to the patient.
• Remove any clothing that may become wet.
• Assist the patient into a comfortable position.
• Ensure adequate pain relief. The wound may need infiltration with LA or the application of a topical anaesthetic gel.

Procedure

- Using the 20mL syringe, push the fluid through the wound to dislodge any dirt or debris. Take care not to cause further damage to the tissue if the water is forced under high pressure.
- Copious amounts of warm tap water are ideal for cleaning dirty wounds. Run the water for ~15s; then cleanse the wound.
- Use a scrubbing brush if there are engrained debris.
- Close and dress the wound, as appropriate.

Discharge advice

▶ Prophylactic antibiotics are not used routinely. Patients should be advised to seek further treatment if the wound is:
- hot;
- red;
- swollen;
- painful;
- odorous;
- not healed in the expected time;
- discharging.

Wound closure: tissue adhesive

Tissue adhesive is a means of closing smaller wounds by the application of specially formulated glue used for medical purposes. It is particularly useful for the management of small wounds in children and wounds where hair is present (scalp and eyebrows). The technique for glue application is relatively easy, provided the right type of wound is selected. There are several products available, and the manufacturer's instructions should always be consulted.

Indications
Wounds suitable for glue:
- clean;
- not over a joint surface or an area prone to excessive movement;
- relatively small, 4–5cm;
- superficial;
- not bleeding;
- edges easily opposed.

Equipment
- Wound-cleansing solution.
- Dressing pack; gauze, sterile gloves, gallipot.
- Glue.
- Sterile dressing.

Patient preparation
Explain the procedure to the patient. There may be a slight sting when the glue is applied.

Procedure
- Hold away any hair that may interfere with the glue application (sometimes the droplet of adhesive can track down the hair shaft).
- Clean the wound; remove any haematoma, and dry it thoroughly.
- Oppose the skin edges.
- Dry the wound again.
- Apply according to the manufacturer's instructions, which will depend on the type of glue applicator.
- Do not apply the glue into the wound.
- Hold the edges of the wound in apposition for 30s to allow the adhesive to dry.
- Apply sterile dressing, if appropriate.

Precautions
- Do not apply too much glue, as excessive adhesive will reduce the tensile strength of the glue.
- ▶ If your glove becomes stuck to the wound, *do not worry*. Trim the glove, so that only the area that is adhered is left. Advise the patient/parent that the glove will fall off as the wound heals.

Discharge advice

- Keep clean, and dry for 4–5 days for a scalp wound, and 5–7 days elsewhere.
- A larger scab may form; this is normal.
- The scab/glue will fall off after the wound is healed.

Steri-Strips™

Steri-Strips™ or 'butterflies' are adhesive strips (usually manufactured in two different widths) that can be used to close superficial wounds of varying lengths.

Indications

Wounds suitable for closure with Steri-Strips™:
- superficial;
- not bleeding profusely;
- edges easily opposed;
- not under tension or excessive movement, i.e. not over a moving extensor surface;
- do not require layered closure (although internal sutures can be applied and the skin closed with Steri-Strips™).

Equipment

- Wound-cleansing solution.
- Dressing pack: gauze; sterile gloves; gallipot.
- Steri-Strips™ of appropriate width.
- Sterile dressing.
- Compound benzoin tincture (e.g. Friars' Balsam). When this is applied to the skin surrounding the wound with a cotton bud, the skin becomes tacky, enabling greater adherence of the Steri-Strips™. (Do not put into the wound or on grazed skin as it will 'sting' until dry.)

Patient preparation

- Explain the procedure to the patient.

Procedure

- Clean the wound; remove any haematoma, and dry it thoroughly.
- Paint the skin around the wound with compound benzoin tincture (e.g. Friars' Balsam), if appropriate.
- Oppose the skin edges.
- Dry the wound again.
- Apply Steri-Strips™, anchoring corners of the wound first, where appropriate.
- Apply with even tension, leaving 3mm gaps between each strip to allow serous fluid to drain from the wound. Ensure that the wound edges are not under too much tension. Undue tension will compromise the blood supply to this part of the wound and may compromise healing. If necessary, strips can be placed parallel to the wound to strengthen closing strips.
- Dress with appropriate dressing. If Steri-Strips™ have been applied about a joint, immobilize the joint to prevent tension on the wound.

Discharge advice

- Keep clean and dry.
- Leave Steri-Strips™ *in situ* for 5–10 days, depending on the site and type of the wound.
- Peel or soak off when the requisite time has elapsed.

Local anaesthetic infiltration of wounds

LA causes a reversible loss of nerve conduction. Lidocaine is available in 1% and 2% concentrations, and is very safe, provided a toxic dose is not given. Allergic reactions are rare.

- The safe maximum dose of lidocaine is 3mg/kg.
- Overdose can occur if >3mg/kg is given or if there is an inadvertent direct intravascular injection. The weaker the solution, the more lidocaine that can be given.
  - 1% lidocaine contains 1g of lidocaine in 100mL.
  - 2% lidocaine contains 2g of lidocaine in 100mL.
  - Therefore, 1mL of 1% contains 10mg of lidocaine (0.1mL = 1mg); 1mL of 2% contains 20mg of lidocaine (0.1mL = 2mg).

There are two techniques for infiltration of the wound with LA: infiltration through the wound edge (➔ see Fig. 21.20a) or a field block (➔ see Fig. 21.20b). Infiltration should be done under the wound edge, as patients cannot usually feel a 25G needle. Pain is felt with tissue distension, and therefore infiltration should be slow and deliberate.

Ensure you have adequate anaesthesia before continuing with the procedure. Onset of action is usually within seconds and lasts 20min.

Digital nerve blocks

It can be painful to inject finger wounds, and LA often distorts the wound margins. A digital nerve block is required. There are a number of techniques that are commonly practised. One technique is described below.

Place the hand flat, palm down, with fingers abducted. Insert a 22G needle at the level of the base of the web. Angle the tip of the needle towards the palmar side. You may feel the needle against the proximal phalanx. Aspirate to ensure that the needle is not in a vessel, and inject 1–2ml of lidocaine. Repeat the procedure on the other side of the finger. Wait 5min for the anaesthesia to develop. (➔ See Fig. 21.21.)

(a)

(b)

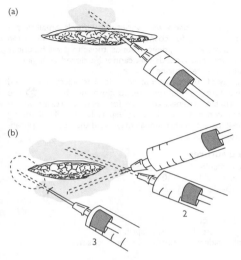

2

3

Fig. 21.20 (a) Infiltration through wound edge. (b) Field block.

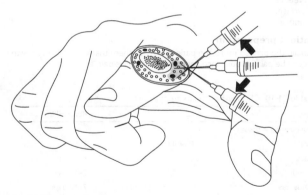

Fig. 21.21 Digital nerve block.

Suturing

Suturing with LA is used to close a wide variety of wounds. Small simple wounds may require suturing for cosmetic reasons, e.g. small vermilion border lacerations. Large wounds, deep wounds, those that will be under some degree of tension, and wounds that cannot be closed with glue or Steri-Strips™ will also require suturing.

There is a vast array of suture material available. The selection is based on the size of the suture material required to close the wound (➔ see Table 21.10). Absorbable materials are used for deep sutures or where there is no cosmetic concern over the scar, e.g. scalp. Rapidly dissolving sutures are also ideal for use in children, as they avoid the need for potentially distressing suture removal.

Commonly used sutures
- Ethilon®: non-absorbable.
- Vicryl Rapide®: absorbable in 7–10 days.
- Monocryl®: absorbable in 7–21 days.

Equipment
- Wound-cleansing solution.
- Dressing pack: gauze; sterile gloves; gallipot.
- Suture set: needle holder; non-toothed forceps; scissors.
- Suture material.
- Sterile dressing.
- Needle.
- Syringe.
- Lidocaine.

Patient preparation
Explain the procedure to the patient. Advise them that the infiltration with LA can be painful, but, once complete, suturing is pain-free.

Table 21.10 Choosing correct size of suture

Site	Size	Removal in
Subcutaneous tissues	6.0	–
Scalp	3.0 or 4.0	7 days
Face	6.0	≤5 days
Hands	4.0 or 5.0	7–10 days
Other area	Dependent on wound	7–10 days
Site over joints	Dependent on wound	10–14 days

Simple sutures

Simple sutures (➋ see Fig. 21.22) are the most commonly used sutures. The aim is to accurately oppose the skin edges and completely close the wound. Deeper wounds may require layered closure (➋ see Deep sutures and mattress sutures, pp. 792–3) to ensure that there is no 'dead space' where a haematoma can develop and act as a focus for infection. Take care not to insert the needle deeper than the visible base of the wound, in case the suture accidentally catches a deep structure, e.g. a tendon or nerve.

Tying knots

This skill is best demonstrated slowly by a competent practitioner.

- Pull the suture through the wound (as shown in ➋ Fig. 21.23), and wrap the long end of the suture (the end with the needle attached) around the tip of the needle holder two or three times.
- Grab the other end of the suture with the needle holder, and pull this end through, pulling the knot tight.
- Repeat two or three more times, wrapping the suture in the opposite direction 2–4 times.

Discharge advice

- Advise about wound care: signs of wound infection; care of the wound; keeping it clean and dry.
- Written and verbal advice about removal of sutures and any follow-up.
- Advise about pain relief and NSAIDs, if appropriate.
- Advise about work/school, contact sport, and other activities that the patient may regularly undertake.
- Advise about how and when to seek further help if problems persist.

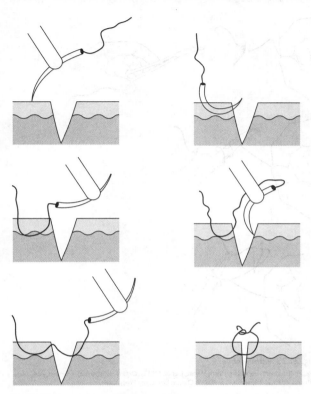

Fig. 21.22 Diagrammatic representation of the stages involved in a basic suture.
(Reproduced with permission from Thomas, J. and Monaghan, T. (2007). *Oxford Handbook of Clinical Examination and Skills*, fig. 17.39, p. 633. Oxford University Press, Oxford.)

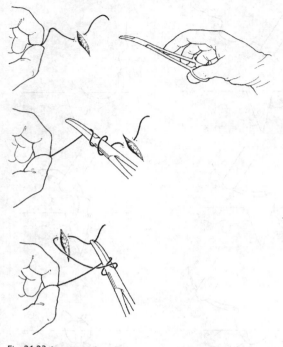

Fig. 21.23 Instrument tie.

(Reproduced with permission from Wyatt, J. et al. (2012). *Oxford Handbook of Emergency Medicine*, 4th edn, figs 9.2, 9.3, and 9.4, p. 408–9. Oxford University Press, Oxford.)

Deep sutures and mattress sutures

Layered closure for deep wounds

If the wound is deep, it may require closure in layers to ensure there is no 'dead space' within the wound (◆ see Fig. 21.24). If all the layers of the wound are not closed, an indentation beneath the scar may affect the final cosmetic outcome. Inserting an accurate layer of deep sutures may also enable the skin to be closed with Steri-Strips™, leading to an improved final result. Tie knots, as described in ◆ Simple sutures on p. 788.

Mattress sutures

Mattress sutures (◆ see Fig. 21.25) are very useful, as they enable inverted skin edges to be more accurately opposed. They are contraindicated on facial wounds. If, after inserting a simple suture, the skin edges are inverted, this indicates that a mattress suture may be more appropriate.

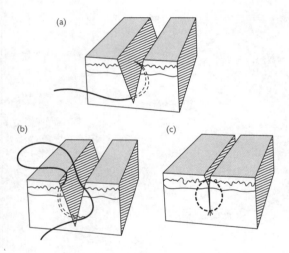

Fig. 21.24 Layered wound closure.

Discharge advice

- Advise about wound care: signs of wound infection; care of the wound; keeping it clean and dry.
- Written and verbal advice about removal of sutures and any follow-up.
- Advise about pain relief and NSAIDs, if appropriate.
- Advise about work/school, contact sport, and other activities that the patient may regularly undertake.
- Advise about how and when to seek further help if problems persist.

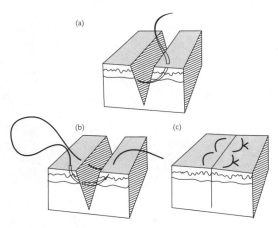

Fig. 21.25 Mattress suture.

Discharge advice

- ...
- ...
- Follow-up ...
- A ...
- Advise ...

Fig. 27.25 ...

Index